Principles of Brain Dynamics

Computational Neuroscience

Terence J. Sejnowski and Tomaso A. Poggio, editors

For a complete list of books in this series, see the back of the book and http://mitpress.mit.edu/Computational_Neuroscience

Principles of Brain Dynamics

Global State Interactions

edited by Mikhail I. Rabinovich, Karl J. Friston, and Pablo Varona

The MIT Press
Cambridge, Massachusetts
London, England

This book was set in Syntax and Times Roman by Toppan Best-set Premedia Limited.

Library of Congress Cataloging-in-Publication Data

Principles of brain dynamics : global state interactions / edited by Mikhail I. Rabinovich, Karl J. Friston, and Pablo Varona.
    p. ; cm. — (Computational neuroscience)
Includes bibliographical references and index.
ISBN 978-0-262-01764-0 (hardcover : alk. paper)
ISBN 978-0-262-54990-5 (paperback)
I. Rabinovich, M. I. II. Friston, K. J. (Karl J.) III. Varona, Pablo, 1968– IV. Series:
Computational neuroscience.
[DNLM: 1. Brain—physiology. 2. Nonlinear Dynamics. WL 300]
612.8′2—dc23
2011048673

Contents

Series Foreword

Computational neuroscience is an approach to understanding the development and function of nervous systems at many different structural scales, including the biophysical, the circuit, and the systems levels. Methods include theoretical analysis and modeling of neurons, networks, and brain systems and are complementary to empirical techniques in neuroscience. Areas and topics of particular interest to this book series include computational mechanisms in neurons, analysis of signal processing in neural circuits, representation of sensory information, systems models of sensorimotor integration, computational approaches to biological motor control, and models of learning and memory. Further topics of interest include the intersection of computational neuroscience with engineering, from representation and dynamics to observation and control.

Terrence J. Sejnowski
Tomaso A. Poggio

Introduction

It is a great pleasure for us to think about how we think and how our thoughts evolve or leap in time.

More than a century ago in 1890, William James articulated a general idea that underlies dynamical descriptions of human consciousness: "Thought is in Constant Change—no state once gone can recur and be identical with what it was before." In other words, we move continuously from one relatively stable thought to another thought [see chapter 9, "The Stream of Thought," in volume 1 of James's classic work (James, 2007)]. After James, many scientists have emphasized the crucial role of itinerant brain activity in human cognition. We recall here the thoughts of two key scientists: the mathematical genius Henri Poincaré, one of the fathers of nonlinear dynamics, and the famous neurophysiologist Thomas Graham Brown.

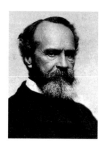 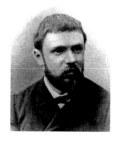 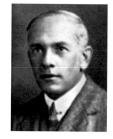

William James (1842-1910)   Henri Poincaré (1854-1912)   Thomas Graham Brown (1882-1965)

In his book *The Foundations of Science*, first published in Paris in 1908, Henri Poincaré wrote: "The genesis of mathematical creation is a problem, which should intensely interest the psychologist. It is the activity in which the human mind seems to take least from the outside world, in which it acts or seems to act only of itself and on itself, so that in studying the procedure of geometric thought we may hope to reach what is most essential in man's mind" (Poincaré, 2009). With a similar perspective, neurophysiologist Thomas Graham Brown, a former student of Sherrington, wrote: "Brain's operations are mainly intrinsic maintenance of information for interpreting, responding and predicting" (Brown, 1914).

Practical applications of nonlinear dynamics to the study of brain activity began in the middle of the past century. However, such efforts only flourished when combined with empirical observations of brain activity from modern morphologic and physiologic experiments. This new perspective was celebrated in a book published by The MIT Press, *Mind as Motion* (Port & van Gelder, 1995). This book reflected the changing views of neuroscientists, psychiatrists, and others trying to understand cognition, mood, and emotions. It promoted a shift of emphasis from anatomic analyses of brain regions to the study of brain activity in time. However, Port and van Gelder's book concentrates mostly on the concept of attractor dynamics (limit cycles, chaotic attractors, and fixed points) and does not consider another important type of neural phenomena: transient brain dynamics.

The consideration of time or dynamics is fundamental for all aspects of mental activity—perception, cognition, and emotion. This is because the main feature of brain activity is the continuous change of the underlying brain states, even in a constant environment. Generally speaking, brain dynamics can be considered as a sequence of controllable *instabilities*. Transient brain states that reflect the stabilization of one instability and, coincidentally, the emergence of another are described as *metastable* states. Learning and generating ordered sequences of metastable states is a core component of mental life, both in living organisms and in artificial systems. This view is supported by novel results in brain imaging, multielectrode recordings, and modeling experiments. In particular, in the past 15 years, three key events have advanced the application of dynamical systems theory to neuroscience: (1) many experiments suggest that macroscopic phenomena in the brain are sequential and transient interactions of mental modes (patterns of activity); (2) joint approaches from complexity theory (dealing with hierarchy and connectivity) and nonlinear dynamics have furnished challenging hypotheses about global brain activity; (3) open questions from research in genetics, ecology, brain sciences, and so forth have led to the discovery of a new dynamical phenomenon; that is, reproducible and robust transients that are at the same time sensitive to informational signals.

An interesting and important feature of robust transients is flexible timing. Timing depends on the sequence of metastable states and is fundamental for adaptive functional responses and cognitive control. Moreover, the sequential instabilities lend themselves to composition within temporal hierarchies and to the possibility of generating "sequence of sequences," which is a natural dynamical mechanism for language.

The book that we present here delivers a privileged view of brain dynamics that draws upon the advances above. This book tries to provide a basis for a closer collaboration between theoreticians and experimentalists and for a further integration of experimental results and levels of analysis. To meet this goal, the editors have invited several authors, whose scientific interests and contributions illuminate the "dynamical brain" from different perspectives, to write the following chapters. We hope that by providing different perspectives and an eclectic treatment of the same, fundamental issues, readers will form their own point of view on brain dynamics.

The book begins with a chapter by Gustavo Deco, Viktor Jirsa, and Karl J. Friston, who consider models of brain dynamics from both a local and global perspective. They present a specific model based on spiking neurons at the local level and large-scale anatomic connectivity matrices at the global level. This approach is used to provide a quantitative example of how to model dynamical mechanisms in the brain. This chapter focuses specifically on the genesis of itinerant dynamics and the role of multistability. It emphasizes the importance of autonomous dynamics in neuroscience and the universal properties that they might possess. Understanding how the human brain produces cognition must ultimately depend on its large-scale organization. Brain areas engaged during cognitive tasks also form coherent large-scale brain networks that can be identified using intrinsic functional connectivity. In chapter 2, Vinod Menon examines how recent research on intrinsic connectivity is beginning to provide new insights into the functional architecture of the human brain. He shows that neurocognitive models help to integrate empirical observations based on functional connectivity into a framework for understanding cognitive function, leading to new avenues for synthesis of disparate findings in the cognitive neuroscience literature. The usefulness of this approach is demonstrated by describing a dynamic neurocognitive network model for saliency detection, attentional capture, and cognitive control.

Human neuroimaging has to date mostly addressed the question of which brain regions are active during specific tasks. Recently, there has been a shift in focus toward more content-based neuroimaging. In chapter 3, John-Dylan Haynes shows, using multivariate decoding techniques, that it is now possible not only to measure the overall activity levels of brain regions but also to assess the amount of information they contain about specific mental representations, such as specific visual images or action plans. *Multidimensional scaling* allows one to construct spaces in which neural representations are coded. The exciting aspect of this work is that it is now possible to use new tools to reconstruct the dynamics of mental states and the interaction between distinct brain regions.

Keeping in mind that one of the main goals of cognitive neuroscience is to understand how the temporal dynamics of the brain are related to perception, emotion, cognition, and behavior, in chapter 4, Mikhail I. Rabinovich and Pablo Varona discuss experimental and computational approaches supporting the view that the brain processes information by forming temporary functional neural networks that exhibit transient states. A new mathematical approach in nonlinear dynamical theory has recently been developed for the rigorous description of transient activity in neural ensembles. These methods have been applied to specific cognitive problems. The authors describe some experiments along with mathematical and computational results that address transient brain dynamics and interactions among macroscopic brain modes.

In chapter 5, Peter beim Graben and Rolland Potthast present a phenomenological modeling of event-related brain potentials in syntactic language processing, which they illustrate in the setting of language processing and phrase structure violations. The authors derive a context-free grammar representation of stimuli and describe phrase structure violation by a prediction error in an interactive left-corner parser that is mapped onto a dynamic field by means of dynamic cognitive modeling.

Stefan J. Kiebel and Karl J. Friston then propose a new approach to speech sound recognition: They formulate recognition in terms of an internal model of how auditory input is generated and its inversion within a Bayesian framework. The model describes *continuous dynamics in the environment as a hierarchy of sequences*, where slower sequences cause faster sequences. The decoding or recognition scheme is illustrated using synthetic sequences of syllables, where syllables are sequences of phonemes and phonemes are sequences of sound-wave modulations. By presenting anomalous stimuli, they show that the ensuing recognition dynamics disclose inference at multiple timescales and are reminiscent of neuronal dynamics seen in the brain.

In chapter 7, Mikhail I. Rabinovich, Christian Bick, and Pablo Varona introduce a novel concept and its corresponding dynamical object to analyze brain activity: the informational flow in phase space (IFPS). This concept is directly related to the sequential dynamics of metastable states that are activated by inputs that do not destroy the origin of a competitive process. For the successful execution of a cognitive function, an IFPS (as a function of time) has to be a laminar (nonchaotic) flow; that is, a stable flow. Such stability guarantees the reproducibility and robustness of cognitive activity. Based on the requirement of IFPS stability, the authors discuss the dynamical origin of finite working memory capacity. They also build a dynamical model of information binding for transients that describes, for example, the interaction of different sensory information flows that are generated concurrently. This approach is used to model speaker–listener dynamics. Finally, they consider the role of noise on the temporal dynamics of sequential decision making.

In chapter 8, and Maxim Bazhenov and Scott Makeig consider the problem of how the electroencephalogram (EEG), electrocorticogram (ECoG), and local field potential (LFP) patterns relate to the activities of contributing neurons and neuronal clusters. Scalp EEG signals sum volume-conducted changes in electrical activity of multiple cortical sources. Thus, such signals represent weighted mixtures of the net electrical activity patterns of portions of cortical neuropile that each exhibit some degree of LFP synchrony. In some cases, these sources can be well localized to near-synchronous activity occurring across square-centimeter–sized or smaller cortical areas. In other circumstances, EEG signals may largely originate in more or less synchronous LFP activity across larger brain areas. Despite decades of studies, the question of how single-neuron activity leads to observed LFP, ECoG, and EEG patterns and how electrical fields in the brain at all spatial scales influence neuronal dynamics remains largely unanswered. Recent advances in both multi-resolution data recordings and large-scale computer modeling bring, however, a hope that combining these powerful approaches may shed a light on the genesis and functions of the large-scale activity patterns generated by the brain.

In chapter 9, Vasily A. Vakorin and Anthony R. McIntosh focus on quantifying the complexity of brain signals as measured by techniques like the EEG or the magnetoencephalogram (MEG). These authors review the definition, interpretation, and applications of sample entropy estimated at different timescales. The relations between sample entropy and other statistics such as spectral power, autocorrelation, nonstationarity, and graph measures are also discussed.

The complex interactions in brain networks, within which neural activity needs to be coordinated, is considered in chapter 10 by Viktor Jirsa and colleagues. These authors review some of the approaches to neural information processing in brain networks and propose a novel concept termed structured flows on manifolds (SFMs), describing function as a low-dimensional dynamic process emerging from coupled neurons. They show how sets of SFMs can capture the dynamic repertoire of complex behaviors and develop novel forms of functional architectures based on hierarchies of timescales. Chapter 11 addresses motor control and the general mechanisms underlying information transfer across the cortex: Andreas Daffertshofer and Bernadette C. M. van Wijk consider the problem of bimanual coordination. This problem requires the functional integration of various cortical, subcortical, spinal, and peripheral neural structures. To describe how this integration is accomplished, the authors use an experimental protocol and a mathematical description of both transient behavior and steady-state performance.

In chapter 12, Karl J. Friston provides a theoretical perspective on global brain dynamics from the point of view of the free-energy principle. This principle has been chosen as a global brain theory that is formulated explicitly in terms of dynamical systems. This principle provides a fairly simple explanation for action and behavior in terms of active inference and the Bayesian brain hypothesis. Within the Bayesian brain framework, the ensuing dynamics can be separated into those serving perceptual inference, learning, and attention. Another general approach, statistical decision theory, is considered in chapter 13 by Samuel J. Gershman and Nathaniel D. Daw. This theory defines the problem of maximizing the utility of one's decisions in terms of two subtasks: inferring the likely state of the world, and tracking the utility that would result from different actions in different states. This computational-level description underpins more process-level research in neuroscience about the brain's dynamic mechanisms for, on the one hand, inferring states and, on the other hand, learning action values. The authors consider the complex interrelationship between perception, action, and utility.

Finally, a short guide to modern nonlinear dynamics (ND) is provided in chapter 14 by Valentin S. Afraimovich, Mikhail I. Rabinovich, and Pablo Varona. This chapter describes the main notations and objects in modern ND, with some comments on their application to neural dynamics. This guide provides a comprehensive and rigorous description (but without theorems) of attractors, bifurcations, and stable transients with examples and illustrations.

We hope you enjoy reading this book as much as we enjoyed editing it and close by thanking all the authors for their marvelous contributions.

References

Brown, T. G. (1914). On the nature of the fundamental activity of the nervous centres; together with an analysis of the conditioning of rhythmic activity in progression, and a theory of the evolution of function in the nervous system. *Journal of Physiology*, *48*(1), 18–46.

James, W. (2007). The stream of thought. In *The Principles of Psychology* (Vol. 1, pp. 224–290). New York: Cosimo, Inc.

Poincaré, H. (2009). *The Foundations of Science*. New York: Cornell University Library.

Port, R. F., & van Gelder, T. (1995). *Mind as Motion: Explorations in the Dynamics of Cognition Description*. Cambridge, MA: MIT Press.

1 The Dynamical and Structural Basis of Brain Activity

Gustavo Deco, Viktor Jirsa, and Karl J. Friston

Summary

Global network dynamics over distributed brain areas emerge from the local dynamics of each brain area. Conversely, global dynamics constrain local activity such that the whole system becomes self-organizing. The implicit coupling between local and global scales induces a form of circular causality that is characteristic of complex, coupled systems that show self-organization, such as the brain. Here we present a network model based on spiking neurons at the local level and large-scale anatomic connectivity matrices at the global level. We demonstrate that this multiscale network displays endogenous or autonomous dynamics of the sort observed in resting-state studies. Our special focus here is on the genesis of itinerant (wandering) dynamics and the role of multistable attractors, which are involved in the generation of empirically known functional connectivity patterns, if the global coupling causes the dynamics to operate in the critical regime. Our results provide once again support for the hypothesis that endogenous brain activity is critical.

1.1 Introduction

Since the inception of experimental brain research, one of the most important objectives of neuroscience has been to understand the neuronal and cortical mechanisms underlying perceptual and cognitive functions. Early approaches to this challenging question originated one of the first influential brain theories, namely *localizationism*, which postulates that the brain is functionally segregated (i.e., that parts of the brain, and not the whole, perform specific functions). Localizationism was motivated by Franz Joseph Gall's theory of phrenology (Gall & Spurzheim, 1809). Although phrenology was not based on rigorous experimental facts, empirical support came from numerous experiments during the 19th century. Anatomists and physiologists such as Pierre Broca, Carl Wernicke, and many others were able to identify specific regions in animals and humans associated with particular brain functions, so that the concept of functional segregation was firmly established by the end of the nineteenth century (for a review, see Feinberg & Farah, 1997). Localizationism enjoyed a renaissance with the advent of functional brain imaging (e.g., functional magnetic resonance imaging; fMRI), which confirmed that specific functions, elicited experimentally, activated particular regions of the brain. However, localizationism is no longer the dominant paradigm in cognitive neuroscience: Many fMRI (and human electroencephalography (EEG) and magnetoencephalography (MEG) as well as animal cell recording) studies support the view that neuronal computations are distributed and engage a network of distributed brain areas (e.g., Cabeza & Nyberg, 2000). This is known as functional integration. This perspective, originally proposed by Flourens (1824) as a response to localizationism, is not inconsistent with functional segregation but emphasizes the interactions among functionally segregated brain areas. Nowadays, there is overwhelming evidence that all representations in the brain are distributed. Perceptions, memories, and even emotions are represented in a distributed manner; hence, a deeper understanding of the mechanisms underlying distributed processing is a central question for neuroscience. The main tools for characterizing distributed brain processing to date include the estimation of functional and effective connectivity from brain-imaging time series (McIntosh & Gonzalez-Lima, 1994; Cordes et al., 2000; Friston, Harrison, & Penny, 2003). Functional connectivity is defined as the statistical dependence between remote neurophysiologic events and is usually assessed with simple correlation or coherence analyses of fMRI or electrophysiologic time series. Conversely, effective connectivity is defined as the influence one system exerts over another and rests explicitly on an underlying model of neuronal dynamics (Friston et al., 2000). These dynamics are fundamental for processing of information at both a local level and a global level. They reconcile the apparently conflicting views of local versus global representation. Global network dynamics over distributed brain areas emerge from the local dynamics of each brain area. Conversely, global dynamics constrain local activity such that the whole system becomes self-organizing. The implicit coupling between local and global scales induces a form of circular causality that is characteristic of complex, coupled systems that show self-organization, like the brain. An important example of this is the slaving principle, where microscopic modes or patterns of activity become enslaved by a small number of macroscopic modes. In this chapter, we will take a look at how the dynamics of neuronal populations within a cortical area are enslaved by large-scale intercortical dynamics.

This chapter comprises two sections. In the first, we will consider models of brain dynamics from both local and global perspectives. We will present a specific model based on spiking neurons at the local level and large-scale anatomic connectivity matrices at the global level. This model is used in the second section to provide a quantitative example of how to model dynamical mechanisms in the brain. The second section focuses on endogenous or autonomous dynamics of the sort observed in resting-state studies. Our special focus here is on the genesis of itinerant (wandering) dynamics and the role of multistable attractors. In brief, we will show that the model described in the first section predicts empirical correlations in the brain when, and only when, global coupling brings it into a critical regime. We conclude with a brief discussion of the importance of autonomous dynamics in neuroscience and the universal properties that they might possess.

1.2   Attractors and Brain Dynamics

Computational neuroscience tries to describe the dynamics of networks of neurons and synapses with realistic models to reproduce emergent properties or predict observed neurophysiology (single- and multiple-cell recordings, local field potentials, optical imaging, EEG, MEG, fMRI) and associated behavior. Recently, a powerful theoretical framework known as *attractor theory* (see, e.g., Brunel & Wang, 2001) was introduced to capture the neural computations inherent in cognitive functions like attention, memory, and decision making. This theoretical framework is based on mathematical models formulated at the level of neuronal spiking and synaptic activity. Analysis of networks of neurons modeled at the integrate-and-fire level enables the study of many aspects of brain function: from the spiking activity of single neurons and the effects of pharmacological agents on synaptic currents, through to fMRI and neuropsychological findings. In the following, we describe the integration of local and global cortical dynamics in the setting of attractor networks.

1.2.1   A Local Model: Spiking Attractor Networks

To model a local brain area (i.e., a node in the global brain network), we will use a biophysically realistic attractor network model consisting of identical integrate-and-fire spiking neurons with synaptic dynamics

(Brunel & Wang, 2001). Extensions to ensembles of nonidentical neurons have been developed for electric (Assisi, Jirsa, & Kelso, 2005; Jirsa, 2007; Stefanescu & Jirsa, 2008) and synaptic (Jirsa & Stefanescu, 2010; Stefanescu & Jirsa, 2011) coupling. Attractor networks of spiking neurons are dynamical systems that have the tendency to settle in stationary states or fixed points called "attractors," typically characterized by a stable pattern of firing. External or even intrinsic noise that manifests in the form of finite size effects can destabilize these fixed-point attractors, inducing transitions among different attractors. The dynamics of these networks can be described by dynamical equations describing each neuron and how they influence each other through their coupling or effective connectivity. Spikes arriving at a given synapse provide an input to the neuron, which induces postsynaptic excitatory or inhibitory potentials. These are described by a low-pass filtering mediated by postsynaptic receptors. For example, the total synaptic current may be assumed to be the sum of glutamatergic (AMPA and NMDA) and GABAergic recurrent inhibitory currents. The parameters describing the biophysics of the neurons and synapses (conductances, latencies, etc.) are generally selected from a biologically realistic range. Each local attractor network typically contains a large number of excitatory pyramidal neurons and inhibitory neurons (100–10,000). We will use local attractor networks whose neurons are organized into two sets of populations (see figure 1.1); namely, an inhibitory population and an excitatory population. The key free parameters controlling the dynamics of the network are the strength of the recurrent excitatory and inhibitory synaptic connections. All neurons in a local network also receive an external background input modeled by uncorrelated Poisson spike trains, whose time-varying rate is given by a noisy Ornstein–Uhlenbeck process representing noisy fluctuations. External sensory or task-dependent inputs can be simulated in the same way, using higher mean input rates.

In what follows, we summarize the mathematical description of spiking and synaptic dynamics. The particular model that we use here is fairly typical of (neural mass) models specified to this level of detail. There are many other forms of model; for example, those based on multiple compartments for each neuron. However, the basic form of the differential equations and the state variables they describe are usually quite similar.

The integrate-and-fire (IF) model of a neuron is specified by the dynamics of its membrane potential $V(t)$. An IF neuron can be described by a basic RC-circuit consisting of a cell membrane capacitance C_m and a membrane resistance R_m. If the membrane potential is below a given

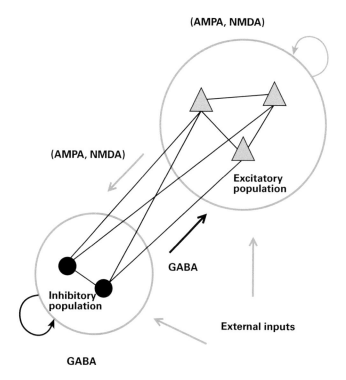

Figure 1.1
A local network. The network consists of spiking neurons with realistic AMPA, NMDA, and GABA synaptic dynamics. The network contains excitatory pyramidal cells and inhibitory interneurons.

threshold V_{thr} (subthreshold dynamics), then the membrane potential of each neuron in the network is given by the equation

$$C_m \frac{dV(t)}{dt} = -g_m[V(t) - V_L] - I_{\text{syn}}(t), \tag{1.1}$$

where $g_m = 1/R_m$ is the membrane leak conductance, V_L is the resting potential, and I_{syn} is the synaptic current. The membrane time constant is defined by $\tau_m = C_m/g_m$. When the voltage across the membrane reaches threshold, the neuron generates a spike, which is then transmitted to other neurons, and the membrane potential is instantaneously reset to V_{reset} and maintained there for a refractory period τ_{ref}, during which time the neuron is unable to produce further spikes.

Input currents from connected neurons or from external inputs drive the membrane potential: The spikes arriving at a synapse induce postsynaptic excitatory or inhibitory potentials. The total synaptic current is given by the sum of glutamatergic AMPA ($I_{AMPA,ext}$) mediated external excitatory currents, AMPA ($I_{AMPA,rec}$) and NMDA ($I_{NMDA,rec}$) mediated recurrent excitatory currents, and GABAergic recurrent inhibitory currents (I_{GABA}):

$$I_{syn} = I_{AMPA,ext} + I_{AMPA,rec} + I_{NMDA,rec} + I_{GABA}, \tag{1.2}$$

where

$$I_{AMPA,ext}(t) = g_{AMPA,ext}[V(t) - V_E]\sum_{j=1}^{N_{ext}} s_j^{AMPA,ext}(t) \tag{1.3}$$

$$I_{AMPA,rec}(t) = g_{AMPA,rec}[V(t) - V_E]\sum_{j=1}^{N_E} w_j s_j^{AMPA,rec}(t) \tag{1.4}$$

$$I_{NMDA,rec}(t) = \frac{g_{NMDA,rec}[V(t) - V_E]}{1 + \gamma e^{-\beta V(t)}}\sum_{j=1}^{N_E} w_j s_j^{NMDA,rec}(t) \tag{1.5}$$

$$I_{GABA}(t) = g_{GABA}[V(t) - V_I]\sum_{j=1}^{N_I} w_j s_j^{GABA}(t). \tag{1.6}$$

Here, $g_{AMPA,ext}$, $g_{AMPA,rec}$, $g_{NMDA,rec}$, and g_{GABA} are the synaptic conductances, and V_E and V_I are the excitatory and inhibitory reversal potentials, respectively. The dimensionless parameters w_j of the connections are the synaptic weights. The NMDA currents are voltage dependent and are modulated by intracellular magnesium concentration. The gating variables $s_j^i(t)$ are the fractions of open channels of neurons and are given by

$$\frac{ds_j^{AMPA,ext}(t)}{dt} = -\frac{s_j^{AMPA,ext}(t)}{\tau_{AMPA}} + \sum_k \delta(t - t_j^k) \tag{1.7}$$

$$\frac{ds_j^{AMPA,rec}(t)}{dt} = -\frac{s_j^{AMPA,rec}(t)}{\tau_{AMPA}} + \sum_k \delta(t - t_j^k) \tag{1.8}$$

$$\frac{ds_j^{NMDA,rec}(t)}{dt} = -\frac{s_j^{NMDA,rec}(t)}{\tau_{NMDA,decay}} + \alpha x_j(t)(1 - s_j^{NMDA,rec}(t)) \tag{1.9}$$

$$\frac{dx_j^{NMDA,rec}(t)}{dt} = -\frac{x_j^{NMDA,rec}(t)}{\tau_{AMPA,rise}} + \sum_k \delta(t - t_j^k) \tag{1.10}$$

$$\frac{ds_j^{GABA}(t)}{dt} = -\frac{s_j^{GABA}(t)}{\tau_{GABA}} + \sum_k \delta(t - t_j^k).$$

(1.11)

The sums over the index k represent all the spikes emitted by the presynaptic neuron j (at times t_j^k). In the equations above, $\tau_{NMDA,rise}$ and $\tau_{NMDA,decay}$ are the rise and decays times for the NMDA synapses, and τ_{AMPA} and τ_{GABA} are the decay times for AMPA and GABA synapses. The rise times of both AMPA and GABA synaptic currents are neglected because they are short (<1 ms). This concludes our description of the local model in terms of differential equations that describe the dynamics of each neuron in the populations considered. We will now turn our attention to the model of macroscopic or global dynamics.

1.2.2   A Global Model: The Connectome

The global brain model considered here is a network of local attractor networks described earlier. Crucially, the between-area (extrinsic) connections between different cortical areas are specified by a neuroanatomic matrix. We assume that the extrinsic connections between two distinct brain areas describe the density of synaptic connections between neurons in those areas. We weight those inter-areal connections by a coupling strength specified in the neuroanatomic matrix (numbers of fibers connecting those regions) and a global factor that plays the role of a control parameter. This control parameter will be used to study the dynamics and fixed points of the global system. Because the global system is defined in terms of its extrinsic connectivity, we can model global dynamics using connectivity data from macaque or humans. In the macaque case, we use the neuroanatomic matrix from the CoCoMac database (Kötter & Wanke, 2005), which describes the connectivity among approximately 40 cortical areas in one hemisphere of the macaque brain. Figure 1.2B shows an example of such a matrix of connection strengths. The center coordinates of each cortical area can be obtained from the geometry defined in the Automatic Anatomic Labeling cortical surface template of a human hemisphere (Kötter & Wanke, 2005). The length of the extrinsic connections (and consequently the delay in the transmission of spikes) can be evaluated from the distance between target and source regions. In the human case, we can use neuroanatomic information obtained by diffusion weighted tensor imaging (DTI) and diffusion spectrum imaging (DSI) tractography. An example is the neuroanatomic matrix of Hagmann et al. (2008: Briefly, after diffusion spec-

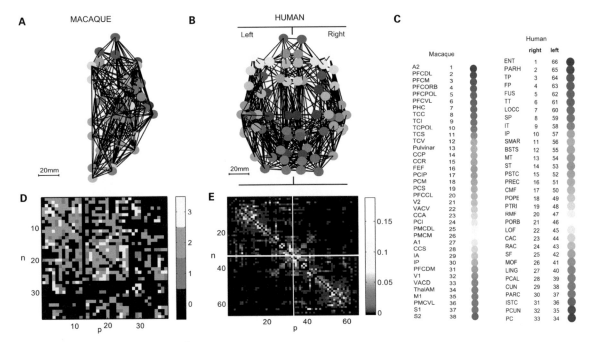

Figure 1.2 (plate 1)
Structural connectivity of the macaque and the human cortex. (A) Three-dimensional representation of the CoCoMac (left) and the human connectome (right) networks (view from above). The nodes representing anatomic regions are placed at their central coordinates. (B) Connection strength matrices for the CoCoMac (left) and the 66 × 66 human connectome (right) where n is the source region and p is the target. The connectome is ordered in such a way that corresponding contralateral regions are arranged symmetrically, with respect to the matrix center; the anti-diagonal reveals the existing connections between these contralateral regions. The white lines separate the two hemispheres. The cortical regions for the CoCoMac and for the human connectome are shown in the left and right subpanels and index the regions in (A).

trum and T1-weighted MRI acquisitions, the segmented gray matter was partitioned into approximately 1000 anatomic regions of interest (ROIs). White matter tractography identified voxel pairs that were connected to specify a neuroanatomic matrix. Note that tractography does not give the directionality of the fibers mediating the connection. This means that the connectivity matrix is symmetric, which may have consequences for the observable network dynamics (Knock et al., 2009; Jirsa, Sporns, Breakspear, Deco, & McIntosh, 2010), but will remain within limits unless the symmetry breaking is large. The resulting structural connectivity (SC) matrices were then averaged across five subjects. To downsample the SC to 66 regions, the connection strength between two regions was calculated by summing all incoming connection strengths to the target region and dividing by its number of ROIs. Clearly, because the number of ROIs depends on the region, the downsampled connectivity matrix is no longer symmetric. As the local dynamical model already models within-area (intrinsic) connectivity, the connection of a region to itself is generally omitted from extrinsic connectivity matrices (see figure 1.2, plate 1). The length of a connection between two regions can be calculated as the average length across all connecting tractography fibers.

In the next section, we will simulate brain responses that arise from spontaneous fluctuations in this dynamical model. At present, most neuroimaging studies of distributed activity of this sort are performed with fMRI. We therefore need to model the mapping between the neuronal dynamics, specified in terms of depolarization, to the sorts of signals observed with fMRI. These are referred to as blood oxygen level–dependent (BOLD) signals. We will model these using a fairly detailed dynamical model of the brain's neurovascular coupling.

Simulating the BOLD Signal

The simulation of fMRI BOLD signals appeals to the Balloon–Windkessel hemodynamic model of Friston et al. (2003). The Balloon–Windkessel model describes the coupling of perfusion to BOLD signal and is augmented with a dynamical model of the transduction of neural activity into perfusion changes. The model assumes that the BOLD signal is a static nonlinear function of normalized total deoxyhemoglobin voxel content, normalized venous volume, resting net oxygen extraction fraction, and resting blood volume fraction. In our model, the input to the hemodynamic model is neuronal activity summed over all neurons in both populations (excitatory and inhibitory populations) in any given area.

In brief, for the ith region, neuronal activity z_i causes an increase in a vasodilatory signal s_i that is subject to autoregulatory feedback. The inflow f_i responds in proportion to this signal with concomitant changes in blood volume v_i and deoxyhemoglobin content q_i. The equations relating these biophysical variables are

$$\frac{\partial s_i(t)}{\partial t} = z_i - k_i s_i - \gamma_1 (f_1 - 1) \tag{1.12}$$

$$\frac{\partial f_i(t)}{\partial t} = s_1 \tag{1.13}$$

$$\frac{\tau_i \partial v_i(t)}{\partial t} = f_i - v_1^{\frac{1}{\alpha}} \qquad (1.14)$$

$$\frac{\tau_i \partial q_i(t)}{\partial t} = \frac{\left\{ f_i [1 - (1 - \rho_i)]^{\frac{1}{f_i}} \right\}}{\rho_i} - \frac{v_1^{\frac{1}{\alpha}} q_1}{v_1}, \qquad (1.15)$$

where ρ is the resting oxygen extraction fraction. The BOLD signal is taken to be a static nonlinear function of volume and deoxyhemoglobin that comprises a volume-weighted sum of extravascular and intravascular signals:

$$y_i = V_0 (7\rho_i (1 - q_i) + 2 \left(1 - \frac{q_i}{v_i} \right) + (2\rho_1 - 0.2)(1 - v_1)), \qquad (1.16)$$

where $V_0 = 0.02$ is the resting blood volume fraction. The biophysical details of this model can be found in Friston et al. (2000).

We have now described a neuronal mass model of populations of neurons within each node of a distributed network. We have also discussed the coupling between these nodes at the macroscopic level in terms of empirically (anatomically) constrained extrinsic connectivity. Finally, we now have a model that maps from hidden neuronal states to observed hemodynamic responses in fMRI. In the next section, we will use this model to study some key emergent properties that illustrate the self-organization of brain dynamics described in the introduction.

1.3   Autonomous Brain Dynamics

Classical accounts of brain function (Hubel & Wiesel, 1968; Barlow, 1990) emphasize the role of feedforward information processing in generating from the "ground up" sensory, cognitive, and motor representations that mediate behavior. Although feedforward sensory analysis can also be modulated by endogenous signals like familiarity, attention, and reward, a central tenet of this view is that any spontaneous or intrinsic activity reflects noise. But internal noise is crucial as it produces random (spike rate) fluctuations that can have a profound effect on the transmission of information. Such feedforward sensorimotor models have been successful in linking activity recorded from single neurons to perceptual decisions (Newsome, Britten, & Movshon, 1989; Shadlen, Britten, Newsome, & Movshon, 1996; Shadlen & Newsome, 1996). However, a different class of models suggests that the brain is not a passive sensorimotor mapping, driven by sensory information, but that it actively generates and maintains predictions (priors) about forthcoming sensory stimuli, cognitive states, and actions (Llinas, Ribary, Contreras, & Pedroarena, 1998; Engel, Fries, & Singer, 2001; Varela, Lachaux, Rodriguez, & Martinerie, 2001; Friston, 2002). This class of models emphasizes the role of spontaneous ongoing activity in maintaining active and itinerant representations that are entrained rather than determined by sensory information. Accordingly, spontaneous ongoing activity should not be random (as often implied by its dismissal as mere "noise") but organized into structured spatiotemporal patterns that reflect the functional architecture of the brain, encode traces of previous behavior, or even predict future decisions. Hence, the study of whole-brain activity during stimulus-free (resting) conditions is a natural forum for examining these itinerant dynamics. The resulting endogenous, self-organized dynamics reflect the activity of the brain that can only arise from its intrinsic properties (neuroanatomic structure, local spontaneous brain areas dynamics, fluctuations, delays).

An increasing number of experimental studies have characterized the dynamics of spontaneous or ongoing activity with a variety of different methods including EEG (Creutzfeldt, Watanabe, & Lux, 1966), optical imaging (Kenet et al., 2003), single unit (Engel et al., 2001), and fMRI (Biswal, Yetkin, Haughton, & Hyde, 1995; Fox & Raichle, 2007). In particular, fMRI measures local changes in magnetic susceptibility (BOLD signal) caused by variations in the capillary concentration of deoxyhemoglobin due to blood flow and blood volume increases in response to neuronal activation (see previous section). In the absence of stimuli, spontaneous fMRI signals are characterized by slow oscillations (< 0.1 Hz). It was noted more than a decade ago that spontaneous BOLD fluctuations are temporally correlated (or coherent) between brain regions with similar functional specialization (Biswal, DeYoe, & Hyde, 1996); see (Fox & Raichle, 2007) for review. The ensuing networks of correlated fluctuations are said to constitute resting-state networks. In what follows, we will look at these endogenous fluctuations using the large-scale model of neocortical dynamics introduced in the previous section (see also Ghosh, Rho, McIntosh, Kötter, & Jirsa, 2008; Deco, Jirsa, McIntosh, Sporns, & Kötter, 2009; Deco, Jirsa, & McIntosh, 2011).

1.3.1   Endogenous Activity and Multistability

We now consider the dynamics of the realistic global attractor spiking network based on the neuroanatomic connectivity matrix of the macaque described earlier. We will see that by placing local dynamics on this macroscopic structure, we can explain many features of resting-state networks as evidenced by fMRI. Specifically, we find that resting-state networks can be accounted for by structured fluctuations around a trivial low-firing equilibrium state (fixed-point attractor). These fluctuations are induced by multistable attractors that correspond to high firing activity in particular brain areas.

We will first look at the stationary fixed points (attractor landscape) of the cortical network. To do this, we can reduce the spiking dynamics of the previous section to a set of mean field equations that describe the stationary states (see Brunel & Wang, 2001; Deco, Jirsa, Robinson, Breakspear, & Friston, 2008). This allows us to identify the fixed points as a function of the parameter W that scales global coupling. Figure 1.3 shows the number of fixed points found in the system as a function of W. These fixed points were found by solving the mean-field equations from a thousand different initial conditions. Figure 1.3 also shows the average uncertainty (entropy) that a given attractor is occupied, when starting from random initial conditions.

This entropy characterizes the variability of cortical activity due to noise-driven transitions among multistable attractors. For very small

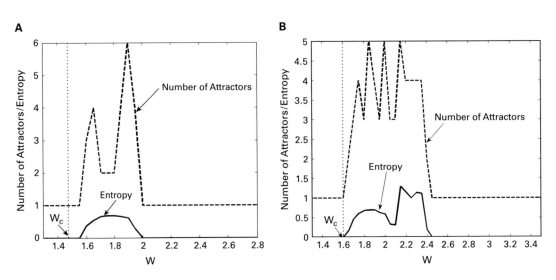

Figure 1.3
Mean field analyses of the attractor landscape of the cortical spiking network as a function of the global inter-areal coupling strength (left, monkey; right, human). The dashed line shows the number of stable attractors, whereas the continuous line shows the entropy of the attractors.

values of W, only one attractor is stable, and therefore the entropy is zero. This fixed-point attractor corresponds to the trivial spontaneous ground state of the system, where all neurons are firing at a low level (excitatory neurons at 3 Hz and inhibitory neurons at 9 Hz). For very large values of W, there is also only one stable attractor, and therefore the entropy is again zero. This attractor corresponds to the epileptiform case, where all excitatory neurons are highly activated in all brain areas. In intermediate regions of W, we find multistability corresponding to distinct foci of high firing activity in particular brain areas. This regime is reported by high entropy and contains many fixed-point attractors. It is this regime that characterizes real brain dynamics and, indeed, the dynamics of self-organized systems that maintain themselves near phase transitions or bifurcations. Similar phenomena are also seen using globally coupled maps based on oscillator models of neuronal dynamics. In these systems, increasingly global coupling takes the system from a completely desynchronized state, through a regime of multistability and itinerant chaos, to a quiescent regime of global synchronization.

To show that the brain may conform to similar principles of self-organization, we tested the hypothesis that simulated global dynamics in the multistable regime were a better predictor of observed fMRI dynamics obtained during resting state in humans: Using the spiking model, we calculated the neuronal activity in all brain areas and then simulated fMRI signals using the Balloon–Windkessel model (Friston et al., 2003). After simulated fMRI signals were downsampled to 2 s (Honey et al., 2007, they were treated in the same way as the empirical data: The global signal (average over all regions) was removed by linear regression (Fox et al., 2005, 2009). Finally, we computed the functional connectivity by calculating the correlation matrix of the BOLD activity among all brain areas. This was repeated for a range of global coupling parameters. To identify the region of the parameter W where the model best reproduces the empirical functional connectivity, we computed the Pearson correlation between the empirical and the simulated functional connectivity matrices. Figure 1.4 shows that this is maximal for the critical values of global coupling found in figure 1.3. This result is important because it suggests the brain might also be exploiting multistability to maintain its rich repertoire of dynamics that are characteristic of endogenous neuronal activity. This repertoire depends upon an intermediate level of overall coupling among brain regions that is not too strong and is not too weak. We conclude with a brief discussion of the larger issues that this type of analysis is designed to address.

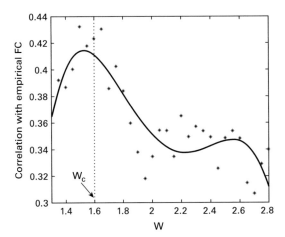

Figure 1.4
Fitting of empirical data in human subjects (as measured by the correlation between simulated and empirical functional connectivity) as a function of the global coupling parameter W. The best fit is achieved at the edge of the bifurcation.

1.4   Conclusion

These analyses above show that, even at rest, endogenous brain activity is self-organizing and highly structured. There are many questions about the genesis of autonomous dynamics and the structures that support them. Some of the more interesting come from computational anatomy and neuroscience. The emerging picture is that endogenous fluctuations are a consequence of dynamics on anatomic connectivity structures with particular scale-invariant and small-world characteristics (Achard, Salvador, Witcher, Suckling, & Bullmore, 2006; Bassett & Bullmore, 2009; Honey, Kötter, Breakspear, & Sporns, 2007; Deco et al., 2009). These are well-studied and universal characteristics of complex systems and suggest that we may be able to understand the brain in terms of universal phenomena (Sporns, 2010). For example, Buice and Cowan (2009) model neocortical dynamics using field-theoretic methods (from nonequilibrium statistical processes) to describe both neural fluctuations and responses to stimuli. In their models, the density and extent of lateral cortical interactions induce a region of state space, in which the effects of fluctuations are negligible. However, as the generation and decay of neuronal activity comes into balance, there is a transition into a regime of critical fluctuations. These models suggest that the scaling laws, found in many measurements of neocortical activity, are consistent with the existence of phase transitions at a critical point. They also speak to larger questions about how the brain maintains itself near phase transitions (i.e., self-organized criticality and gain control; Abbott, Varela, Sen, & Nelson, 1997; Kitzbichler, Smith, Christensen, & Bullmore, 2009). This is an important issue, because systems near phase transitions show universal phenomena (Jirsa, Friedrich, Haken, & Kelso, 1994; Jirsa & Haken, 1996; Jirsa & Kelso, 2000; Tschacher & Haken, 2007; Tognoli & Kelso, 2009). Although many people argue for criticality and power-law effects in large-scale cortical activity (e.g., Linkenkaer-Hansen, Nikouline, Palva, & Ilmoniemi, 2001; Stam & de Bruin, 2004; Freyer, Aquino, Robinson, Ritter, & Breakspear, 2009; Kitzbichler et al., 2009), other people do not (Bedard, Kroger, & Destexhe, 2006). It may be that slow (electrophysiologic) frequencies contain critical oscillations, whereas high-frequency coherent oscillations may reflect other dynamical processes. In short, endogenous fluctuations are an important example of dynamics and structure and may disclose fundamental principles of self-organization that underwrite the brain's remarkable capacity to support itinerant and adaptive dynamics.

References

Abbott, L. F., Varela, J. A., Sen, K., & Nelson, S. B. (1997). Synaptic depression and cortical gain control. *Science*, *275*(5297), 220–224.

Achard, S., Salvador, R., Whitcher, B., Suckling, J., & Bullmore, E. (2006). A resilient, low-frequency, small-world human brain functional network with highly connected association cortical hubs. *Journal of Neuroscience*, *26*(1), 63–72.

Assisi, C. G., Jirsa, V. K., & Kelso, J. A. S. (2005). Synchrony and clustering in heterogeneous networks with global coupling and parameter dispersion. *Physical Review Letters*, *94*, 018106.

Barlow, H. (1990). What the brain tells the eye. *Scientific American*, *262*, 90–95.

Bassett, D. S., & Bullmore, E. T. (2009). Human brain networks in health and disease. *Current Opinion in Neurology*, *22*(4), 340–347.

Bedard, C., Kroger, H., & Destexhe, A. (2006). Model of low-pass filtering of local field potentials in brain tissue. *Physical Review E: Statistical, Nonlinear, and Soft Matter Physics*, *73*(5 Pt 1), 051911.

Biswal, B., DeYoe, A. E., & Hyde, J. S. (1996). Reduction of physiological fluctuations in fMRI using digital filters. *Magnetic Resonance in Medicine*, *35*, 107–113.

Biswal, B., Yetkin, F., Haughton, V., & Hyde, J. (1995). Functional connectivity in the motor cortex of resting human brain using echo-planar MRI. *Magnetic Resonance in Medicine*, *34*, 537–541.

Brunel, N., & Wang, X. J. (2001). Effects of neuromodulation in a cortical network model of object working memory dominated by recurrent inhibition. *Journal of Computational Neuroscience*, *11*, 63–85.

Buice, M. A., & Cowan, J. D. (2009). Statistical mechanics of the neocortex. *Progress in Biophysics and Molecular Biology*, *99*(2–3), 53–86.

Cabeza, R., & Nyberg, L. (2000). Imaging cognition II: empirical review of 275 PET and fMRI studies. *Journal of Cognitive Neuroscience*, *12*, 1–47.

Cordes, D., Haughton, V., Arfanakis, K., Wendt, G., Turski, W., Moritz, C., et al. (2000). Mapping functionally related regions of brain with functional connectivity MR imaging. *AJNR. American Journal of Neuroradiology, 21,* 1636–1644.

Creutzfeldt, O., Watanabe, S., & Lux, H. (1966). Relations between EEG phenomena and potentials of single cortical cells. *Electroencephalography and Clinical Neurophysiology, 20,* 19–37.

Deco, G., Jirsa, V., & McIntosh, A. R. (2011). Emerging concepts for the dynamical organization of resting-state activity in the brain. *Nature Reviews. Neuroscience, 12,* 43–56.

Deco, G., Jirsa, V., McIntosh, A. R., Sporns, O., & Kötter, R. (2009). Key role of coupling, delay, and noise in resting brain fluctuations. *Proceedings of the National Academy of Sciences of the United States of America, 106,* 10302–10307.

Deco, G., Jirsa, V., Robinson, P., Breakspear M., and Friston, K. (2008). The dynamic brain: From spiking neurons to neural masses and cortical fields. *PLoS Computational Biology 4* (8), e1000092.

Engel, A., Fries, P., & Singer, W. (2001). Dynamic predictions: oscillations and synchrony in top-down processing. *Nature Reviews. Neuroscience, 2,* 704–716.

Feinberg, T. E., & Farah, M. J. (1997). The development of modern behavioral neurology and neuropsychology. In T. E. Feinberg & M. J. Farah (Eds.), *Behavioral Neurology and Neuropsychology.* New York: McGraw Hill.

Flourens, M. J. P. (1824). *Recherches expérimentales sur les propriétés et les fonctions du système nerveux, dans les animaux vertébrés* (1st ed., Vol. 26, p. 20). Paris: Chez Crevot.

Fox, M. D., Snyder, A. Z., Vincent, J. L., Corbetta, M., Van Essen, D. C., et al. (2005). The human brain is intrinsically organized into dynamic, anticorrelated functional networks. *Proceedings of the National Academy of Sciences USA, 102,* 9673–9678.

Fox, M., & Raichle, M. (2007). Spontaneous fluctuations in brain activity observed with functional magnetic resonance imaging. *Nature Reviews. Neuroscience, 8,* 700–711.

Fox, M. D., Zhang, D., Snyder, A. Z., & Raichle, M. E. (2009). The global signal and observed anticorrelated resting state brain networks. *Journal of Neurophysiology, 101,* 3270–3283.

Freyer, F., Aquino, K., Robinson, P. A., Ritter, P., & Breakspear, M. (2009). Non-Gaussian statistics in temporal fluctuations of spontaneous cortical activity. *Journal of Neuroscience, 29,* 8512–8524.

Friston, K. J., Mechelli, A., Turner, R., & Price, C. J. (2000). Nonlinear responses in fMRI: The Balloon model, Volterra kernels, and other hemodynamics. *Neuroimage, 12,* 466–477.

Friston, K. (2002). Beyond phrenology: what can neuroimaging tell us about distributed circuitry? *Annual Review of Neuroscience, 25,* 221–250.

Friston, K., Harrison, L., & Penny, W. (2003). Dynamic causal modelling. *NeuroImage, 19,* 1273–1302.

Gall, F. J., & Spurzheim, J. G. (1967). *Recherches sur le Systeme Nerveux.* Amsterdam: Bonset. Originally published in 1809.

Ghosh, A., Rho, Y., McIntosh, A. R., Kötter, R., & Jirsa, V. K. (2008). Noise during rest enables the exploration of the brain's dynamic repertoire. *PLoS Computational Biology, 4,* e1000196.

Hagmann, P., Cammoun, L., Gigandet, X., Meuli, R., Honey, C. J., Wedeen, V. J., & Sporns, O. (2008). Mapping the structural core of human cerebral cortex. *PLoS Biology, 6,* e159.

Honey, C. J., Kötter, R., Breakspear, M., & Sporns, O. (2007). Network structure of cerebral cortex shapes functional connectivity on multiple time scales. *Proceedings of the National Academy of Sciences of the United States of America, 104,* 10240–10245.

Hubel, D. H., & Wiesel, T. N. (1968). Receptive fields and functional architecture of monkey striate cortex. *Journal of Physiology, 195,* 215–243.

Jirsa, V. K. (2007). Dispersion and time-delay effects in synchronized spike-burst networks. *Cognitive Neurodynamics, 2*(1), 29–38.

Jirsa, V. K., & Haken, H. (1996). Field theory of electromagnetic brain activity. *Physical Review Letters*, *77*, 960–963.

Jirsa, V. K., & Kelso, J. A. (2000). Spatiotemporal pattern formation in neural systems with heterogeneous connection topologies. *Physical Review E: Statistical Physics, Plasmas, Fluids, and Related Interdisciplinary Topics*, *62*(6 Pt B), 8462–8465.

Jirsa, V. K., Friedrich, R., Haken, H., & Kelso, J. A. (1994). A theoretical model of phase transitions in the human brain. *Biological Cybernetics*, *71*(1), 27–35.

Jirsa, V. K., & Stefanescu, R. A. (2010). Neural population modes capture biologically realistic large scale network dynamics. *Bulletin of Mathematical Biology, 73*, 325–343.

Jirsa, V. K., Sporns, O., Breakspear, M., Deco, G., & McIntosh, A. R. (2010). Towards the virtual brain: network modeling of the intact and the damaged brain. *Archives Italiennes de Biologie*, *148*, 189–205.

Kenet, T., Bibitchkov, D., Tsodyks, M., Grinvald, A., & Arieli, A. (2003). Spontaneously emerging cortical representations of visual attributes. *Nature*, *425*, 954–956.

Kitzbichler, M. G., Smith, M. L., Christensen, S. R., & Bullmore, E. (2009). Broadband criticality of human brain network synchronization. *PLoS Computational Biology*, *5*(3), e1000314.

Knock, S. A., McIntosh, A. R., Sporns, O., Kötter, R., Hagmann, P., & Jirsa, V. K. (2009). The effects of physiologically plausible connectivity structure on local and global dynamics in large scale brain models. *Journal of Neuroscience Methods*, *183*, 86–94.

Kötter, R., & Wanke, E. (2005). Mapping brains without coordinates. *Philosophical Transactions of the Royal Society of London. Series B*, *360*, 751–766.

Linkenkaer-Hansen, K., Nikouline, V. V., Palva, J. M., & Ilmoniemi, R. J. (2001). Long-range temporal correlations and scaling behavior in human brain oscillations. *Journal of Neuroscience*, *21*, 1370–1377.

Llinas, R., Ribary, U., Contreras, D., & Pedroarena, C. (1998). The neuronal basis for consciousness. *Philosophical Transactions of the Royal Society of London. Series B, Biological Sciences*, *353*, 1841–1849.

McIntosh, R., & Gonzalez-Lima, F. (1994). Structural equation modeling and its application to network analysis in functional brain imaging. *Human Brain Mapping*, *2*, 2–22.

Newsome, W. T., Britten, K. H., & Movshon, J. A. (1989). Neuronal correlates of a perceptual decision. *Nature*, *341*, 52–54.

Shadlen, M., & Newsome, W. (1996). Motion perception: seeing and deciding. *Proceedings of the National Academy of Sciences of the United States of America*, *93*, 628–633.

Shadlen, M., Britten, K., Newsome, W., & Movshon, J. A. (1996). Computational analysis of the relationship between neuronal and behavioral responses to visual motion. *Journal of Neuroscience*, *16*, 1486–1510.

Sporns, O. (2010). *Networks of the Brain*. Cambridge, MA: MIT Press.

Stam, C. J., & de Bruin, E. A. (2004). Scale-free dynamics of global functional connectivity in the human brain. *Human Brain Mapping*, *22*, 97–109.

Stefanescu, R., & Jirsa, V. K. (2008). A low dimensional description of globally coupled heterogeneous neural networks of excitatory and inhibitory neurons. *PLoS Computational Biology*, *4*(11), e1000219.

Stefanescu, R., & Jirsa, V. K. (2011). *Reduced neural population dynamics with synaptic coupling*. PRE.

Tognoli, E., & Kelso, J. A. (2009). Brain coordination dynamics: true and false faces of phase synchrony and metastability. *Progress in Neurobiology*, *87*(1), 31–40.

Tschacher, W., & Haken, H. (2007). Intentionality in non-equilibrium systems? The functional aspects of self-organised pattern formation. *New Ideas in Psychology*, *25*, 1–15.

Varela, F., Lachaux, J., Rodriguez, E., & Martinerie, J. (2001). The brainweb: phase synchronization and large-scale integration. *Nature Reviews. Neuroscience*, *2*, 229–239.

2 Functional Connectivity, Neurocognitive Networks, and Brain Dynamics

Vinod Menon

Summary

Understanding how the human brain produces cognition must ultimately depend on knowledge of its large-scale organization. Brain areas engaged during cognitive tasks also form coherent large-scale brain networks that can be readily identified using intrinsic functional connectivity. We examine how recent research on intrinsic connectivity is beginning to provide new insights into the functional architecture of the human brain. We show that neurocognitive models help to synthesize extant findings of functional connectivity into a framework for understanding cognitive function, leading to new avenues for synthesis of disparate findings in the cognitive neuroscience literature. We demonstrate the usefulness of this approach by illustrating a dynamic neurocognitive network model for saliency detection, attentional capture, and cognitive control.

2.1 A Connectivity and Network Perspective on Cognition

Functional magnetic resonance imaging (fMRI) has contributed greatly to our understanding of the neural basis of perception, cognition, and emotion in humans (Huettel, Song, & McCarthy, 2008). The first two decades of fMRI research were largely focused on localization of brain responses in relation to specific experimental manipulations (Cabeza & Kingstone, 2006). It has become increasingly apparent, however, that even the most basic behavioral processes are implemented by multiple distributed brain regions, and the original goal of mapping cognitive and psychological constructs onto individual brain areas is now widely considered implausible (Fuster, 2006). As a result, researchers have increasingly turned their attention to characterizing the interaction of multiple brain regions. Functional connectivity analyses based on temporal coupling of fMRI responses are now widely used to examine context- and stimulus-dependent interactions between brain regions (Friston, 1994,

2005; Jirsa & McIntosh, 2007). Although these studies have provided insights into the interaction of multiple brain regions activated by particular tasks, a principled understanding of functional brain circuits has remained elusive.

The functions of a cortical area are determined by its intrinsic properties and its extrinsic connections (Passingham, Stephan, & Kotter, 2002). Each brain region likely has a unique fingerprint of connectivity that distinguishes it from other brain regions, endowing it with specific functional properties. Understanding the function of any specific brain region therefore requires analysis of how its connectivity differs from the pattern of connections in other functionally related brain areas. In recent years, the interests of neuroscientists have shifted toward developing a deeper understanding of how intrinsic functional and structural connectivity influences cognitive and affective information processing (Greicius, Krasnow, Reiss, & Menon, 2003; Fox & Raichle, 2007; Dosenbach, Fair, Cohen, Schlaggar, & Petersen, 2008), and network approaches are becoming increasingly useful for understanding the neural underpinnings of cognition (Bressler & Menon, 2010). Such an approach affords the possibility of building a more systematic and principled understanding of the concerted coordination between multiple brain regions during cognition.

The human brain undergoes protracted structural and functional changes (Sowell et al., 2003; Barnea-Goraly et al., 2005; Supekar, Musen, & Menon, 2009) during which it constructs dedicated large-scale brain networks composed of discrete, interconnected brain regions (Fair et al., 2007; Supekar et al., 2009). In this chapter, we discuss how functional connectivity measures can be used to identify and characterize core large-scale brain networks in the human brain. We develop the notion of neurocognitive networks and then illustrate how such networks allow us to construct models that provide new insights into the dynamical basis of fundamental cognitive processes. We demonstrate the usefulness of this approach by illustrating a network model for attention and cognitive control.

2.2 Identifying Major Cognitive Networks

A formal characterization of core neurocognitive networks was first enunciated by Mesulam, who proposed that the human brain contains at least five major core networks, each dedicated to a more or less distinct cognitive function (Mesulam, 1998):

1. A spatial attention network anchored in posterior parietal cortex and frontal eye fields.

2. A language network anchored in the middle temporal gyrus and Wernicke's and Broca's areas.

3. An explicit memory network anchored in the hippocampal–entorhinal complex and inferior parietal cortex.

4. A face-object recognition network anchored in the ventral temporal cortex and anterior temporal lobe.

5. A working memory–executive function network anchored in the dorsolateral prefrontal and inferior parietal cortices.

The nodes of such neurocognitive networks were initially identified using lesion studies (Damasio & Damasio, 1989). Although these studies have taken on increasing sophistication over the years with voxel-based lesion-symptom mapping (Bates et al., 2003), their anatomic precision remains poor. Further, lesion mapping does not lend itself to identification of common patterns of distributed brain processes associated with precise cognitive functions. More recently, fMRI activations have been used more precisely to demarcate nodes of individual functional circuits associated with specific cognitive processes. However, regions of interest identified in this manner tend to vary considerably with task demands and the specific control or baseline condition used to identify them. As a result, uncovering the nodes of these neurocognitive networks in a principled and reliable manner has turned out to be elusive. A full characterization of functional brain networks has required novel methods for specifying network nodes and edges in a more principled manner, and considerable effort is now being devoted to this from multiple fronts both functional and anatomic (Zilles & Amunts, 2010).

A more general approach is afforded by analysis of the large-scale brain organization (Bressler & Menon, 2010). Recent research suggests that brain networks may be more readily characterized on the basis of intrinsic anatomic and functional connectivity (Fox & Raichle, 2007; Uddin, Supekar, & Menon, 2010). Although neuronal populations have a variety of different internal circuitry configurations, they may be represented as network nodes if they have a uniquely identifiable local structural organization, large-scale structural connectivity pattern, or local functional activity pattern that allows them to be distinguished from their neighbors (Bressler & Menon, 2010). The analysis of intrinsic functional connectivity has facilitated the discovery of core brain networks that cannot yet be captured with more sophisticated tract-tracing techniques such as diffusion spectrum imaging and autoradiography (Schmahmann et al., 2007; Wedeen et al., 2008). Functional connectivity analyses can be used reliably to identify several large-scale networks in the human brain (Greicius et al., 2003; Damoiseaux et al., 2006; Seeley et al., 2007). Both model-based regression analysis and model-free independent component analysis (ICA) of temporal fluctuations in fMRI signals have proved to be useful techniques for investigating functionally coupled networks (Seeley et al., 2007). Although both methods rely on analysis of low-frequency fMRI signals, cortical potentials demonstrate a correlation structure similar to that of spontaneous fMRI fluctuations (He, Snyder, Zempel, Smyth, & Raichle, 2008; Nir et al., 2008; Popa, Popescu, & Pare, 2009; Dastjerdi et al., 2011).

2.3   Intrinsic Connectivity Networks

Since the discovery of coherent fluctuations within the somatomotor system (Biswal et al., 1995), a growing number of studies have shown that many of the brain areas engaged during various cognitive tasks also form coherent large-scale brain networks that can be readily identified using intrinsic functional connectivity (Greicius & Menon, 2004; Smith et al., 2009). The underlying premise of these studies is that intrinsic brain connectivity constrains perception and cognition in fundamental ways. Task-free "resting-state" fMRI (rsfMRI) has emerged as a novel tool for characterizing functional brain networks. Model-free analysis of intrinsic connectivity using ICA (Beckmann & Smith, 2004) has turned out to be an important tool for identifying intrinsic connectivity networks (ICNs) from rsfMRI data (Damoiseaux et al., 2006; Seeley et al., 2007). ICNs reflect strong spontaneous fluctuations in ongoing activity that remains robust under different mental states including sleep, anesthesia, and loss of consciousness (Greicius et al., 2008; Horovitz et al., 2009; Vanhaudenhuyse et al., 2010). Some examples include a sensorimotor ICN anchored in bilateral somatosensory and motor cortices; a lower-order visual network anchored in the striate and extrastriate cortex; a visuospatial network anchored in intraparietal sulci and frontal eye fields; and a higher-order visual network anchored in lateral occipital and inferior temporal cortices (Damoiseaux et al., 2006; Shirer, Ryali, Rykhlevskaia, Menon, & Greicius, 2011) (figure 2.1, plate 2). ICNs have been implicated not only in sensory processing but also in higher cognitive functions, including working memory, attention, episodic memory, autobiographical memory, and self-referential processing (Greicius et al., 2003). Critically,

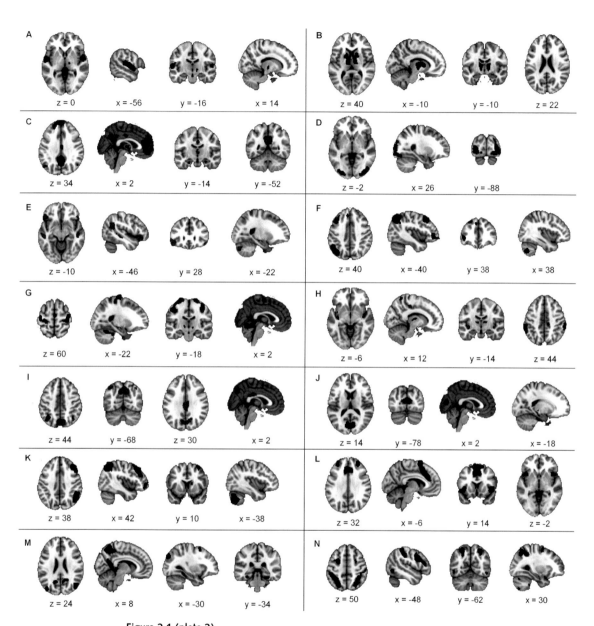

Figure 2.1 (plate 2)
Fourteen intrinsic connectivity networks (ICNs) identified in resting-state fMRI (rsfMRI) data. Figure highlights regions of interest (ROIs) contained within each ICN identified using independent component analysis (ICA): (A) auditory; (B) basal ganglia; (C) posterior cingulate cortex (PCC)/ventromedial prefrontal cortex (VMPFC); (D) secondary visual cortex (V2); (E) language; (F) left dorsolateral prefrontal cortex (left DLPFC)/left parietal lobe; (G) sensorimotor; (H) posterior insula; (I) precuneus; (J) primary visual cortex (V1); (K) right dorsolateral prefrontal cortex (right DLPFC)/right parietal lobe; (L) insula/dorsal anterior cingulate cortex (dACC); (M) retrosplenial cortex (RSC)/medial temporal lobe (MTL); (N) intraparietal sulcus (IPS)/frontal eye field (FEF). From Shirer et al. (2011).

these networks show close correspondence in independent analyses of resting and task-related connectivity patterns (Smith et al., 2009), suggesting that network nodes identified using intrinsic functional connectivity are also, for the most part, simultaneously engaged during cognition. Indeed, studies of intrinsic brain connectivity are useful only insofar as they clarify the architecture of brain networks involved in cognition, a topic that we turn to next.

2.4   Three Core Neurocognitive Networks

Of the many stable ICNs identified to date, three have turned out to be particularly useful for understanding higher cognitive function in fundamental ways—hence use of the term *core neurocognitive networks*. In this section, we describe their network structure and the principal cognitive functions they serve. The three core networks are the central-executive network (CEN) anchored in dorsolateral prefrontal cortex (DLPFC) and posterior parietal cortex (PPC); the salience network (SN) anchored in anterior insula (AI), adjoining fronto-insular cortex (FIC) and anterior cingulate cortex (ACC); and the default mode network (DMN) anchored in the posterior cingulate cortex (PCC), medial prefrontal cortex (mPFC), medial temporal lobe (MTL), and angular gyrus (AG) (Greicius et al., 2003; Fox & Raichle, 2007; Seeley et al., 2007). Importantly, these ICNs allow intrinsic (figure 2.2, plate 3) and task-related (figure 2.3, plate 4) fMRI activation patterns to be identified and studied in a common framework. These three networks can be readily identified across a wide range of cognitive tasks, and their responses increase and decrease proportionately with task demands. The CEN and SN typically show increases in activation, whereas the DMN shows decreases in activation during cognitive tasks in which self-referential processing is not required (Raichle et al., 2001; Greicius et al., 2003; Greicius & Menon, 2004). CEN nodes that show strong intrinsic functional coupling also show strong coactivation during cognitively challenging tasks. In particular, the CEN is critical for actively maintaining and manipulating information in working memory and for judgment and decision making in the context of goal-directed behavior (Petrides, 2005; Koechlin & Summerfield, 2007).

In task-based functional imaging, it has been difficult to isolate AI responses because it is often coactivated with the ACC, the DLPFC, and the ventrolateral prefrontal cortex (VLPFC). To circumvent this problem, Dosenbach and colleagues used functional connectivity analysis to show

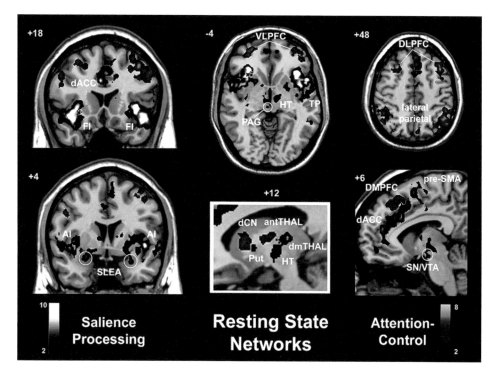

Figure 2.2 (plate 3)

Two core neurocognitive networks. The salience network (SN; shown in red) is important for monitoring the saliency of external inputs and internal brain events, and the central-executive network (CEN; shown in blue) is engaged in higher-order cognitive control. The SN is anchored in the fronto-insular (FI) cortex and dorsal anterior cingulate cortex (dACC) and features extensive connectivity with subcortical and limbic structures involved in reward and motivation. The CEN links the dorsolateral prefrontal cortex (DLPFC) and lateral parietal cortex and has subcortical coupling that is distinct from that of the SN. AI, anterior insula; antTHAL, anterior thalamus; dCN, dorsal caudate nucleus; dmTHAL, dorsomedial thalamus; HT, hypothalamus; PAG, periaqueductal gray; pre-SMA, pre-supplementary motor area; Put, putamen; SLEA, sublenticular extended amygdala; SN/VTA, substantia nigra/ventral tegmental area; TP, temporal pole. From Seeley et al. (2007).

that these regions can be grouped into distinct fronto-parietal and cin-gulo-opercular components (Dosenbach et al., 2007). Similarly, Seeley and colleagues used region of interest and ICA of rsfMRI data to demonstrate the existence of an ICN comprising the AI, dorsal ACC, and subcortical structures, including the amygdala, substantia nigra/ventral tegmental area, and thalamus (Seeley et al., 2007). The distinction between these two networks is therefore robust and reliable, and it can be used to gain new insights into their distinct cognitive functions, a topic we turn to in the following section.

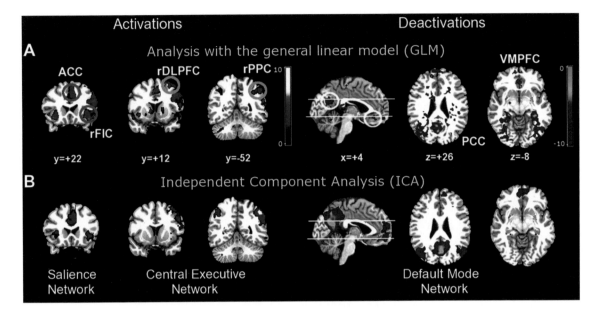

Figure 2.3 (plate 4)
Task-related activation and deactivation in three major neurocognitive networks. Task-related activation patterns in the central-executive network (CEN) and salience network (SN) and deactivation patterns in the default mode network (DMN) during an auditory attention task. Activation and deactivation patterns can be decomposed into distinct sub-patterns. (A) Analysis with the general linear model revealed regional activations (left) in the right anterior insula (rAI) and anterior cingulate cortex (ACC) (blue circles), right dorsolateral prefrontal cortex (rDLPFC) and right posterior parietal cortex (rPPC) (green circles), and deactivations (right) in the ventromedial prefrontal cortex (VMPFC) and posterior cingulate cortex (PCC). (B) ICA provided converging evidence for spatially distinct networks. From left to right: SN (rAI and ACC), CEN (rDLPFC and rPPC), and DMN (PCC and VMPFC). From Sridharan et al. (2008).

Of the three networks, the DMN was the first ICN to be identified using rsfMRI (Greicius et al., 2003). A variety of functions has been ascribed to these areas in the classical lesion and functional imaging literatures. For example, the PCC is activated during tasks that involve autobiographical memory and self-referential processes (Buckner & Carroll, 2007); the mPFC is associated with social cognitive processes related to self and others (Amodio & Frith, 2006); the MTL is engaged in episodic and autobiographical memory (Cabeza et al., 2004); and the AG is implicated in semantic processing (Binder, Desai, Graves, & Conant, 2009). Even though a unique task-based function cannot be assigned to each of its nodes (Spreng, Mar, & Kim, 2009), the DMN collectively comprises an integrated system for autobiographical memory, self-monitoring, value judgments, and other cognitive functions associated with self-referential mental processes.

The CEN, SN, and DMN are unique in that they can be readily identified across an extremely wide range of cognitive tasks, and their responses increase and decrease proportionately, and often antagonistically, with general cognitive task demands. The CEN and SN typically show increases in activation during stimulus-driven cognitive and affective information processing, whereas the DMN shows decreases in activation during tasks in which self-referential and stimulus-independent memory recall is not critical (Raichle et al., 2001; Greicius et al., 2003; Greicius & Menon, 2004). Dynamic engagement and disengagement of these three core neurocognitive networks is prominent in many cognitive tasks (Greicius & Menon, 2004; Sridharan, Levitin, & Menon, 2008).

2.5   Dynamics of Signaling in the CEN, SN, and DMN

Although intrinsic connectivity is useful in demarcating functional circuits, the critical question is how the underlying patterns of interdependency inform and constrain models of cognitive information processing in the human brain. In this section, we describe how the identification and characterization of distinct ICNs has helped to provide a framework for systematically examining key control processes in the brain. These control processes turn out to be critical for a wide range of cognitive tasks. As noted above, the three core ICNs, which were originally identified using rsfMRI data, can also be consistently identified in task-related data. ICA of fMRI data acquired during performance of auditory and visual attention tasks has revealed distinct activations and deactivations in the CEN, DMN, and SN (Sridharan et al., 2008), extending recent discovery of similar networks in task-free, resting-state conditions. This approach is particularly useful for identification of network nodes in an unbiased manner. Once the key nodes of these networks are identified using rsfMRI, the neural mechanisms underlying common patterns of task-related activation and deactivation as well as stimulus-driven attentional capture can be examined in a more principled manner than has been previously possible. Significant activation of the CEN and deactivation of the DMN nodes, along with co-activation of the SN comprising the right FIC and ACC, is a common feature across many different cognitive domains.

Chronometric techniques and dynamic causal analysis provide further insights into the temporal dynamics and causal interactions underlying dynamic changes in task-related activation and deactivation driven by the cognitive demands of attending to salient task- and goal-related stimuli. Sridharan and colleagues used regions of interest in six key nodes of the SN, CEN, and DMN derived from ICA analysis of rsfMRI data (Sridharan et al., 2008). They extracted time series from the six key nodes of the SN, CEN, and DMN and examined the temporal latency and causal interactions in two tasks involving reflexive attention. Onset latency analysis of fMRI response in these regions showed that the right FIC onsets significantly earlier than all of the nodes in the CEN and DMN. Latency analysis of event-related responses across the entire brain provided converging evidence that signals in the right FIC and ACC peak earlier compared with the signal in the nodes of the CEN and DMN, indicating that the neural responses in the right FIC and ACC precede those of the CEN and DMN (figure 2.4). In summary, these results confirm that activity in the right FIC onsets earlier compared with the activation in the CEN and deactivation in the DMN nodes. Dynamic causal analysis provides additional insights into the temporal dynamics

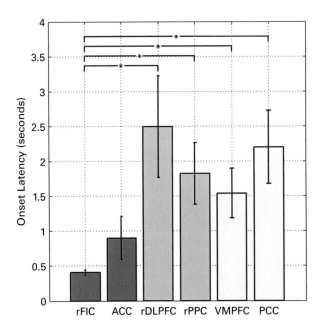

Figure 2.4
Onset latencies in the key nodes of the central-executive, saliency, and default mode networks. Onset latencies of the event-related responses in the six key nodes of the SN (blue bars), CEN (green bars), and DMN (yellow bars) during an auditory attention task. The right fronto-insular cortex (rFIC) onset significantly earlier than each of the nodes in the CEN and DMN. Error bars denote standard error of the mean across subjects. From Sridharan et al. (2008).

and functional interactions between the key nodes of the three networks. This analysis detects causal interactions between brain regions by assessing the predictability of signal changes in one brain region based on the time course of responses in another brain region (Roebroeck, Formisano, & Goebel, 2005, 2011; Seth, 2010). Network analysis on the causal flow network revealed that the right FIC has the highest number of causal outflow connections (out-degree), the lowest number of causal inflow connections (in-degree), and the shortest path length among all regions examined in this model (figure 2.5). The right FIC also had a significantly higher net causal outflow (out–in degree) among all of the nodes of the CEN and DMN. These results suggest that the right FIC is an outflow hub at the junction of the CEN and DMN. This analysis indicates that the right FIC, a key node of the SN, plays a critical, and causal, role in switching between the CEN and the DMN. The striking similarity of significant causal outflow from the right FIC across tasks, involving different stimulus modalities, indicates a general role for the right FIC in switching between the CEN and the DMN (figure 2.6, plate 5). These results indicate that the right FIC is likely to play a major role in engaging and disengaging distinct brain networks across task paradigms and stimulus modalities.

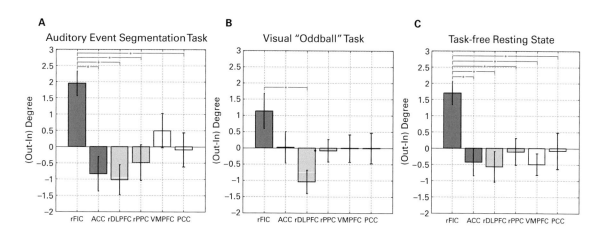

Figure 2.5
Net causal outflow in the central-executive, saliency, and default mode networks. Comparison of the net causal outflow (out–in degree) for six key nodes of the SN, CEN, and DMN as assessed by Granger causal analysis revealed that the right fronto-insular cortex (rFIC) has a significantly higher net causal outflow than the CEN and DMN nodes across (A) auditory and (B) visual attention tasks and in (C) the resting state. From Sridharan et al. (2008).

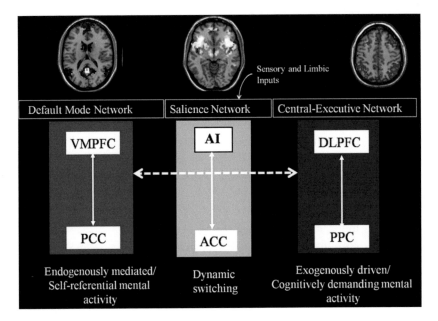

Figure 2.6 (plate 5)
Multinetwork switching initiated by the SN. The SN is hypothesized to initiate dynamic switching between the CEN and DMN and to mediate between attention to endogenous and exogenous events. In this model, sensory and limbic inputs are processed by the anterior insula (AI), which detects salient events and initiates appropriate control signals to regulate behavior via the anterior cingulate cortex (ACC) and homeostatic state via the mid and posterior insular cortex. Key nodes of the SN: AI and ACC. Key nodes of the DMN: ventral medial prefrontal cortex (VMPFC) and posterior cingulate cortex (PCC). Key nodes of the CEN: dorsolateral prefrontal cortex (DLPFC) and the posterior parietal cortex (PPC). From Bressler and Menon (2010).

2.6   A Dynamical Network Model of Saliency, Attention, and Control

These functional connectivity and dynamical analyses suggest a dynamic network model of cognitive control with the FIC as a key hub mediating salience detection and attentional capture. Although classically considered a limbic region, brain imaging studies have consistently found that the FIC is activated in a wide range of cognitive and affective tasks. Anatomically, the insula is a functionally heterogeneous brain region involved in visceral sensory and somatic sensory processes as well as autonomic and physiologic regulation (Augustine, 1996). This early viewpoint has given rise to a much more complex and multifaceted view of insular cortex function, as reviewed in a special issue of *Brain Structure & Function* on insular cortex function (Craig, 2010). Functional neuroimaging studies have shown that the right AI is active during a wide variety of tasks involving the subjective awareness of both positive and negative feelings, including studies of anger, disgust, and judgments of trustworthiness (for review, see Craig, 2002). The AI has also been implicated in high-level social cognitive processes such as deception. It was recently demonstrated that the breach of a promise can be predicted by brain activity patterns including activations in the AI, ACC, and VLPFC, implicating the AI and associated circuits in the representation of malevolent intentions before dishonest or deceitful acts are actually committed (Baumgartner, Fischbacher, Feierabend, Lutz, & Fehr, 2009). The AI is also implicated in empathy, or the "capacity to understand emotions of others by sharing their affective states" (Singer, 2006). Although these studies suggest an important role for the insula in social, affective, and higher-order mental processes guiding behavior, a more parsimonious account of its core functions is suggested by paradigms that have used far more simple stimuli and experimental manipulations. Specifically, across visual, tactile, and auditory modalities, the insula responds strongly to deviant stimuli embedded in a stream of continuous stimuli (Linden et al., 1999; Downar, Crawley, Mikulis, & Davis, 2001; Crottaz-Herbette, & Menon, 2006). Furthermore, once unfamiliar deviants replace familiar deviants, the latter engages the AI to a greater extent in each one of these modalities (Downar, Crawley, Mikulis, & Davis, 2000, 2002). Studies such as these suggest that the insula plays a major role in detection of novel salient stimuli across multiple modalities (Sterzer & Kleinschmidt, 2010). In our view, this represents a useful starting point for synthesizing the wide range of complex functions that have been ascribed to the insula. Critically, however, what has been missing from these studies is the lack of a systematic framework for interpreting these disparate findings. The insula's complex and as yet only partially characterized pattern of structural connectivity highlights the need for a more principled understanding of its functional connectivity. The crucial insight that neurocognitive network analysis has afforded is to place the AI as a major hub mediating dynamic interactions between other large-scale brain networks involved in externally oriented attention and internally oriented, or self-related, cognition (figure 2.5).

Within the framework of a network model, the disparate functions ascribed to the AI and adjoining FIC can be conceptualized by a few basic mechanisms:

1. Bottom-up detection of salient events.

2. Switching between other large-scale networks to facilitate access to attention and working memory resources when a salient event occurs.

3. Interaction of the anterior and posterior insula to modulate autonomic reactivity to salient stimuli.

4. Strong functional coupling with the ACC that facilitates rapid access to the motor system.

In this model, with the AI as its integral hub, the SN assists target brain regions in the generation of appropriate behavioral responses to salient stimuli. We have proposed that this framework provides a parsimonious account of insula function in neurotypical adults and may provide novel insights into the neural basis of disorders of affective and social cognition (Menon & Uddin, 2010). Previous studies have suggested that the inferior frontal gyrus and ACC are involved in a variety of monitoring, decision-making, and cognitive control processes (Crottaz-Herbette & Menon, 2006; Cole & Schneider, 2007; Johnston, Levin, Koval, & Everling, 2007; Posner & Rothbart, 2007; Dosenbach et al., 2008; Eichele et al., 2008). However, the AI has not been a particular focus of most of these studies. Our model posits that the core function of the proposed SN, and the AI in particular, is first to identify stimuli from the vast and continuous stream that impacts the senses. Once such a stimulus is detected, the AI facilitates task-related information processing by initiating appropriate transient control signals. These signals engage brain areas that mediate attentional, working memory, and higher-order cognitive processes while disengaging the DMN via mechanisms that have been described in the previous section.

These crucial switching mechanisms help focus attention on external stimuli; as a result, they take on added significance or saliency. The large-scale network switching mechanisms we have described here can be thought of as the culmination of a hierarchy of saliency filters. In these filters, each successive stage helps to differentially amplify a stimulus sufficiently to engage the AI. The precise pathways and filters underlying the transformation of external stimuli, and the manner in which the AI is activated, remain to be investigated. Of critical importance, our model suggests that, once a stimulus activates the AI, it will have preferential access to the brain's attentional and working memory resources.

Although dynamical systems analysis of fMRI connectivity data can help capture aspects of causal interactions between distributed brain areas, a more complete characterization of bottom-up and top-down attentional control requires access to temporal dynamics on the 30- to 70-ms timescale. Analysis of combined EEG and fMRI data provides

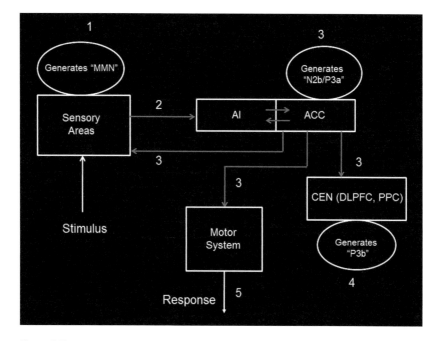

Figure 2.7
Schematic model of dynamic bottom-up and top-down interactions underlying attentional
control. Stage 1: About 150 ms poststimulus, primary sensory areas detect a deviant stimulus as indexed by the mismatch negativity (MMN) component of the evoked potential.
Stage 2: This "bottom-up" MMN signal is transmitted to other brain regions, including the
anterior insula (AI). The AI provides selective amplification of salient events and triggers
a strong response in the anterior cingulate cortex (ACC). Stage 3: About 200–300 ms
poststimulus, the ACC generates a "top-down" control signal as indexed by the N2b/P3a
component of the evoked potential. This signal is simultaneously transmitted to primary
sensory and association cortices, as well as to the CEN. Stage 4: About 300–400 ms poststimulus, neocortical regions, notably the premotor cortex and temporoparietal areas,
respond to the attentional shift with a signal that is indexed by the time-average P3b evoked
potential. *Stage 5*: The ACC also facilitates response selection and motor response via its
links to the midcingulate cortex, supplementary motor cortex, and other motor areas. From
Crottaz-Herbette and Menon (2006) and Menon and Uddin (2010).

additional insights into how the SN plays an important role in attentional
control (Crottaz-Herbette & Menon, 2006). Figure 2.7 is a schematic
model of bottom-up and top-down interactions that underlie attentional
control. This model was suggested by the relative timing of responses in
the AI and ACC, versus other cortical regions, based on our dynamic
source-imaging study and by lesion studies of the P3a complex (Soltani
& Knight, 2000). The spatiotemporal dynamics underlying this process
has five distinct stages:

- *Stage 1* Approximately 150 ms poststimulus, primary sensory areas detect a deviant stimulus, as indexed by the mismatch negativity (MMN) component of the evoked potential.

- *Stage 2* This bottom-up MMN signal is transmitted to other brain regions, notably the AI and the ACC.

- *Stage 3* Approximately 200–300 ms poststimulus, the AI and ACC generate a top-down control signal, as indexed by the N2b/P3a component of the evoked potential. This signal is simultaneously transmitted to primary sensory areas, as well as to other neocortical regions.

- *Stage 4* Approximately 300–400 ms poststimulus, neocortical regions, notably the premotor cortex and temporoparietal areas, respond to the attentional shift with a signal that is indexed by the time-average P3b evoked potential.

- *Stage 5* The ACC facilitates response selection and motor response via its links to the midcingulate cortex, supplementary motor cortex, and other motor areas (Rudebeck et al., 2008; Vogt, 2009).

Within the framework of the network model described earlier, we suggest that the AI plays a more prominent role in detecting salient stimuli, whereas the ACC plays a more prominent role in modulating responses in the sensory, motor, and association cortices. A wide range of functional imaging studies and theoretical models has suggested that the ACC plays a prominent role in action selection (Rushworth, 2008). Together, as part of a functionally coupled network, the AI and ACC help to integrate bottom-up attention switching with top-down control and biasing of sensory input. This dynamic process enables an organism to sift through many different incoming sensory stimuli and to adjust gain for task-relevant stimuli—processes central to attention (Yantis, 2008).

An examination of the differential pattern of input–output connectivity of the AI and the ACC yields further insights into the dynamical functions of the AI and SN. Whereas the AI receives multimodal sensory input, the ACC and associated dorsal mPFC receive very little sensory input (Averbeck & Seo, 2008). Conversely, whereas the ACC and associated dorsal mPFC send strong motor output, there is very little direct motor input to or output from the AI. Furthermore, the ACC and dorsal mPFC have direct connections to the spinal cord and subcortical oculomotor areas (Fries, 1984), giving them direct control over action. With these differential anatomic pathways and von Economo neurons, which facilitate rapid signaling between the AI and the ACC, the SN is well positioned to influence not only attention but also motor responses to salient sensory stimuli. In this manner, the AI plays both a direct and an indirect role in attention, cognition, and behavioral control. In the context of our model, this critical input–output pattern suggests that the AI may generate the signals to trigger hierarchical control. Consistent with this view, among patients with frontal lobe damage, those with lesions in the AI were the most impaired in altering their behavior in accordance with the changing rules of an oculomotor-switching task (Hodgson et al., 2007). Our model further suggests that when the ACC is dysfunctional (Fellows & Farah, 2005; Baird et al., 2006), the AI is well positioned to trigger alternative cognitive control signals via other lateral cortical regions such as the VLPFC and the DLPFC (Johnston et al., 2007). Thus, our network model helps to clarify an important controversy regarding the primacy and uniqueness of control signals in the prefrontal cortex (Fellows & Farah, 2005).

2.7   Conclusion

In this chapter, we have discussed how functional connectivity can be used to characterize and identify major neurocognitive networks in the human brain. The human brain is a complex network of interconnected regions, thus network approaches have become increasingly useful for understanding how functionally connected systems engender, and constrain, cognitive functions. Conceptualizing ongoing brain activity in terms of interacting networks provides a systematic framework for understanding fundamental aspects of human brain organization, independent of specific cognitive and experimental manipulations and individual differences in behavior. Intrinsic connectivity analysis when combined with dynamic network modeling provides a powerful tool for examining brain systems dedicated to distinct processes that underlie complex cognitive functions. Neurocognitive models help synthesize extant findings of functional connectivity into a common dynamical framework, and they suggest new avenues for synthesis of disparate findings in the cognitive neuroscience literature. Such an approach has led to the identification of fundamental mechanisms underlying the dynamics of attentional capture and cognitive control. More generally, we have illustrated the power of a unified neurocognitive network approach— wherein we first specify intrinsic brain networks and then analyze interactions among anatomically discrete regions within these networks during cognitive information processing—for understanding fundamental aspects of human brain function.

References

Amodio, D. M., & Frith, C. D. (2006). Meeting of minds: the medial frontal cortex and social cognition. *Nature Reviews. Neuroscience, 7*(4), 268–277.

Augustine, J. R. (1996). Circuitry and functional aspects of the insular lobe in primates including humans. *Brain Research. Brain Research Reviews, 22*(3), 229–244.

Averbeck, B. B., & Seo, M. (2008). The statistical neuroanatomy of frontal networks in the macaque. *PLoS Computational Biology, 4*(4), e1000050.

Baird, A., Dewar, B. K., Critchley, H., Gilbert, S. J., Dolan, R. J., & Cipolotti, L. (2006). Cognitive functioning after medial frontal lobe damage including the anterior cingulate cortex: a preliminary investigation. *Brain and Cognition, 60*(2), 166–175.

Barnea-Goraly, N., Menon, V., Eckert, M., Tamm, L., Bammer, R., Karchemskiy, A., et al. (2005). White matter development during childhood and adolescence: a cross-sectional diffusion tensor imaging study. *Cerebral Cortex, 15*(12), 1848–1854.

Bates, E., Wilson, S. M., Saygin, A. P., Dick, F., Sereno, M. I., Knight, R. T., et al. (2003). Voxel-based lesion-symptom mapping. *Nature Neuroscience, 6*(5), 448–450.

Baumgartner, T., Fischbacher, U., Feierabend, A., Lutz, K., & Fehr, E. (2009). The neural circuitry of a broken promise. *Neuron, 64*(5), 756–770.

Beckmann, C. F., & Smith, S. M. (2004). Probabilistic independent component analysis for functional magnetic resonance imaging. *IEEE Transactions on Medical Imaging, 23*(2), 137–152.

Binder, J. R., Desai, R. H., Graves, W. W., & Conant, L. L. (2009). Where is the semantic system? A critical review and meta-analysis of 120 functional neuroimaging studies. *Cerebral Cortex, 19*, 2767–2796.

Biswal, B., Yetkin, F. Z., Haughton, V. M., & Hyde, J. S. (1995). Functional connectivity in the motor cortex of resting human brain using echo-planar MRI. *Magnetic Resonance Medicine, 34*(4), 537–541.

Bressler, S. L., & Menon, V. (2010). Large-scale brain networks in cognition: emerging methods and principles. *Trends in Cognitive Sciences, 14*, 277–290.

Buckner, R. L., & Carroll, D. C. (2007). Self-projection and the brain. *Trends in Cognitive Sciences, 11*(2), 49–57.

Cabeza, R., & Kingstone, A. (Eds.). (2006). *Handbook of Functional Neuroimaging of Cognition* (2nd ed.). Cambridge, MA: MIT Press.

Cabeza, R., Prince, S. E., Daselaar, S. M., Greenberg, D. L., Budde, M., Dolcos, F., et al. (2004). Brain activity during episodic retrieval of autobiographical and laboratory events: an fMRI study using a novel photo paradigm. *Journal of Cognitive Neuroscience, 16*(9), 1583–1594.

Cole, M. W., & Schneider, W. (2007). The cognitive control network: Integrated cortical regions with dissociable functions. *NeuroImage, 37*(1), 343–360.

Craig, A. D. (2002). How do you feel? Interoception: the sense of the physiological condition of the body. *Nature Reviews. Neuroscience, 3*(8), 655–666.

Craig, A. D. (2010). Once an island, now the focus of attention. *Brain Structure & Function, 214*(5–6), 395–396.

Crottaz-Herbette, S., & Menon, V. (2006). Where and when the anterior cingulate cortex modulates attentional response: combined fMRI and ERP evidence. *Journal of Cognitive Neuroscience, 18*(5), 766–780.

Damasio, H., & Damasio, A. R. (1989). *Lesion Analysis in Neuropsychology*. New York: Oxford University Press.

Damoiseaux, J. S., Rombouts, S. A., Barkhof, F., Scheltens, P., Stam, C. J., Smith, S. M., et al. (2006). Consistent resting-state networks across healthy subjects. *Proceedings of the National Academy of Sciences of the United States of America, 103*(37), 13848–13853.

Dastjerdi, M., Foster, B. L., Nasrullah, S., Rauschecker, A. M., Dougherty, R. F., Townsend, J. D., et al. (2011). Differential electrophysiological response during rest, self-referential, and non-self-referential tasks in human posteromedial cortex. *Proceedings of the National Academy of Sciences of the United States of America, 108*(7), 3023–3028.

Dosenbach, N. U., Fair, D. A., Cohen, A. L., Schlaggar, B. L., & Petersen, S. E. (2008). A dual-networks architecture of top-down control. *Trends in Cognitive Sciences, 12*(3), 99–105.

Dosenbach, N. U., Fair, D. A., Miezin, F. M., Cohen, A. L., Wenger, K. K., Dosenbach, R. A., et al. (2007). Distinct brain networks for adaptive and stable task control in humans. *Proceedings of the National Academy of Sciences of the United States of America, 104*(26), 11073–11078.

Downar, J., Crawley, A. P., Mikulis, D. J., & Davis, K. D. (2000). A multimodal cortical network for the detection of changes in the sensory environment. *Nature Neuroscience, 3*(3), 277–283.

Downar, J., Crawley, A. P., Mikulis, D. J., & Davis, K. D. (2001). The effect of task relevance on the cortical response to changes in visual and auditory stimuli: an event-related fMRI study. *NeuroImage, 14*(6), 1256–1267.

Downar, J., Crawley, A. P., Mikulis, D. J., & Davis, K. D. (2002). A cortical network sensitive to stimulus salience in a neutral behavioral context across multiple sensory modalities. *Journal of Neurophysiology, 87*(1), 615–620.

Eichele, T., Debener, S., Calhoun, V. D., Specht, K., Engel, A. K., Hugdahl, K., et al. (2008). Prediction of human errors by maladaptive changes in event-related brain networks. *Proceedings of the National Academy of Sciences of the United States of America, 105*(16), 6173–6178.

Fair, D. A., Dosenbach, N. U., Church, J. A., Cohen, A. L., Brahmbhatt, S., Miezin, F. M., et al. (2007). Development of distinct control networks through segregation and integration. *Proceedings of the National Academy of Sciences of the United States of America, 104*(33), 13507–13512.

Fellows, L. K., & Farah, M. J. (2005). Is anterior cingulate cortex necessary for cognitive control? *Brain, 128*(Pt 4), 788–796.

Fox, M. D., & Raichle, M. E. (2007). Spontaneous fluctuations in brain activity observed with functional magnetic resonance imaging. *Nature Reviews. Neuroscience, 8*(9), 700–711.

Fries, W. (1984). Cortical projections to the superior colliculus in the macaque monkey: a retrograde study using horseradish peroxidase. *Journal of Comparative Neurology, 230*(1), 55–76.

Friston, K. J. (1994). Functional and effective connectivity in neuroimaging: A synthesis. *Human Brain Mapping, 2*, 56–78.

Friston, K. J. (2005). Models of brain function in neuroimaging. *Annual Review of Psychology, 56*, 57–87.

Fuster, J. M. (2006). The cognit: a network model of cortical representation. *International Journal of Psychophysiology, 60*(2), 125–132.

Greicius, M. D., & Menon, V. (2004). Default-mode activity during a passive sensory task: uncoupled from deactivation but impacting activation. *Journal of Cognitive Neuroscience, 16*(9), 1484–1492.

Greicius, M. D., Kiviniemi, V., Tervonen, O., Vainionpaa, V., Alahuhta, S., Reiss, A. L., et al. (2008). Persistent default-mode network connectivity during light sedation. *Human Brain Mapping, 29*(7), 839–847.

Greicius, M. D., Krasnow, B., Reiss, A. L., & Menon, V. (2003). Functional connectivity in the resting brain: a network analysis of the default mode hypothesis. *Proceedings of the National Academy of Sciences of the United States of America, 100*(1), 253–258.

He, B. J., Snyder, A. Z., Zempel, J. M., Smyth, M. D., & Raichle, M. E. (2008). Electrophysiological correlates of the brain's intrinsic large-scale functional architecture. *Proceedings of the National Academy of Sciences of the United States of America*, *105*(41), 16039–16044.

Hodgson, T., Chamberlain, M., Parris, B., James, M., Gutowski, N., Husain, M., et al. (2007). The role of the ventrolateral frontal cortex in inhibitory oculomotor control. *Brain*, *130* (Pt 6), 1525–1537.

Horovitz, S. G., Braun, A. R., Carr, W. S., Picchioni, D., Balkin, T. J., Fukunaga, M., et al. (2009). Decoupling of the brain's default mode network during deep sleep. *Proceedings of the National Academy of Sciences of the United States of America*, *106*(27), 11376–11381.

Huettel, S. A., Song, A. W., & McCarthy, G. (2008). *Functional Magnetic Resonance Imaging* (2nd ed.). Sunderland, MA: Sinauer Associates.

Jirsa, V. K., & McIntosh, A. R. (2007). *Handbook of Brain Connectivity*. New York: Springer.

Johnston, K., Levin, H. M., Koval, M. J., & Everling, S. (2007). Top-down control-signal dynamics in anterior cingulate and prefrontal cortex neurons following task switching. *Neuron*, *53*(3), 453–462.

Koechlin, E., & Summerfield, C. (2007). An information theoretical approach to prefrontal executive function. *Trends in Cognitive Sciences*, *11*(6), 229–235.

Linden, D. E., Prvulovic, D., Formisano, E., Vollinger, M., Zanella, F. E., Goebel, R., et al. (1999). The functional neuroanatomy of target detection: an fMRI study of visual and auditory oddball tasks. *Cerebral Cortex*, *9*(8), 815–823.

Menon, V., & Uddin, L. Q. (2010). Saliency, switching, attention and control: a network model of insula function. *Brain Structure & Function*, *214*(5–6), 655–667.

Mesulam, M. M. (1998). From sensation to cognition. *Brain: A Journal of Neurology*, *121* (Pt 6), 1013–1052.

Nir, Y., Mukamel, R., Dinstein, I., Privman, E., Harel, M., Fisch, L., et al. (2008). Interhemispheric correlations of slow spontaneous neuronal fluctuations revealed in human sensory cortex. *Nature Neuroscience*, *11*(9), 1100–1108.

Passingham, R. E., Stephan, K. E., & Kotter, R. (2002). The anatomical basis of functional localization in the cortex. *Nature Reviews. Neuroscience*, *3*(8), 606–616.

Petrides, M. (2005). Lateral prefrontal cortex: architectonic and functional organization. *Philosophical Transactions of the Royal Society of London. Series B, Biological Sciences*, *360*(1456), 781–795.

Popa, D., Popescu, A. T., & Pare, D. (2009). Contrasting activity profile of two distributed cortical networks as a function of attentional demands. *Journal of Neuroscience*, *29*(4), 1191–1201.

Posner, M. I., & Rothbart, M. K. (2007). Research on attention networks as a model for the integration of psychological science. *Annual Review of Psychology*, *58*, 1–23.

Raichle, M. E., MacLeod, A. M., Snyder, A. Z., Powers, W. J., Gusnard, D. A., & Shulman, G. L. (2001). A default mode of brain function. *Proceedings of the National Academy of Sciences of the United States of America*, *98*(2), 676–682.

Roebroeck, A., Formisano, E., & Goebel, R. (2005). Mapping directed influence over the brain using Granger causality and fMRI. *NeuroImage*, *25*(1), 230–242.

Roebroeck, A., Formisano, E., & Goebel, R. (2011). The identification of interacting networks in the brain using fMRI: model selection, causality and deconvolution. *Neuroimage*, *58*, 296–302.

Rudebeck, P. H., Behrens, T. E., Kennerley, S. W., Baxter, M. G., Buckley, M. J., Walton, M. E., et al. (2008). Frontal cortex subregions play distinct roles in choices between actions and stimuli. *Journal of Neuroscience*, *28*(51), 13775–13785.

Rushworth, M. F. (2008). Intention, choice, and the medial frontal cortex. *Annals of the New York Academy of Sciences*, *1124*, 181–207.

Schmahmann, J. D., Pandya, D. N., Wang, R., Dai, G., D'Arceuil, H. E., de Crespigny, A. J., et al. (2007). Association fibre pathways of the brain: parallel observations from diffusion spectrum imaging and autoradiography. *Brain*, *130*(Pt 3), 630–653.

Seeley, W. W., Menon, V., Schatzberg, A. F., Keller, J., Glover, G. H., Kenna, H., et al. (2007). Dissociable intrinsic connectivity networks for salience processing and executive control. *Journal of Neuroscience*, *27*(9), 2349–2356.

Seth, A. K. (2010). A MATLAB toolbox for Granger causal connectivity analysis. *Journal of Neuroscience Methods*, *186*(2), 262–273.

Shirer, W. R., Ryali, S., Rykhlevskaia, E., Menon, V., & Greicius, M. D. (2011). Decoding subject-driven cognitive states with whole-brain connectivity patterns. *Cerebral Cortex* (in press).

Singer, T. (2006). The neuronal basis and ontogeny of empathy and mind reading: Review of literature and implications for future research. *Neuroscience and Biobehavioral Reviews*, *30*(6), 855–863.

Smith, S. M., Fox, P. T., Miller, K. L., Glahn, D. C., Fox, P. M., Mackay, C. E., et al. (2009). Correspondence of the brain's functional architecture during activation and rest. *Proceedings of the National Academy of Sciences of the United States of America*, *106*(31), 13040–13045.

Soltani, M., & Knight, R. T. (2000). Neural origins of the P300. *Critical Reviews in Neurobiology*, *14*(3–4), 199–224.

Sowell, E. R., Peterson, B. S., Thompson, P. M., Welcome, S. E., Henkenius, A. L., & Toga, A. W. (2003). Mapping cortical change across the human life span. *Nature Neuroscience*, *6*(3), 309–315.

Spreng, R. N., Mar, R. A., & Kim, A. S. (2009). The common neural basis of autobiographical memory, prospection, navigation, theory of mind, and the default mode: a quantitative meta-analysis. *Journal of Cognitive Neuroscience*, *21*(3), 489–510.

Sridharan, D., Levitin, D. J., & Menon, V. (2008). A critical role for the right fronto-insular cortex in switching between central-executive and default-mode networks. *Proceedings of the National Academy of Sciences of the United States of America*, *105*(34), 12569–12574.

Sterzer, P., & Kleinschmidt, A. (2010). Anterior insula activations in perceptual paradigms: often observed but barely understood. *Brain Structure & Function*, *214*(5–6), 611–622.

Supekar, K., Musen, M., & Menon, V. (2009). Development of large-scale functional brain networks in children. *PLoS Biology*, *7*(7), e1000157.

Uddin, L. Q., Supekar, K., & Menon, V. (2010). Typical and atypical development of functional human brain networks: insights from resting-state FMRI. *Frontiers in Systems Neuroscience*, *4*, 21.

Vanhaudenhuyse, A., Noirhomme, Q., Tshibanda, L. J., Bruno, M. A., Boveroux, P., Schnakers, C., et al. (2010). Default network connectivity reflects the level of consciousness in non-communicative brain-damaged patients. *Brain: A Journal of Neurology*, *133*(Pt 1), 161–171.

Vogt, B. A. (2009). *Cingulate Neurobiology and Disease*. New York: Oxford University Press.

Wedeen, V. J., Wang, R. P., Schmahmann, J. D., Benner, T., Tseng, W. Y., Dai, G., et al. (2008). Diffusion spectrum magnetic resonance imaging (DSI) tractography of crossing fibers. *NeuroImage*, *41*(4), 1267–1277.

Yantis, S. (2008). The neural basis of selective attention: cortical sources and targets of attentional modulation. *Current Directions in Psychological Science*, *17*(2), 86–90.

Zilles, K., & Amunts, K. (2010). Centenary of Brodmann's map—conception and fate. *Nature Reviews. Neuroscience*, *11*(2), 139–145.

3 Decoding Mental States from Patterns of Brain Activity

John-Dylan Haynes

Summary

Human neuroimaging has to date mostly addressed the question of which brain regions are active during specific tasks. Recently, there has been a shift in focus toward more content-based neuroimaging. Using multivariate decoding techniques, it is now possible not only to measure the overall activity levels of brain regions but also to assess the amount of information they contain about specific mental representations, such as specific visual images or specific action plans. Several extensions to the basic multivariate decoding framework have now been proposed. *Multidimensional scaling* allows assessment of the spaces in which neural representations are coded. *Model-based classification* uses computational models to capture the mapping between mental states and brain responses and can generalize to novel cases. Finally, it is possible to use classifiers to reconstruct dynamic time series of mental states and the dynamics of interaction between distinct brain regions.

3.1 Introduction

Traditionally, neuroimaging has been dominated by mass-univariate analyses based on the general linear model (GLM; see Friston et al., 1995). In this approach, univariate statistical tests are applied at each location of the brain individually, and the statistical parameters are then plotted at each position of the brain (hence *statistical parametric mapping*; SPM). Importantly, in this approach any interaction between voxels is neglected.

The GLM/SPM approach is highly suitable when the aim of a study is to assess whether the activity level at a single location in the brain is modulated by a specific mental operation. However, an important question has frequently remained unclear: How and where is information about specific mental contents represented in the brain? To date, content-specific research has typically relied on markers for content-specific processing such as frequency tags (Tononi, Srinivasan, Russell, & Edelman, 1998) or semantic tags like activity in the fusiform face area during processing of faces or activity in the parahippocampal place area during processing of visual scenes and buildings (Kanwisher, McDermott, & Chun, 1997; Epstein & Kanwisher, 1998; Tong, Nakayama, Vaughan, & Kanwisher, 1998; Moutoussis & Zeki, 2002).

It has long been established that the brain encodes most mental contents using entire populations of cells (Georgopoulos, Schwartz, & Kettner, 1986; Tanaka, 1996) and that the covariance structure between multiple individual units is of essential importance in neural coding (Averbeck, Latham, & Pouget, 2006). For example, in motor cortex the direction of movement of a cursor is coded in the population vector that is a sum of the preferred movement directions of each individual motor cortex cell (Georgopoulos, Schwartz, & Kettner, 1986). Similarly, it is possible to decode the object a person is currently viewing by applying classifiers to multiple unit recordings in the temporal lobe of monkeys (Hung, Kreiman, Poggio, & DiCarlo, 2005). There are two basic types of multivariate code that can be used: a sparse code and a distributed code (Haynes, 2009; see figure 3.1). The sparseness of neural representations has been a matter of constant debate (Kanwisher, McDermott, & Chun, 1997; Haxby et al., 2001), but it is important to note that even a population code can be sparse (Quiroga, Kreiman, Koch, & Fried, 2008) (see figure 3.1).

The importance of population activity is paralleled by findings from human neuroimaging. In functional magnetic resonance imaging (fMRI), the presentation of a single object will frequently activate extended regions of object-selective lateral occipital complex cortex rather than a single location (Haxby et al., 2001). In an important study, Haxby and colleagues (2001) presented subjects with images of objects. These images were different exemplars taken from eight different categories (faces, houses, cats, chairs, scissors, shoes, bottles, and phase-scrambled noise). The fMRI responses in object-selective cortex were determined for each category and accumulated separately for odd and even acquisition runs. They found that each category of object evoked a spatial pattern of fMRI activity that was unique for this category only (figure 3.2). They then attempted to classify the objects viewed during even runs based on the knowledge of patterns of responses for the different categories during odd runs. The classification rule was to assign a given fMRI response pattern in the even runs to the category that had evoked the most similar response pattern in

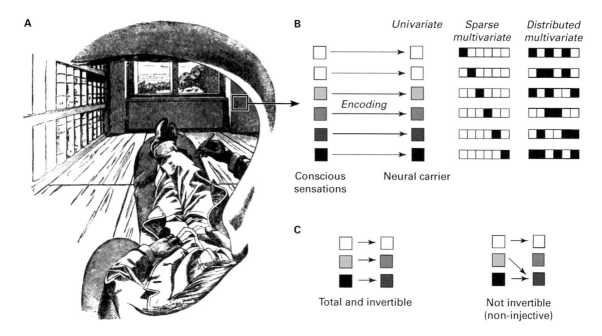

Figure 3.1
Encoding of contents in neural carrier signals. (A) Ernst Mach's (1886) famous image
showing his subjective experiences while looking through his left eye into his study. The
different perceived shades of brightness constitute a class of mental states. (B) The perceived brightness could be encoded in a neural carrier in different ways. A *univariate* code
would assign one activity level of a single neuron to each mental content. A *sparse multivariate* code assigns one neuron that responds if and only if a specific mental content is
present. A *distributed multivariate* code represents each mental content with a specific
distributed pattern of population activity. The sparse multivariate code can be thought of
as a labeled line, with each neuron signaling a different content. In contrast, in a distributed
multivariate code, individual neurons cannot be linked to specific mental contents. (C)
Mapping criteria: Two important criteria have to hold for the mapping of mental states to
neural states in order for a mental content to be represented in that neural state (Haynes,
2009): First, the mapping has to be total, meaning that each mental state is assigned to a
neural state. Second, the mapping has to be invertible, meaning that each neural state is
only assigned to maximally one mental content. Otherwise, it would not be possible to read
out the mental state from the corresponding neural state. From Haynes (2009).

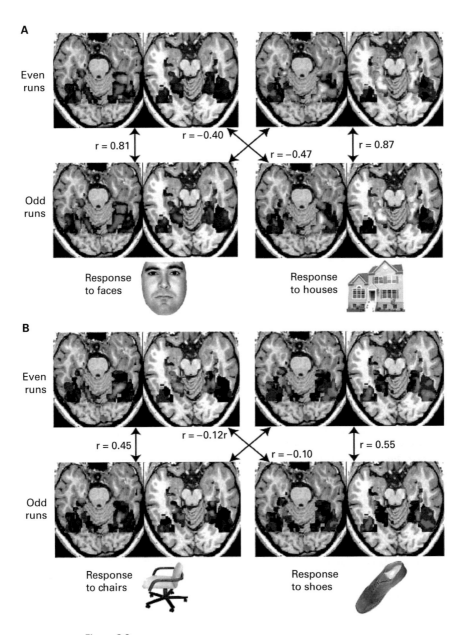

Figure 3.2
fMRI pattern responses in the lateral occipital cortex encode the identity of visually presented objects. The patterning of the fMRI response to visual presentation of (A) faces and houses and (B) chairs and shoes. The top rows show average responses during even runs, and the bottom rows show average responses during odd runs. The pattern responses to the different objects are highly reproducible across odd and even runs and selective for the corresponding category. To decode which category a person was viewing, the response pattern in an even run is correlated with the response patterns of all categories in an odd run. The object is then assigned to the category with the highest similarity. Modified from Haxby et al. (2001).

the odd runs (k-nearest neighbor classification with $k = 1$). Following this approach, they were able to determine which object the subject had been viewing with an accuracy of 96% (based on pairwise classifications). Notably, there was only a minor reduction in accuracy if the classification was based on voxels that did not respond maximally to the corresponding objects. This is an important finding because it suggests the existence of category-specific information outside the regions that would be considered most relevant for this category in a conventional GLM analysis.

3.2 Multivariate Decoding

One fruitful framework for understanding the link between distributed brain response patterns and mental states is multivariate decoding (Haxby et al., 2001; Haynes & Rees, 2006; Kriegeskorte, Goebel, & Bandettini, 2006; Norman, Polyn, Detre, & Haxby, 2006; Pereira, Mitchell, & Botvinick, 2009). The idea is that a classifier learns to assign labels (i.e., the mental states) to measurements of brain activity patterns. First a *training data set* is required that provides samples of the brain activity patterns for each mental state of interest. A classifier is trained to correctly assign the labels to brain patterns in this training data set. Then, the classifier is tested by predicting the labels of a new and independent *test data set* (see figure 3.3). The accuracy with which the labels for the test data can be correctly assigned can be used as a measure of the mental state–related information that is encoded in the multivariate signal. Applying machine-learning techniques to fMRI is a nontrivial endeavor. Hence, the following sections will provide a brief overview of the main concepts and technical issues. Then, some important experimental findings will be presented.

The measured pattern signals define repeated measures x_i of response vectors in an N-dimensional space where N is the number of voxels considered. There are several possible ways to perform classification in this space (for full details, see, e.g., Pereira et al., 2009; Lemm, Blankertz, Dickhaus, & Müller, 2011; Misaki, Kim, Bandettini, & Kriegeskorte, 2010). The simplest classifier is a *split-half correlation*. The data set is split in two equal sections, and the average response patterns to each category are determined separately for both halves. Then, one of the halves plays the role of a labeled "training" set and the remaining half provides the "test" patterns that are compared with each training pattern in turn, and the label is assigned that has the highest correlation. This classification

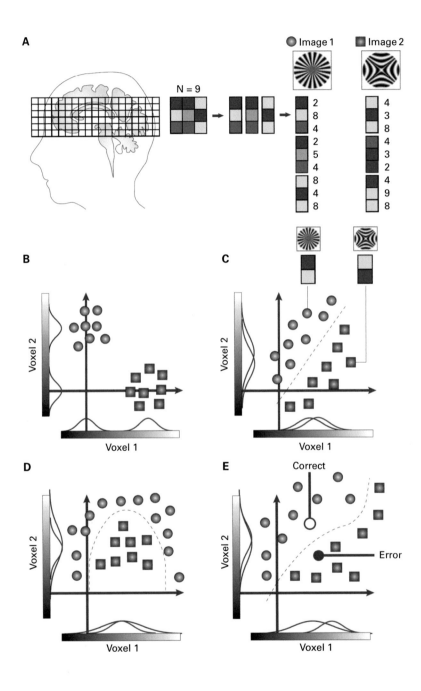

Figure 3.3
Multivariate decoding of perceptual states from brain signals. (A) A sample 3×3 multivariate fMRI measurement of brain activity from visual cortex. A measurement is coded as a pattern vector with as many dimensions as measurement channels (here, nine voxels). Repeated measurements are made for two different visual stimuli ("image 1," "image 2"). (B) The different dimensions of the vector can be considered as axes of an N-dimensional coordinate system where N is the number of channels (here, nine channels). The figure shows the first two dimensions plotted as the two axes of a Cartesian coordinate system. In the easiest case shown here, it is possible to separate the repeated measurements of both stimulus classes (shown here as circles and squares) on either of the two axes, as can be seen from the fact that the marginal distributions do not overlap. (C) In this case, the marginal distributions are largely overlapping, and thus classification would not be possible based on one channel alone. However, by taking into account the activity in both channels, it is possible fully to separate the multivariate responses to both stimuli using a linear decision boundary. (D) In some cases, a linear decision boundary is not sufficient, and a nonlinear decision boundary is required. (E) After learning the decision boundary on a training data set, a new measurement can be made that can be used to test the ability of the classifier correctly to predict the label of an independent measurement. If the multivariate response falls on the correct side of the decision boundary, this will result in a hit ("correct"); if it falls on the wrong side, this will result in a miss ("error"). From Haynes and Rees (2006).

approach is very similar to the *k-nearest neighbor classifier* where the label is determined as the most frequent label occurring in the k-nearest training samples. Another simple classifier is a Gaussian naive Bayes classifier that makes a simplifying assumption that each feature is independent. Computationally, this approach has the advantages that it can operate on a small amount of training data and that the covariance matrix does not have to be estimated because covariance is not taken into account.

Another frequently used type are linear classifiers that use a hyperplane to separate distributions of patterns from two classes. One approach that takes covariances into account is the linear discriminant analysis (LDA), which assumes two classes to have an equal covariance matrix. Similarly, the linear support vector classifier uses a hyperplane that is placed to yield maximal margin from the nearest patterns of each class (for details, see Lemm et al., 2011). Nonlinear classifiers can use more complex decision boundaries such as polynomials or radial basis functions. However, there is some disagreement as to whether their performance is routinely better than that of linear classifiers (Misaki et al., 2010; Tusche, Bode, & Haynes, 2010). Importantly, different classifiers implicitly make different assumptions about the distribution of the patterns of different classes, a phenomenon known as *inductive bias* (Kriegeskorte, 2011). For example, a split half or nearest neighbor classifier makes the assumption of contiguity; that is, that similar labels occupy a contiguous region of pattern space. Recursive feature elimination (De Martino et al., 2008; see later) makes the assumption that only a small number of features contain discriminative information.

Another important question is which measure of multivariate information to use. Several measures are routinely computed. If the focus is on classification, then the measure of interest is typically the classification accuracy (i.e., the proportion of correctly labeled samples in an independent test data set). One problem is that this measure is not very sensitive because it is bound by 100% accuracy corresponding with perfect classification. The response patterns of two classes could be separated to different degrees even beyond the point to which they can be perfectly separated. Thus, a more useful measure can be a distance measure such as a Euclidean distance or a Mahalanobis distance that takes the covariance between features into account.

3.2.1 The Variables of Classification

Neuroimaging data sets are highly complex, and thus there are multiple choices to be made in their analysis (Haxby et al., 2001; Kjems et al., 2002; Haynes & Rees, 2006; Kriegeskorte et al., 2006; Norman, Polyn, Detre, & Haxby, 2006; Pereira et al., 2009; Misaki et al., 2010). The two main choices to be made are *spatial* and *temporal*: The spatial selection defines the voxels (also referred to as features) that are going to be entered into the classification. This defines the dimensionality of the patterns under investigation. Routinely there are three different approaches:

1. *Whole-brain classification* The voxels of the whole brain are used, and thus the pattern vectors have as many dimensions as there are voxels in the brain (up to 10^5, depending on resolution). This approach has the advantage that it makes no assumptions about which brain regions carry information pertaining to a specific mental state classification. However, this comes at the expense of lacking neurobiological plausibility. Information that can be decoded from whole-brain activity patterns is available to the experimenter, but it might not be available within the brain itself because there is no single location in the brain that receives input from all over the brain, which would be necessary in order to decode this information.

2. *Region-of-interest classification* The voxels of a specific, independently defined subregion of the brain are used as pattern vectors, thus

reducing dimensionality and achieving higher regional specificity. This requires that some method is available for defining the subset of voxels that is independent from the classification task, otherwise the analysis could be circular (Kriegeskorte et al., 2009). For regions where independent anatomic or functional markers exist, for example for the hippocampus or the primary visual cortex, this can be a very powerful approach.

3. *Searchlight classification*   Here, the classification assesses the information stored in the local neighborhood surrounding each voxel (Kriegeskorte et al., 2006; Haynes et al., 2007). For a given voxel, a local searchlight is defined as a spherical cluster of voxels in its immediate surround. The classification is performed for this local cluster of voxels, and the classification accuracy is entered into a resulting accuracy map. The procedure is repeated each time using a different voxel as the searchlight center. This way, it is possible to obtain a map of the brain that plots the mental state–related information contained in each local neighborhood of voxels. This approach provides a combination of spatial specificity and whole-brain assessment of information. Recently, searchlight classification approaches have been developed that operate on the two-dimensional cortical surface (Chen et al., 2011; Oosterhof, Wiestler, Downing, & Diedrichsen, 2011) rather than the three-dimensional volume. This leads to increased spatial specificity and less distortion of informative brain patterns.

Feeding large regions of the brain with many voxels into a classifier involves a "curse of dimensionality," meaning that it can be difficult to determine the decision boundary that will yield optimal performance in the test data set due to the many noninformative "noisy" channels some of which might spuriously correlate with the training labels. There are several approaches to ameliorate this problem. Besides dimensionality reduction using principal component analysis (PCA) or independent component analysis (ICA), one common approach is to preselect voxels (or features) based on specific criteria, a procedure that is known as *feature selection*. For example, one can restrict the classification to voxels that are activated by all conditions of the task (versus baseline) or that are discriminative as assessed by a univariate *t*- or *F*-test. However, this preselection of features has to be performed only on the training data set to avoid circularity and overfitting (see later). Whereas the previous feature-selection techniques only assess the univariate information for each individual voxel, recursive feature elimination (RFE; De Martino et al., 2008) starts with a classifier with full dimensionality and then progressively eliminates the least contributing voxels resulting in sparse classifiers. It should be noted that despite the power of feature selection algorithms, the only ultimate solution to the dimensionality problem is to obtain a larger training data set.

Besides the spatial selection of classifier input and thus the dimensionality, there are also several approaches to the *temporal* selection and accumulation of measurements that define the number of available samples. The simplest approach is to use the raw signal of each fMRI volume within the selected region. This allows for classification with high temporal precision, but at the expense of accuracy for each time point. Another approach is to compute an estimate of the activity throughout either a specific trial or block, for instance by averaging activity across several volumes or by fitting a hemodynamic response function(HRF) model. The next level of accumulation is to use a GLM as a first stage of analysis that provides parameter estimates for each condition and each run. The pattern then consists of the parameter estimates at each position, and the number of samples is equal to the number of runs. Finally, it is possible to obtain a single average spatial pattern for each subject and to use the measurements of different subjects as the samples. This requires that the pattern information be coded in a similar fashion in each subject, which can be the case (Shinkareva et al., 2008) but is often not (Kamitani & Tong, 2005).

3.2.2   Independence of Training and Test Data

It is of vital importance in classification to ensure that the training and test data sets are independent (Kriegeskorte et al., 2009; Pereira et al., 2009; Lemm et al., 2011). Otherwise, overfitting would occur, and the classifier's performance on the test data set is not a measure of the true information. This can for example happen due to the autocorrelation in the neural signals, especially in fMRI signals. In these cases, consecutive trials are not independent. Similarly, a feature selection based on the entire data set including training and test data would be a violation of such independence because the classifier would select a subset of voxels that are known to allow for classification in the test data. A preselection of voxels based on a data set that involves the test data or is correlated with the test data would result in above-chance classification accuracy even in random surrogate data.

3.2.3 Biased Sampling

Notably, using pattern classification it is possible to decode mental states that only differ at the columnar level of neural representation (Haynes & Rees, 2005a; Kamitani & Tong, 2005). The prime example is orientation encoding in primary visual cortex, although there are now also hints that similar pattern signals in other areas can be linked to neural population signals (Kahnt, Heinzle, Park, & Haynes, 2010). For a long time, it was believed to be impossible to study the processing of specific orientations in V1 because the columnar grid in which different orientations are coded is much finer than the measurement grid of fMRI (figure 3.4, plate 6). One should expect that stimuli with different orientations would evoke the same net responses in V1 due to the intertwined columnar representation. However, when human subjects view different orientation stimuli, a clear bias of individual fMRI voxels toward specific orientations can be observed (Haynes & Rees, 2005a; Kamitani & Tong, 2005; Swisher et al., 2010). This bias is reproducible across repeated measurements. One potential explanation is that each voxel samples a slightly different proportion of cells with different tuning preferences and thus has a slightly variable response to different orientations. The effect is also termed the *biased sampling* effect. These biases are very small and typically not statistically significant at the single voxel level. However, using multivariate pattern recognition, it is possible to show that a larger set of V1 voxels has a different population response to different orientations. This information that is available at the voxel population level is considerable and can allow for classification accuracies up to around 90% based on single fMRI volumes (Haynes & Rees, 2005a). Subsequently, there has been considerable debate on the nature of the orientation biases of single voxels and on the nature of the pattern signals used for orientation decoding (Sasaki et al., 2006; Chaimow, Yacoub, Ugurbil, & Shmuel, 2011; Gardner, 2010; Kamitani & Sawahata, 2010; Op de Beeck, 2010; Swisher et al., 2010). It has been proposed that orientation decoding might reflect large-scale radial biases in the large-scale topography of V1 rather than sampling of irregular columnar grids (Sasaki et al., 2006; Op de Beeck, 2010). However, closer examination using fMRI signals filtered into different spatial frequency bands (Swisher et al., 2010) and computational modeling (Chaimow et al., 2011) revealed a large contribution of information from a millimeter-scale of resolution, while not excluding the possibility of additional information from

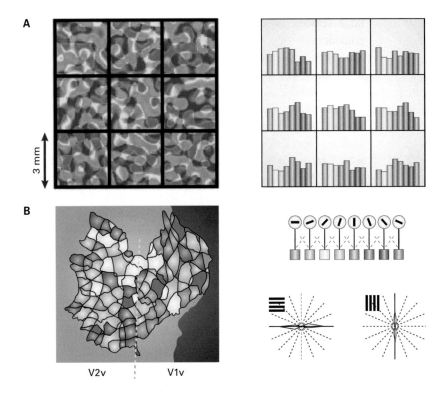

Figure 3.4 (plate 6)
The biased sampling model attempts to explain the patterning of fMRI signals by a selective sampling of the underlying columnar architecture in the brain. (A) Left: A pattern of cortical columns schematically reproducing the surface of early visual cortex. Each color corresponds with a different orientation tuning preference of cells. The columnar structure is too fine to be resolved with the standard resolution of fMRI (approximately 1.5–3 mm). Right: Because of small fluctuations in the density of different cell types, each voxel (black grid) will sample a slightly different proportion of cells with different tuning preferences. The top right voxel will sample more cells with horizontal tuning, and the top left voxel will sample more cells with vertical orientation tuning. This would predict a small but reproducible patterning of the fMRI signal in V1 when stimulated with different orientations (Boynton, 2005). (B) Left: A single subject map of orientation tuning preferences of individual voxels in the region of V1/V2. Right: An ensemble of linear support vector machine (SVM) classifiers is trained such that they each provide a peak response for a different orientation. The class corresponds with the orientation of the classifier with the strongest output. From Kamitani and Tong (2005), Boynton (2005), and Haynes and Rees (2006).

large-scale topographies. Importantly, the role of vasculature has to be considered as well given that fMRI reflects vascular signals. Gardner (2010) postulated a close link between columns and functional vascular units that could lead to additional feature biases. This has been developed further in the model of a complex spatiotemporal filter with which the fMRI signal samples the underlying cortical architecture (Kriegeskorte, Cusack, & Bandettini, 2010).

3.2.4 Multidimensional Scaling

One interesting use of multivariate analyses is to investigate the space in which the individual patterns are coded. In a pioneering study, Edelman and colleagues (1998) recorded fMRI-response patterns in object-selective cortex while subjects viewed objects from multiple categories (planes, fish, figures, cars, four-legged animals). After applying multidimensional scaling (MDS) to the patterns of brain activity evoked by the different objects, the exemplars of different categories group together, suggesting a similarity in their neural representation in object-selective regions of the human brain (figure 3.5). Using a similar approach, Kriegeskorte and colleagues (2008) have shown that the representational spaces of human and primate object-selective cortex are highly similar.

3.2.5 Model-Based Classification

In the approaches mentioned earlier, the mapping between multivariate responses and mental states is learned using brute-force classification techniques. This means that a classifier is trained optimally to distinguish between *each different* mental state based on the corresponding brain response pattern. Only mental states with known brain response patterns can be decoded. To overcome this limitation, it can be useful to investigate the mapping between mental states and brain activity patterns more systematically, based on encoding models (Nevado, Young, & Panzeri, 2004; Thirion et al., 2006; Kay, Naselaris, Prenger, & Gallant, 2008; Mitchell et al., 2008; Miyawaki et al., 2008). The idea is to provide a model that captures the relationship between a whole set of mental states and the corresponding brain activity patterns. One example is to use receptive field models to predict the responses in primary visual cortex from visual input stimuli (Thirion et al., 2006; Kay et al., 2008; Miyawaki et al., 2008). Then, the model can be inverted to estimate the unknown visual input to a novel pattern of brain activity. This can make it possible to generalize

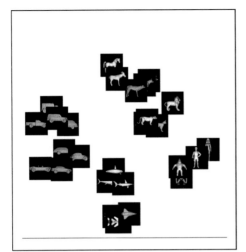 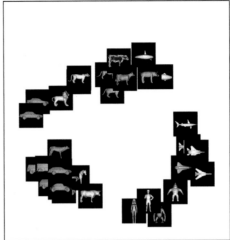

Figure 3.5
Psychophysical and cortical shape space (Edelman et al., 1998). The left panel shows a set of objects grouped according to a multidimensional scaling (MDS) algorithm based on psychophysical similarity ratings. The right panel shows the same set of objects grouped with a MDS based on the similarity of their corresponding spatial patterns of brain activity in lateral occipital object selective cortex. The MDS plot of brain activity patterns shows that similar objects are clustered together, even if they are spatially dissimilar (e.g., the different animals).

and decode many mental states based only on a limited set of training samples. Using such approaches, it has been possible to decode which abstract shape, natural scene, or letter a subject was currently viewing (Thirion et al., 2006; Kay et al., 2008; Miyawaki et al., 2008). Similary, it has been possible to reconstruct which of 1001 words was currently being presented to a subject based on a data set with brain responses to only 25 intermediate features (Mitchell et al., 2008; figure 3.6).

3.3   Decoding Dynamics

An interesting approach in multivariate classification and regression is to predict continuously time-varying signals. For example, in a visual study on a phenomenon known as *binocular rivalry*, we demonstrated that it is possible to decode a time series of perception that is stochastically fluctuating between two states (Haynes & Rees, 2005b; see figure 3.7). Decoding was based on fMRI images focused on the early visual cortex (V1, V2, V3) that could be measured every 1.3 s. The high accuracies in reconstructing these time series show that fMRI decoding

Predictive model

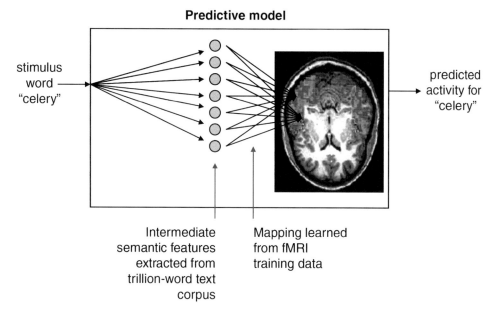

stimulus word "celery"

Intermediate
semantic features
extracted from
trillion-word text
corpus

Mapping learned
from fMRI
training data

predicted
activity for
"celery"

Figure 3.6
Generalization of classification to many new test cases. A study by Mitchell et al. (2008)
investigated whether it is possible to decode a large number of stimulus words using a
classifier that has learned the brain activity for only a small subset of these words. They
use a trillion-word text corpus to assess the similarity between each word and a set of 25
intermediate features. The similarity structure obtained from the text database can then be
used to reconstruct a large number of novel candidate words, thus allowing classification
of which word out of 1001 was presented. From Mitchell et al. (2008).

approaches have sufficient power to decode mental states on a sample-
by-sample basis. Similar time-series decoding has also been observed for
other cases of multistable perception (Brouwer & van Ee, 2007).

In another study, we investigated to which degree the dynamics between
individual brain regions can be captured using pattern classification techniques (Heinzle, Kahnt, & Haynes, 2011; see figure 3.8). The aim was to
capture the "information flow" between two topographically organized
cortical regions by training a classifier to predict signals in one region
based on a weighted sum of signals in another region. We chose the link
between V1 and V3 as a testing case because both regions exhibit a clear
topographical representation of visual input, but they are not adjacent,
and thus any findings cannot be due to shared local vasculature.

We trained a support vector regression to predict fMRI signal fluctuations in V3 based on a weighted sum of signals in V1. One key piece of
information was the weight map that describes the linear weights for

A

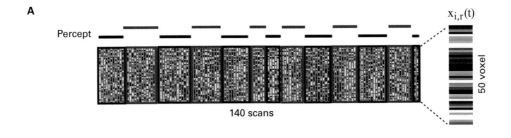

B

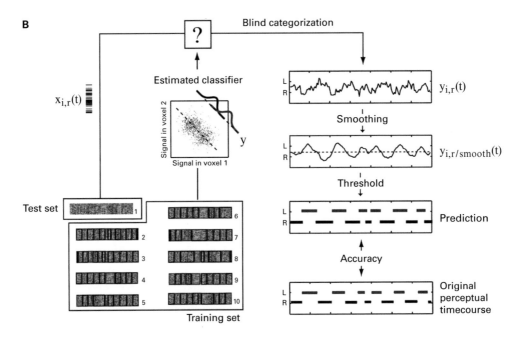

Figure 3.7
Multivariate decoding of continuous perceptual time series. (A) A stochastically alternating time course of perception during binocular rivalry. The left and right eyes are stimulated with conflicting orthogonal red and blue grating stimuli (not reproduced in this b/w figure), thus causing perceptual alternations between phases where either one or the other color is perceived (the two time series in the top of the figure). Parallel to this, fMRI signals are recorded from early visual areas (V1 to V3). The rows correspond with the 50 most strongly stimulus-driven voxels from one brain region (e.g., V1). The columns are the total 140 individual fMRI scans of 1.3 s each. The pattern vectors for each time point are labeled according to the dominant percept at that time point (using a canonical HRF model to compute a time shift to account for the hemodynamic latency). (B) A pattern classifier is trained on data from all but one run. A linear discriminant classifier learns the projection from 50-dimensional space onto a single dimension that maximizes the distance between the two distributions. The individual pattern vectors of an independent test data set are fed into the estimated classifier resulting in a graded classification of the perceptual state. This time series is then low pass–filtered and finally thresholded resulting in a predicted perceptual time course that closely matches the original time course. From Haynes and Rees (2005b).

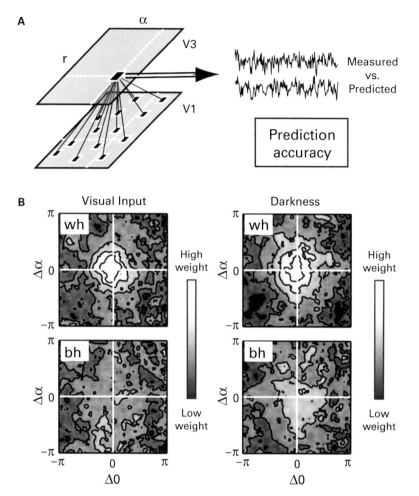

Figure 3.8

Cortico-cortical receptive fields and topographic connectivity structure between visual areas. (A) The cortico-cortical receptive field (CCRF) of a voxel in V3 is given by the weight distribution of the optimal linear combination of voxels in V1 that best predicts the signal fluctuations of the voxel in V3. Whereas prediction accuracy measures how well the predicted time course of the V3 voxel matches the true measured time course, the weights of the linear model indicate how important different parts of V1 are for the prediction. (B) Individual CCRFs can be averaged to yield the topographic connectivity structure between V1 and V3. Average connectivity structures over several subjects are shown for two conditions: when the subjects saw a visual input (left, $n = 4$) and when they were blindfolded and did not see any visual input (right, $n = 8$). The connectivity structure was calculated within hemispheres (wh) and, as a control, between hemispheres (bh). Note that the connectivity structure is a function of the relative difference of eccentricity (Δr) and visual angle ($\Delta \alpha$) between V1 and V3. Weights are coded as grayscale values (see color bar) between the lowest and highest weight over both average topographic connectivity structures (TCS). Black lines show contours of equal weight and are positioned at the same weight values in both wh and bh illustrations. Adapted from Heinzle, Kahnt, and Haynes (2011).

each position in V1. We found that the weight map topology had similarity with a Gaussian input field and clearly conserved the retinotopic organization of the two visual areas. Importantly, we showed that this tight link between the dynamics of signals in V3 and V1 holds not only under conditions of visual stimulation but also in complete darkness in the absence of visual input. This points toward a highly specific co-fluctuation between signals in V1 and V3 that precisely follows the known anatomic connectivity pattern. This means that "background" or "resting" signals in fMRI are influenced by the anatomic connectome in a very detailed fashion.

In a related approach, we investigated whether information about mental states can be decoded from seemingly unspecific "background" signals (Soon, Brass, Heinze, & Haynes, 2008). We asked subjects freely to decide between two response buttons while lying in an MRI scanner. We used a multivariate decoder to predict how a subject was going to decide from their brain activity. For this purpose, we examined for each time point preceding the intention whether a given brain region carried information related to the specific outcome of a decision; that is, the urge to press either a left or a right button. We found that indeed, brain activity in two regions partially predicted prior to the conscious decision whether the subject was about to choose the left or right response, even though the subject did not consciously know yet which way they were about to decide. The regions were frontopolar cortex (FPC) and precuneus/parietal cortex. Importantly, the predictive information in the fMRI signals from this brain region was present already 7 s prior to the subject's decision. This period of 7 s is a conservative estimate that does not yet take into account the delay of the fMRI response with respect to neural activity. Because this delay is several seconds, the predictive neural information will have preceded the conscious decision by up to 10 s. An important next step will now be to establish whether early predictive signals are decision-related at all. This might sound strange given that they predict the choices. However, this early information could hypothetically also be the consequence of stochastic, fluctuating background activity in the decision network, similar to the known fluctuations of signals in early visual cortex (Haynes, 2011; see also Leopold, Murayama, & Logothetis, 2003). In this view, the processes relevant for the decision could occur late, say in the last second before the decision. In the absence of any "reasons" for deciding for one or the other option, the decision network might need to break the symmetry, for example by using stochastic background fluctuations in the network.

If the fluctuations in the network are say in one subpartition, the decision could be biased toward "left," and if the fluctuations are in a different subpartition, the decision could be biased toward "right." But how could fluctuations at the time of the conscious decision be reflected already 7 s before? One reason could be that the temporal autocorrelation of neural signals includes very slow fluctuations (Leopold et al., 2003). To assess whether these early signals are indeed decision-generating or merely decision-predictive, it will be interesting to compare situations in which the subject does or does not know what an upcoming decision is going to be about. The study by Soon et al. (2008) again highlights the power of classification approaches to reveal information in brain signals that are believed to be mere "background" fluctuations.

3.4   Conclusion

Taken together, multivariate decoding and related approaches open a new window on large-scale brain signals that emphasizes the role of representation. It is now possible to track the storage of specific mental contents in brain activity, to understand the spaces in which they are encoded, to track their dynamics, and to reconstruct many different mental states based on encoding models.

Acknowledgments

The author would like to thank Dr. Jakob Heinzle for valuable comments and discussions on the manuscript. This work was funded by the Bernstein Computational Neuroscience Program of the German Federal Ministry of Education and Research (BMBF Grant 01GQ0411), the Excellence Initiative of the German Federal Ministry of Education and Research (DFG Grant GSC86/1–2009), and the Max Planck Society.

References

Averbeck, B. B., Latham, P. E., & Pouget, A. (2006). Neural correlations, population coding and computation. *Nature Reviews. Neuroscience*, 7(5), 358–366.

Boynton, G. M. (2005). Imaging orientation selectivity: decoding conscious perception in V1. *Nature Neuroscience*, 8(5), 541–542.

Brouwer, G. J., & van Ee, R. (2007). Visual cortex allows prediction of perceptual states during ambiguous structure-from-motion. *Journal of Neuroscience*, 27(5), 1015–1023.

Chaimow, D., Yacoub, E., Ugurbil, K., & Shmuel, A. (2011). Modeling and analysis of mechanisms underlying fMRI-based decoding of information conveyed in cortical columns. *NeuroImage*, 56(2), 627–642.

Chen, Y., Namburi, P., Elliott, L. T., Heinzle, J., Soon, C. S., Chee, M. W., et al. (2011). Cortical surface-based searchlight decoding. *NeuroImage, 56*(2), 582–592.

De Martino, F., Valente, G., Staeren, N., Ashburner, J., Goebel, R., & Formisano, E. (2008). Combining multivariate voxel selection and support vector machines for mapping and classification of fMRI spatial patterns. *NeuroImage, 43*(1), 44–58.

Edelman, S., Grill-Spector, K., Kushnir, R., & Malach, R. (1998). Towards a direct visualization of the internal shape representation space by fMRI. *Psychbiology, 26*, 309.

Epstein, R., & Kanwisher, N. (1998). A cortical representation of the local visual environment. *Nature, 392*(6676), 598–601.

Friston, K. J., Holmes, A. P., Poline, J. B., Grasby, P. J., Williams, S. C., Frackowiak, R. S., et al. (1995). Analysis of fMRI time-series revisited. *NeuroImage, 2*(1), 45–53.

Gardner, J. L. (2010). Is cortical vasculature functionally organized? *NeuroImage, 49*(3), 1953–1956.

Georgopoulos, A. P., Schwartz, A. B., & Kettner, R. E. (1986). Neuronal population coding of movement direction. *Science, 233*(4771), 1416–1419.

Haynes, J. D. (2009). Decoding visual consciousness from human brain signals. *Trends in Cognitive Sciences, 13*(5), 194–202.

Haynes, J. D. (2011). Decoding and predicting decisions. *Annals of the New York Academy of Sciences, 1224*, 9–21.

Haynes, J. D., & Rees, G. (2005a). Predicting the orientation of invisible stimuli from activity in human primary visual cortex. *Nature Neuroscience, 8*(5), 686–691.

Haynes, J. D., & Rees, G. (2005b). Predicting the stream of consciousness from activity in human visual cortex. *Current Biology, 15*(14), 1301–1307.

Haynes, J. D., & Rees, G. (2006). Decoding mental states from brain activity in humans. *Nature Reviews. Neuroscience, 7*(7), 523–534.

Haynes, J. D., Sakai, K., Rees, G., Gilbert, S., Frith, C., & Passingham, R. E. (2007). Reading hidden intentions in the human brain. *Current Biology, 17*(4), 323–328.

Haxby, J. V., Gobbini, M. I., Furey, M. L., Ishai, A., Schouten, J. L., & Pietrini, P. (2001). Distributed and overlapping representations of faces and objects in ventral temporal cortex. *Science, 293*(5539), 2425–2430.

Heinzle, J., Kahnt, T., & Haynes, J. (2011). Topographically-specific functional connectivity between visual field maps in the human brain. *Neuroimage, 56*(3), 1426–36.

Hung, C. P., Kreiman, G., Poggio, T., & DiCarlo, J. J. (2005). Fast readout of object identity from macaque inferior temporal cortex. *Science, 310*(5749), 863–866.

Kahnt, T., Heinzle, J., Park, S. Q., & Haynes, J. D. (2010). The neural code of reward anticipation in human orbitofrontal cortex. *Proceedings of the National Academy of Sciences of the United States of America, 107*(13), 6010–6015.

Kamitani, Y., & Sawahata, Y. (2010). Spatial smoothing hurts localization but not information: pitfalls for brain mappers. *NeuroImage, 49*(3), 1949–1952.

Kamitani, Y., & Tong, F. (2005). Decoding the visual and subjective contents of the human brain. *Nature Neuroscience, 8*(5), 679–685.

Kanwisher, N., McDermott, J., & Chun, M. M. (1997). The fusiform face area: a module in human extrastriate cortex specialized for face perception. *Journal of Neuroscience, 17*(11), 4302–4311.

Kay, K. N., Naselaris, T., Prenger, R. J., & Gallant, J. L. (2008). Identifying natural images from human brain activity. *Nature, 452*(7185), 352–355.

Kjems, U., Hansen, L. K., Anderson, J., Frutiger, S., Muley, S., Sidtis, J., et al. (2002). The quantitative evaluation of functional neuroimaging experiments: mutual information learning curves. *NeuroImage, 15*(4), 772–786.

Kriegeskorte, N. (2011). Pattern-information analysis: from stimulus decoding to computational-model testing. *NeuroImage*, *56*(2), 411–421.

Kriegeskorte, N., Cusack, R., & Bandettini, P. (2010). How does an fMRI voxel sample the neuronal activity pattern: compact-kernel or complex spatiotemporal filter? *NeuroImage*, *49*(3), 1965–1976.

Kriegeskorte, N., Goebel, R., & Bandettini, P. (2006). Information-based functional brain mapping. *Proceedings of the National Academy of Sciences of the United States of America*, *103*(10), 3863–3868.

Kriegeskorte, N., Mur, M., Ruff, D. A., Kiani, R., Bodurka, J., Esteky, H., et al. (2008). Matching categorical object representations in inferior temporal cortex of man and monkey. *Neuron*, *60*(6), 1126–1141.

Kriegeskorte, N., Simmons, W. K., Bellgowan, P. S., & Baker, C. I. (2009). Circular analysis in systems neuroscience: the dangers of double dipping. *Nature Neuroscience, 12*(5), 535–40.

Lemm, S., Blankertz, B., Dickhaus, T., & Müller, K. R. (2011). Introduction to machine learning for brain imaging. *NeuroImage*, *56*(2), 387–399.

Leopold, D. A., Murayama, Y., & Logothetis, N. K. (2003). Very slow activity fluctuations in monkey visual cortex: implications for functional brain imaging. *Cerebral Cortex*, *13*, 422–433.

Misaki, M., Kim, Y., Bandettini, P. A., & Kriegeskorte, N. (2010). Comparison of multivariate classifiers and response normalizations for pattern-information fMRI. *NeuroImage*, *53*(1), 103–118.

Mach, E. (1886). *Beiträge zur Analyse der Empfindungen*. Jena: Fischer.

Mitchell, T. M., Shinkareva, S. V., Carlson, A., Chang, K. M., Malave, V. L., Mason, R. A., et al. (2008). Predicting human brain activity associated with the meanings of nouns. *Science*, *320*(5880), 1191–1195.

Miyawaki, Y., Uchida, H., Yamashita, O., Sato, M. A., Morito, Y., Tanabe, H. C., et al. (2008). Visual image reconstruction from human brain activity using a combination of multiscale local image decoders. *Neuron*, *60*(5), 915–929.

Moutoussis, K., & Zeki, S. (2002). The relationship between cortical activation and perception investigated with invisible stimuli. *Proceedings of the National Academy of Sciences of the United States of America*, *99*(14), 9527–9532.

Nevado, A., Young, M. P., & Panzeri, S. (2004). Functional imaging and neural information coding. *NeuroImage*, *21*(3), 1083–1095.

Norman, K. A., Polyn, S. M., Detre, G. J., & Haxby, J. V. (2006). Beyond mind-reading: multi-voxel pattern analysis of fMRI data. *Trends in Cognitive Sciences*, *10*(9), 424–430.

Oosterhof, N. N., Wiestler, T., Downing, P. E., & Diedrichsen, J. (2011). A comparison of volume-based and surface-based multi-voxel pattern analysis. *NeuroImage*, *56*(2), 593–600.

Op de Beeck, H. P. (2010). Against hyperacuity in brain reading: spatial smoothing does not hurt multivariate fMRI analyses? *NeuroImage*, *49*(3), 1943–1948.

Pereira, F., Mitchell, T., & Botvinick, M. (2009). Machine learning classifiers and fMRI: a tutorial overview. *NeuroImage*, *45*(1 Suppl), S199–S209.

Quiroga, R. Q., Kreiman, G., Koch, C., & Fried, I. (2008). Sparse but not "grandmother-cell" coding in the medial temporal lobe. *Trends in Cognitive Sciences*, *12*(3), 87–91.

Sasaki, Y., Rajimehr, R., Kim, B. W., Ekstrom, L. B., Vanduffel, W., & Tootell, R. B. (2006). The radial bias: a different slant on visual orientation sensitivity in human and nonhuman primates. *Neuron*, *51*(5), 661–670.

Shinkareva, S. V., Mason, R. A., Malave, V. L., Wang, W., Mitchell, T. M., & Just, M. A. (2008). Using FMRI brain activation to identify cognitive states associated with perception of tools and dwellings. *PLoS ONE*, *3*(1), e1394.

Soon, C. S., Brass, M., Heinze, H. J., & Haynes, J. D. (2008). Unconscious determinants of free decisions in the human brain. *Nature Neuroscience, 11*(5), 543–545.

Swisher, J. D., Gatenby, J. C., Gore, J. C., Wolfe, B. A., Moon, C. H., Kim, S. G., et al. (2010). Multiscale pattern analysis of orientation-selective activity in the primary visual cortex. *Journal of Neuroscience, 30*(1), 325–330.

Tanaka, K. (1996). Inferotemporal cortex and object vision. *Annual Review of Neuroscience, 19*, 109–139.

Thirion, B., Duchesnay, E., Hubbard, E., Dubois, J., Poline, J. B., Lebihan, D., et al. (2006). Inverse retinotopy: inferring the visual content of images from brain activation patterns. *NeuroImage, 33*(4), 1104–1116.

Tong, F., Nakayama, K., Vaughan, J. T., & Kanwisher, N. (1998). Binocular rivalry and visual awareness in human extrastriate cortex. *Neuron, 21*(4), 753–759.

Tononi, G., Srinivasan, R., Russell, D. P., & Edelman, G. M. (1998). Investigating neural correlates of conscious perception by frequency-tagged neuromagnetic responses. *Proceedings of the National Academy of Sciences of the United States of America, 95*(6), 3198–3203.

Tusche, A., Bode, S., & Haynes, J. D. (2010). Neural responses to unattended products predict later consumer choices. *Journal of Neuroscience, 30*(23), 8024–8031.

4 Transient Brain Dynamics

Mikhail I. Rabinovich and Pablo Varona

Summary

One of the main goals of modern neuroscience is to understand how the dynamics of the brain is related to perception, emotion, cognition, and behavior. In the past decade, experimental and computational approaches support the point of view that the brain processes information by forming temporary functional neural networks that display transient states. Recently, a new mathematical approach in nonlinear dynamical theory has been developed for the rigorous description of the transient activity of neural ensembles, and the associated methods have been applied to specific cognitive problems. In this chapter, we describe some of these experiments and some of the mathematical and computational results that address transient brain dynamics and interactions among the brain's modes.

4.1 Transients versus Attractors in Perception

Neuroscience is often based on the assumption that neural mechanisms underlying perception and other brain functions can be inferred by steady-state measurements of neural activity or by models in which the behavior of the network is at steady state or periodic. Computing with "attractors" is a concept familiar to the neuroscience community. Upon the arrival of a stimulus, a neural network gradually changes its pattern of activation until it settles into one pattern—an attractor state. Thus, the input—a visual stimulus, a voice, an odor, or something more abstract—is associated with properties of the entire network in a particular attractor state. Such patterns of neural activity might be established, learned, and recalled during perception, memorization, and retrieval, respectively. However, recent experimental evidence and theoretical work show that transient states—ones in which no stable equilibrium is reached—can better represent several types of neural activity.

These two perspectives provide very different views of the dynamics produced by neural networks. The first emphasizes stable attractors, with memories as possible interpretations (Hopfield, 1982). The other, newer and possibly less intuitive, emphasizes nonclassical, transient dynamics, in which computation proceeds over time without the need for a classical attractor state. Because neural phenomena often occur on very short timescales, classical attractor states—fixed points or limit cycles—cannot be realistically reached. Behavioral and neurophysiologic experiments reveal the existence and functional relevance of dynamics that, although deterministic, do not require classical attractor states (Baeg et al., 2003; Uchida & Mainen, 2003; Lin et al., 2005; Jones, Fontanini, Sadacca, Miller, & Katz, 2007; Rabinovich, Huerta, & Laurent, 2008). In many cases, the conditions required to reach such attractors are often implausible for known biological circuits. Furthermore, fixed-point attractor dynamics express a somewhat restricted dynamics: Only the state the network settles into, given by its initial conditions (and characterized mathematically by, for example, a minimum in an energy function), matters, not the path taken to reach that state (see figure 4.1A).

In this context, an alternative theoretical framework can explain some forms of neural network dynamics that are consistent both with experiments and with transient dynamics. Transient dynamics have two main features. First, they can be resistant to noise and reliable even in the face of small variations in initial conditions; the succession of states visited by the system (its trajectory, or transient) is then stable. Second, the transients are input-specific and thus contain information about what caused

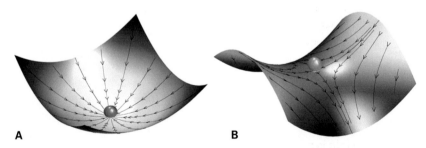

A   B

Figure 4.1
Intuitive illustration of the mathematical concepts that describe attractor and transient dynamics. (A) Representation of a simple attractor in the phase space of a dynamical system. (B) Representation of a saddle with two stable and two unstable separatrices (a separatrix is a surface or curve that refers to the boundary separating two modes of behavior in the phase space of a dynamical system). Illustrations kindly provided by R. Huerta.

them in the first place. Systems with few degrees of freedom do not, as a rule, express transient dynamics with such properties. Therefore, they are not good models for developing the kind of intuition required here. Nevertheless, stable transient dynamics can be understood from within the existing framework of nonlinear dynamical systems.

There are two fundamental contradictions regarding the use of transient dynamics for the description of brain activity. First of all, transient dynamics are inherently unstable. Any transient depends on initial conditions and cannot be reproduced from arbitrary initial conditions. Second, dynamical robustness precludes sensitivity to informative perturbations. If transients are reproducible in spite of the presence of noise, how can they also be sensitive to small informative signals? In section 4.2, we will explain how these contradictions can be resolved through the concept of metastability. This concept was introduced to cognitive science at the end of the past century (Scott Kelso, 1995; Friston, 1997, 2000; Fingelkurts & Fingelkurts, 2006; Oullier & Scott Kelso, 2006; Gros, 2007; Ito, Nikolaev, & van Leeuwen, 2007).

Let us first describe the results of several experiments addressing sensory dynamics. Sensory signals are processed in animals through the activation of specific groups of neurons, which are determined by both the quality and the quantity of the stimulus. The intrinsic dynamics of neural networks produces firing patterns that encode informative inputs, which then are relayed to higher processing centers. In general, this code is spatiotemporal and sequential. Experimental observations in the olfactory systems of locust (Laurent & Davidowitz, 1994) and zebrafish (Friedrich & Laurent, 2001) support this view. Odors generate distributed (in time and space) odor- and concentration-specific patterns of activity in principal neurons (see figure 4.2). Hence, odor representations can be described as successions of states, or trajectories, each corresponding to one stimulus and one concentration (Stopfer et al., 2003). Only when a stimulus is sustained does its corresponding trajectory reach a stable fixed-point attractor (Mazor & Laurent, 2005). However, stable transients are observed whether a stimulus is sustained or not; that is, even when a stimulus is sufficiently short that no fixed-point attractor state is reached. When the responses to several stimuli are compared, the distances between the trajectories corresponding to each stimulus are larger during the transients, not between the fixed points (Mazor & Laurent, 2005). Because transients and fixed points represent states of neuronal populations, and because these states are themselves read out or "decoded" by other neuronal populations, stimulus identification by

A   B   C

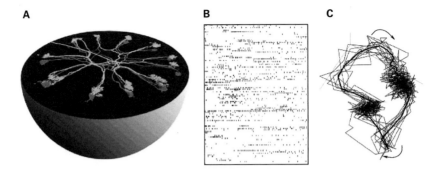

Figure 4.2
Experimental evidence for transient sequential dynamics. The panels illustrate the spatiotemporal representation of sensory information in the olfactory system of a locust (antennal lobe). (A) Schematic of an insect antennal lobe sectioned through its equatorial plane.
(B) Response of 110 neurons of the antennal lobe to an odorant that lasted 1.5 s. (C)
Projection of neural activity on three-dimensional principal component space (black trajectory is the average of 10 different experiments). Adapted from Rabinovich et al. (2008a).

such decoders should be more reliable with transient than with fixed-
point states. This conclusion is supported by the observation that a population of neurons that receives signals from the principal neurons
responds mostly during transients, when the separation between inputs
is optimized. In response to these observations, a theoretical framework
needs to explain the system's sensitivity to incoming signals, its stability
against noise (external noise and intrinsic pulsations of the system), and
its minimal dependence on the initial conditions (reproducibility).

In mammals, a remarkable example of transient neural dynamics has
been described in the analysis of the response in the rat's gustatory
cortex to prototype tastes. This study revealed that reproducible taste-
specific switching patterns are triggered shortly after the stimulus is
presented (Jones et al., 2007). Figure 4.3 shows representative single
trials of the neural response of gustatory cortex neurons to each basic
taste stimulus. Numbers within each grayscale region label the state
number. The activity sequences are reproducible in spite of the irregularity in their switching times.

To describe transient dynamics, we need a mathematical image (function or mathematical map) that is consistent with existing observations.
Once we have this mathematical tool, we can build models that can be
used to reveal and understand the properties of this type of dynamics
and generate testable predictions. One plausible image is a stable heteroclinic channel (Rabinovich et al., 2001; Rabinovich et al., 2008a,
2008b) (see figure 4.4). A stable heteroclinic channel is defined by a

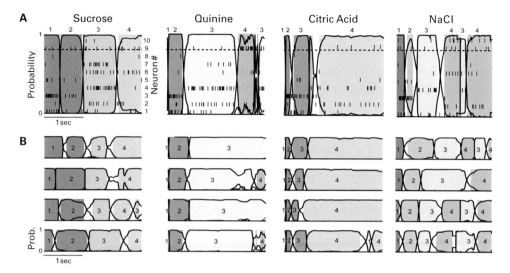

Figure 4.3
Experimental evidence for transient sequential dynamics in mammals. Neurons in the rat's gustatory cortex generate a taste-specific sequential pattern (Jones et al., 2007). (A) Panels show the sequential activations among 10 cortex neurons in response to four taste stimuli (sucrose, quinine, citric acid, and NaCl). (B) Four additional sequences for the same neuron ensemble showing the reliability of the sequences. The sequences are reproducible in spite of the irregularity in their switching times. Adapted from Jones et al. (2007).

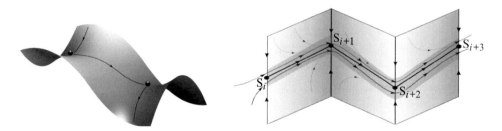

Figure 4.4
Representation of a simple heteroclinic chain (left) and a robust sequence of metastable states (right); a useful mathematical concept to describe transient dynamics that we discuss in this chapter.

sequence of successive metastable ("saddle") states (cf. figure 4.1B). Under proper conditions, all trajectories in the neighborhood of these saddle points remain in the channel, ensuring robustness and reproducibility over a wide range of control parameters. These saddles can be pictured as successive and temporary winners in a never-ending competitive game (see right panel in figure 4.4) as we discuss in the next section.

4.2   Robustness through Metastability: Winnerless Competition

In this section, we will use the mathematical image that we have just introduced to discuss a paradigm of sequence generation that does not depend on the geometric structure of the neural ensemble in physical space. This paradigm can explain and predict many dynamical phenomena in neural networks with excitatory and inhibitory synaptic connections. The paradigm is called winnerless competition (WLC).

The study of competitive dynamics has a long tradition. "Survival of the fittest" is a cliché that is often associated with the term *competition*. However, competition is not merely a means of determining the winner, as in a winner-take-all network with attractor dynamics. It is also a multifunctional instrument that nature uses at all levels of the neuronal hierarchy. Competition is also a mechanism that maintains the highest level of variability and stability of neural dynamics, even under transient behaviors. More than 200 years ago, the mathematicians Borda and de Condorcet were interested in the process of plurality elections at the French Royal Academy of Sciences. They considered voting dynamics in a case of three candidates A, B, and C. If A beats B and B beats C in a head-to-head competition, we might reasonably expect A to beat C. Thus, predicting the results of the election is easy. However, this is not always the case. It may happen that C beats A, resulting in a so-called Condorcet triangle, and there is no real winner in such a competitive process (Borda, 1781; Saari, 1995). This example is also called a *voting paradox*. The dynamical image of this phenomenon is a robust heteroclinic cycle like the one depicted in figure 4.5. In some specific cases, the heteroclinic cycle is even structurally stable (Guckenheimer & Holmes, 1988; Krupa, 1997; Stone & Armbruster, 1999; Ashwin et al., 2003; Postlethwaite & Dawes, 2005).

Competition without a winner is also a known phenomenon in physics: Busse and Heikes discovered that convective roll patterns in a rotating plane layer exhibit sequential changes of the roll's direction as a result of the competition between patterns with different roll orientations. No pattern wins, and the system exhibits periodic or chaotic switching

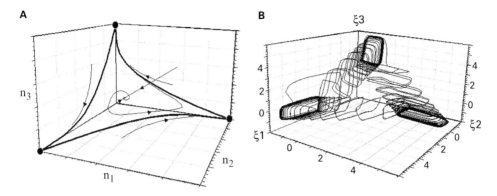

Figure 4.5
Illustration of WLC dynamics. (A) Phase portrait corresponding to autonomous WLC dynamics of a three-dimensional case. (B) Projection of a nine-dimensional heteroclinic orbit of three inhibitory coupled FitzHugh–Nagumo spiking model neurons in a three-dimensional space (the variables $\xi1$, $\xi2$, $\xi3$ are linear combinations of the actual phase variables of the system. Adapted from Rabinovich et al. (2006).

dynamics (Busse & Heikes, 1980; for a review, see Rabinovich et al., 2000). The same phenomenon has also been discovered in a genetic system; that is, in experiments with a synthetic network of three transcriptional regulators (Elowitz & Leibler, 2000). Specifically, these authors described three repressor genes A, B, and C organized in a closed chain with unidirectional inhibitory connections such that A, B, and C beat each other. This network behaves like a clock: It periodically induces synthesis of green fluorescent proteins as an indicator of the state of individual cells in a timescale of hours.

Before we introduce a basic model for the analysis of reproducible transient dynamics, it is important to discuss two general features of the stable heteroclinic channel that do not depend on the model (cf. figure 4.5 and figure 4.6, plate 7). These are (i) the origin of the structural stability of the stable heteroclinic channel and (ii) the long passage time in the vicinity of saddles in the presence of moderate noise. The conditions of existence and the dynamical features of stable heteroclinic channels can be implemented in a wide variety of models: from simple Lotka–Volterra descriptions to complex Hodgkin–Huxley models, and from small networks to large ensembles of many elements.

Thus, nonlinear dynamical theory has furnished the concept of stable transients that are robust against noise yet sensitive to external signals (Afraimovich et al., 2004; Rabinovich et al., 2008b). We have already described the mathematical object that corresponds to such stable

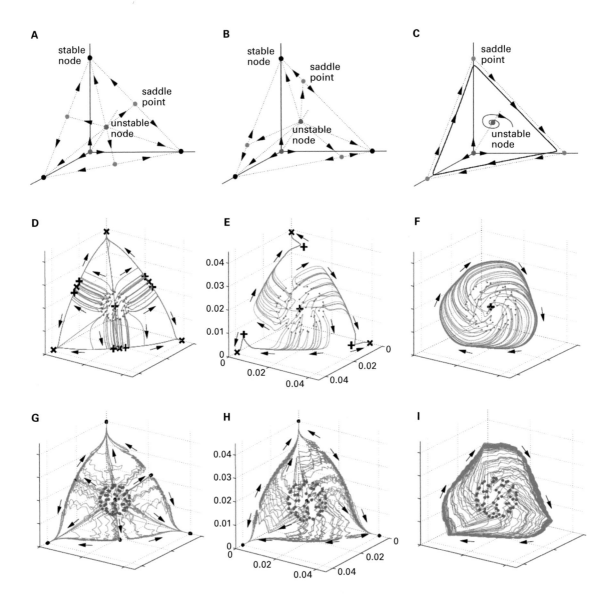

Figure 4.6 (plate 7)
Bifurcation toward a heteroclinic chain in different models. The Lotka–Volterra model with three units (A–C) undergoes a simultaneous saddle-node bifurcation in the three corners of the shown phase-space simplex, with increasing asymmetry of the inhibitory connections [red points, stable fixed points (FPs); blue points, saddles; green points, unstable FPs]. Numerical evidence for a similar bifurcation can be found in a system of realistic Hodgkin–Huxley neurons (G–I) coupled by inhibitory synapses. This is confirmed by a systematic reduction of the biophysical Hodgkin–Huxley model to an equivalent rate model (D–F) and a subsequent numerical bifurcation analysis [red and black crosses in D–F denote the calculated FPs; red crosses are stable FPs and black markers are FPs with at least one unstable direction (saddles or unstable FPs)]. Adapted from Nowotny and Rabinovich (2007).

transients: a sequence of metastable states that are connected by separatrices (see figure 4.4). Under proper conditions, all trajectories in the neighborhood of metastable states that form the chain remain in their vicinity, ensuring robustness and reproducibility over a wide range of control parameters. Such sequence is possibly the only dynamical object that satisfies the dynamical principles that were formulated earlier. To understand the conditions of the stability of heteroclinic channels, we have to take into account that an elementary phase volume in the neighborhood of a saddle is compressed along the stable separatrices, and it is stretched along an unstable separatrix. Let us order the eigenvalues of the Jacobian at the ith saddle point as

$$\lambda_1^{(i)} > 0 > \operatorname{Re} \lambda_2^{(i)} \ge \operatorname{Re} \lambda_3^{(i)} \ge \ldots \ge \operatorname{Re} \lambda_d^{(i)}.$$

The number $v_i = -\operatorname{Re} \lambda_2^{(i)} / \lambda_1^{(i)}$ is called the saddle value. If $v_i > 1$ (the compressing is larger than the stretching), the saddle is named as a dissipative saddle. Intuitively, it is clear that the trajectories do not leave the heteroclinic channel if all saddles in the heteroclinic chain are dissipative. A rigorous analysis of the structural stability of the heteroclinic channel supports this intuition (Rabinovich et al., 2008b).

The temporal characteristics of transients are related to the "exit problem" for small random perturbations of dynamical systems with saddle sets. A local stability analysis in the vicinity of a saddle fixed point allows estimation of the time that the system spends in the vicinity of the saddle $\tau(p) = 1/\lambda_1^{(i)} \ln (1/|\eta|)$, where $\tau(p)$ is the mean passage time, $|\eta|$ is the level of noise, and $\lambda_1^{(i)}$ is an eigenvalue corresponding to the unstable separatrix of the saddle.

To understand fully such structurally stable transient dynamics, we need further to describe the mathematical image of a stable heteroclinic channel (cf. figure 4.4). A stable heteroclinic channel is defined by a sequence of successive metastable ("saddle") states. Under appropriate conditions, all the trajectories in the neighborhood of these saddle points remain in the channel, ensuring robustness and reproducibility in a wide range of control parameters. Such dynamical objects are rare in low-dimensional systems but common in complex ones. A simple model to describe these objects is a generalized Lotka–Volterra equation, which expresses and predicts the fate of an ongoing competition between N interactive elements:

$$\frac{dA_i(t)}{dt} A_i(t) F\left(\sigma_i(S_k) - \sum_{j=1}^{N} \rho_{ij} A_j(t) \right) + A_i(t) \eta_i(t) \quad i = 1, \ldots, N \qquad (4.1)$$

where $A(t)$ is the activity rate of element i, σ_i is the gain function that controls the impact of the stimulus, S_k is an environmental stimulus, ρ_{ij} determines the interaction between the variables, η_i represents the noise level, and F is a function, in the simplest case a linear function.

When N is small (e.g., two species competing for the same food source, or predator–prey interactions), limit cycles are often seen, consistent with observations. When N is large, the state portrait of the system often contains a heteroclinic sequence linking saddle points. These saddles can be pictured as successive and temporary winners in a never-ending competitive game. In neural systems, because a representative model must produce sequences of connected neuronal population states (the saddle points), neural connectivity must be asymmetric, as determined by theoretical examination of a basic "coarse grain" model (Huerta & Rabinovich, 2004). Although many connection statistics probably work for stable heteroclinic-type dynamics, it is likely that connectivity within biological networks is, to some extent at least, the result of optimization by evolution and synaptic plasticity.

Models like the generalized Lotka–Volterra equations allow one to establish the conditions necessary for transient stability. Consider a three-dimensional autonomous inhibitory circuit with asymmetric connections. Such a system displays stable, sequential, and cyclic activation of its components, the simplest variant of winnerless competition (Rabinovich et al., 2001). High-dimensional systems with asymmetric connections can generate structurally stable sequences—transients, each shaped by one input (Nowotny & Rabinovich, 2007). A stable heteroclinic channel is the dynamical image of this behavior.

Asymmetric inhibitory connectivity also helps to solve the apparent paradox that sensitivity and reliability can coexist in a network (Huerta & Rabinovich, 2004; Nowotny & Rabinovich, 2007; Rabinovich et al. 2008b; Rabinovich & Varona, 2011). To be reliable, a system must be both sensitive to the input and insensitive to perturbations and initial conditions. To solve this paradox, one must realize that the neurons participating in a stable heteroclinic channel are assigned by the stimulus, by virtue of their direct and/or indirect input from the neurons activated by that stimulus. The joint action of the external input and a stimulus-dependent connectivity matrix defines the stimulus-specific heteroclinic channel. In addition, asymmetric inhibition coordinates the sequential activity of the neurons and keeps a heteroclinic channel stable.

Within this framework, neural networks can be viewed as nonequilibrium systems and their associated computations as unique patterns of

transient activity, controlled by incoming input. The results of these computations must be reproducible, robust against noise, and easily decoded.
Because a stable heteroclinic channel is possibly the only dynamical
object that satisfies all the requisite conditions, it is plausible that these
networks are dynamical systems with stable heteroclinic channels, based
on the principle of winnerless competition discussed earlier. Thus, using
asymmetric inhibition appropriately, the space of possible states of large
neural systems can be restricted to connected saddle points, forming
stable heteroclinic channels. These channels can be thought of as underlying reliable transient brain dynamics.

4.3 Hierarchical Competition: Canonical Models

In the previous section, we argued that from the dynamical point of view,
neural competition can be implemented through a sequence of metastable states. The following is a formulation of the desired features of a
hierarchical competition model: The model must be dissipative with an
unstable trivial state (origin) in the phase space, and the corresponding
linear increments must be stabilized by the nonlinear terms organized
by self-inhibition and mutual inhibition (mode competition); the phase
space of the system must include metastable states that represent the
activity of an individual mode when other modes are passive; and finally
these metastable states must be connected by separatrices to build a
sequence. Well-known rate models in neuroscience satisfy these conditions in some regions of control parameter space (Huerta & Rabinovich,
2004; Rabinovich, Varona, Selverston, & Abarbanel, 2006). Thus, the
canonical model describing the mode dynamics that we describe in this
section uses the nonlinear rate equations (Rabinovich, Muezzinoglu,
Strigo, & Bystritsky, 2010):

$$\tau_{A_i} \frac{d}{dt} A_i(t) = A_i(t) \cdot F_i(\mathbf{A}, \mathbf{B}, \mathbf{R}, \mathbf{S})$$

$$\tau_{B_i} \frac{d}{dt} B_j(t) = B_j(t) \cdot \Phi_j(\mathbf{A}, \mathbf{B}, \mathbf{R}, \mathbf{S}) \qquad (4.2)$$

$$\theta_k \frac{d}{dt} R_k(t) = R_k(t) \cdot Q_k(\mathbf{A}, \mathbf{B}, \mathbf{R}, \mathbf{S})$$

where A_i, $B_j \geq 0$ ($i = 1,\dots, N; j = 1,\dots, M$) represent two competitive families of modes, and R_k, $k = 1,\dots, K$, represents the resources consumed by
these neural processes. F_i, Φ_j, and Q_k are functions of A_i, B_j, and R_k,
respectively. The collections of N, M neural modes and K resource items

are encapsulated in **A**, **B**, and **R**, respectively. When initiated properly, this set of equations ensures that all the variables remain non-negative. The vector **S** represents the external and/or internal inputs to the system, and τ_A, τ_B, and θ are the time constants.

In what follows, we will associate the modes above with patterns of distributed activity in the brain. There are several efficient ways to extract empirical modes from experimental data, for example, by principal or independent components analyses of temporal brain activity (McKeown et al., 1998; Friston et al., 2000; Koenig et al., 2001) as recorded in electroencephalography (EEG) or functional magnetic resonance imaging (fMRI) setups. First, let us apply model (4.2) to just one form of neural activity when mode $A–B$ interaction is negligible. Let us imagine a situation where A changes over time while B remains more or less constant. Keeping in mind that the competition between the different modes of neural activity can be described in the simplest form of the functions on the right side of equation (4.2), that is, $F(A,S)$ is linear, we can present the first set of equations (4.2) in a form of the generalized Lotka–Volterra (GLV) model (Lotka, 1925):

$$\tau_A \frac{d}{dt} A_i = A_i \left[\mu_i(\mathbf{S}) - \sum_{j=1}^{N} \rho_{ij} A_j \right] + A_i \eta(t) \qquad (4.3)$$

Here, $\mu_i(\mathbf{S})$ is the increment that represents both intrinsic and external excitation, ρ_{ij} is the competition matrix between the modes, $\eta(t)$ is a multiplicative noise perturbing the system, and **S** is the input that captures the sources of internal or external effects on the increment.

Model (4.3) has several remarkable features, which we will use to build and understand the canonical model; depending on the control parameters, it can describe a vast array of behaviors. In particular, when connections are nearly symmetric, that is, $\rho_{ij} \approx \rho_{ji}$, two or more stable states can coexist, yielding multistable dynamics where the initial condition determines the final state. When the connections are strongly nonsymmetric, a stable sequence of the metastable states can emerge (Afraimovich et al., 2004) (cf. figure 4.4). The nonsymmetric inhibitory interaction between the modes helps to solve an apparent paradox related to the notion that sensitivity and reliability in a network can coexist: The joint action of the external input and a stimulus-dependent connectivity matrix defines the stimulus-specific sequence. Dynamical chaos can also be observed in this case (Muezzinoglu et al., 2010). Furthermore, a specific kind of the dynamical chaos, where the order of the switching is deterministic but the lifetime of the metastable states is irregular, is possible (Varona et al., 2002; Venaille et al., 2005). Similar "timing chaos with serial order" has been observed in vivo in the gustatory cortex example that we discussed earlier (Jones et al., 2007). For model (4.3), the area in parameter space with structural stability of the transients has been formulated in Afraimovich et al. (2004).

When describing the interaction between the different neural modes and the resources consumed by these processes, we are particularly interested in a structurally stable transient neural activity. This can effectively describe the reproducible activation patterns during normal brain states and identify specific instabilities that correspond to pathologic dynamics. Based on the GLV model (4.3), we introduce the system (4.2) as follows:

$$\tau_{A_i} \frac{d}{dt} A_i(t) = A_i(t) \cdot \left[\sigma_i(\mathbf{S}, \mathbf{B}, \mathbf{R}_A) - \sum_{j=1}^{N} \rho_{ij} A_j(t) \right] + A_i(t)\eta_A(t), \ i = 1,\dots, N \tag{4.4}$$

$$\tau_{B_i} \frac{d}{dt} B_i(t) = B_i(t) \cdot \left[\zeta_i(\mathbf{S}, \mathbf{A}, \mathbf{R}_B) - \sum_{j=1}^{M} \xi_{ij} B_j(t) \right] + B_i(t)\eta_B(t), \ i = 1,\dots, M \tag{4.5}$$

$$\theta_A^i \frac{d}{dt} R_A^i(t) = R_A^i(t) \cdot \left[\sum_{j=1}^{N} A_j(t) - \sum_{m=1}^{K_A} R_A^m - \phi_A \sum_{m=1}^{K_B} R_B^m + d_A(t) \right], \ i = 1,\dots, K_A \tag{4.6}$$

$$\theta_B^i \frac{d}{dt} R_B^i(t) = R_B^i(t) \cdot \left[\sum_{j=1}^{M} B_j(t) - \sum_{m=1}^{K_B} R_B^m - \phi_B \sum_{m=1}^{K_A} R_A^m + d_B(t) \right], \ i = 1,\dots, K_B. \tag{4.7}$$

The model (4.4)–(4.7) reflects a mutual inhibition and excitation within and among the two modes (see table 4.1). These modes depend on the inputs through parameter $\mathbf{S}$ (which may represent, for example, stress, cognitive load, physical state of the body). The variables R_A^i and R_B^i characterize the K_A and K_B resource items that are allocated to different modes, and the vectors $\mathbf{R}_A$ and $\mathbf{R}_B$ are the collections of these items that gate incremental expression of the modes during competition. The characteristic times θ of the different resources may vary. The coefficients ϕ_A and ϕ_B determine the level of competition for these resources. Each process is open to the multiplicative noise denoted by η and d terms in the equations.

The values of the increments σ_i and ζ_i depend on the stimuli and/or the intensity of the modes, respectively. The only design constraint that we can impose on the increments σ_i and ζ_i is that they must be positive.

Table 4.1
Model parameters and their values in the simulations

Parameter	Role	Range of Values in Simulations
τ_{A_i}	Time constants for neural A modes	1e–2 to1e–1
τ_{B_i}	Time constants for neural B modes	1e–2 to 1e–1
θ_A^i, θ_B^i	Time constants for resource dynamics	1
ρ, ξ	Competition matrices — inducing metastable state sequence	Selected according to the inequalities in Rabinovich et al. (2010), assuming all increment values equal unity
σ_i	Increments to the A modes — locating the metastable states	Dependent variable within 0 and 1: proportional to exogenous input S, inversely proportional to either a specific mode or the total B mode activity, i.e., $\Sigma \, B_i$
ζ_i	Increments to the B modes	Dependent variable within 0 and 1: either a constant of 1 or inversely proportional to $\Sigma \, A_i$
η_A, η_B, d_A, d_B	Noise components	Uniform random terms within 0 and u, where u is set between 1e–6 and 1e–3
ϕ_A, ϕ_B	Regulate the resource modes competition	Constants set to 1, except in hysteresis simulation, where $\phi_A = 0.33$ and $\phi_B = 1.0$

Three types of interactions are described by the model (4.4)–(4.7): (i) a competitive interaction within each set of modes; (ii) interaction through excitation (increments); and (iii) competition for resources. For the latter, mediated via variables R_A and R_B, one only needs appropriate values of the parameters ϕ_A and ϕ_B. The values of the control parameters, which ensure stability of the transients, can be obtained from the inequalities that describe the ratio between the compressing and stretching of the phase volume in the vicinity of the metastable states (Afraimovich et al., 2004).

The brain imaging data currently available does not allow us to specify the detailed structure of the modes or constrain the values of parameters precisely. However, the model has a large dynamical repertoire and can exhibit different behaviors and transitions among them (i.e., bifurcations that are reminiscent of those observed empirically). This capability, together with their success in representing some key phenomena observed in the brain, may be useful when trying to understand the origin of cognitive phenomena such as working memory and decision making in a changing environment (Huber et al., 1999, 2000). First, we will focus on modeling physiologic modes observed in the brain.

4.4   Modulation Instability and Resting-State Dynamics

Spontaneous neural dynamics can be analyzed when the brain is not engaged in a particular task (i.e., resting-state brain dynamics). In the resting state, a prevalent pattern of mode of activity is the default mode network (DMN). This network comprises a set of specific brain regions whose activity is predominant during the resting state. We chose control parameters of the model (4.4)–(4.7) so that it exhibits simple rhythmic activity (oscillations with a characteristic time scale of 2–3 s), which is in the range of slow fluctuations observed empirically. When competition becomes larger than a critical value, this simple rhythmic activity becomes unstable due to modulation instability, and a stable limit cycle appears on the phase plane of the mean activity:

$$\tilde{A}(t) = \frac{1}{N}\sum_{i=1}^{N} A_i$$

$$\tilde{B}(t) = \frac{1}{M}\sum_{i=1}^{M} B_i.$$

This leads to stable low-frequency oscillations (LFOs), as shown in figure 4.7 (plate 8). The averaged-in-time time series indicates that the modulation process is close to a quasi-periodic LFO that is reminiscent of the ultraslow fluctuations seen in the resting brain.

An increasing number of EEG and resting-state fMRI studies in humans and animals indicate that spontaneous low-frequency fluctuations in cerebral activity at 0.01–0.1 Hz represent a fundamental characteristic of spontaneous physiologic dynamics. In particular, resting-state fMRI measures show the stable properties of LFOs. In general, the LFO fluctuations observed with fMRI are not the same as the underlying neuronal fluctuations because they have been passed through a hemodynamic response function. However, several studies (Lörincz, Geall, Bao, Crunelli, & Hughes, 2009; Taylor, Seminowicz, & Davis, 2009; Tomasi & Volkow, 2010; Buckner, 2010) support the hypothesis that LFOs are correlated with neuronal activity; that is, cooperative dynamics (due to their modulation or synchronization). The modulation instability that we have observed in computer experiments discloses a plausible dynamical origin of low-frequency mode dynamics in resting states, possibly related to the "cortical-subcortical cross-talk" (Salvador et al., 2005). Characterizing changes in resting-state dynamics in various psychiatric disorders may provide a tool for the diagnosis of psychopathology or for identify-

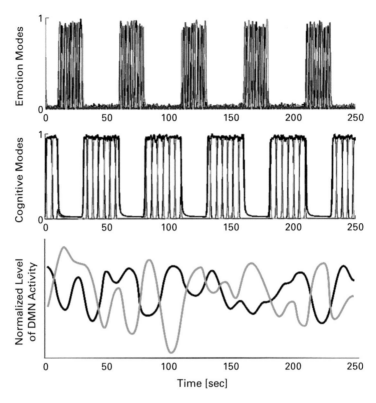

Figure 4.7 (plate 8)
Anti-phase low-frequency oscillations displayed by the model (4.4)–(4.7). In the resting
state, these are a result of competition—modulation instability [S is constant, $N = M = 5$
in the model (4.4)–(4.7)]. The black envelope on the middle panel is the total activity as
predicted by the model. Its competition with the second mode (top panel) results in a
pulsation as observed in many EEG and fMRI studies. The bottom panel, reconstructed
based on the data presented in Taylor et al. (2009), shows empirical observations in the
brain's resting state. Adapted from Rabinovich et al. (2010).

ing individual variations in physiologic arousal (Baliki, Geha, Apkarian,
& Chialvo, 2008; Broyd et al., 2009; Fornito & Bullmore, 2010; Mannell
et al., 2010).

4.5   Modeling Psychopathology

Although we have described equations (4.4)–(4.7) as representing the
interaction between neural modes representing distributed patterns of
activity, these modes can be associated with specific functional roles, such
as emotion (e.g., salience modes) and cognition (e.g., attention modes)

(Rabinovich et al., 2010). The objects in phase space representing these processes are influenced by intrinsic brain dynamics and external stimuli. For example, during sequential decision-making, sequential working memory or navigation, the image of the implicit cognitive dynamics is a stable transient, whereas other cognitive functions, such as those pertaining to music or linguistic processing, may be represented by recurrent dynamics. One might even consider emotional modes that can demonstrate a range of dynamical behaviors, such as the transient regimes considered under cognitive processes, recurrent regular or irregular dynamics corresponding to mood changes, and long-lasting equilibria associated with clinical cases of deep depression or hypomania. The canonical model presented earlier might also be applied to anxiety disorders that have been associated with abnormal brain activity. Although there is large symptomatic overlap between different anxiety disorders, each can be characterized by specific symptoms that, in principle, can be associated with particular values of the model's control parameters.

Psychopathology, like panic attacks and obsessive-compulsive disorder (OCD), are associated with irregular dynamical behavior that is often consistent with chaotic dynamics (see, e.g., Masterpasqua & Perna, 1997; Kubota & Sakai, 2002; Katerndahl et al., 2007; Zor et al., 2009). Mathematical images of such dynamics are transient chaos or strange attractors (Ott, 1993). The canonical model allows us to understand and depict the main types of dynamics that might be observed in such pathologic states. We are still far from a clinical use of these dynamical models. However, the dynamics they support exhibit rhythmic cycles of sequential activity that are characteristic of these pathologic states.

OCD is a type of anxiety disorder that traps people in an endless cycle of repetitive feelings, unwanted thoughts and acts, which the sufferer realizes are undesirable but is unable to resist; for example, compulsive rituals (Huppert & Franklin, 2005; Hollander et al., 2007). The compulsive rituals characteristic of OCD are performed in an attempt to prevent obsessive thoughts or make them go away. Although ritualistic behavior may suppress anxiety temporarily, the person must perform the ritualistic behavior again when the obsessive thoughts return. People with OCD may be aware that their obsessions and compulsions are senseless or unrealistic, but they cannot stop themselves. An attractor-based description of these features of OCD has been attempted recently by Rolls et al. (2008). To model OCD with equations (4.4)–(4.7), we can introduce a sequence of saddles, that is, metastable states, in the cognitive (faster) subspace. Each saddle in this sequence has, by construction, a two-dimensional unstable manifold as described in Rabinovich et al. (2010). One of these dimensions forms the separatrix leading to the next (cognitive) metastable state along a sequence, whereas the second unstable separatrix targets a saddle that represents the entry to the ritual, modeled as a stable chain of emotional (slower) metastable states. The ritual terminates at a saddle that has many unstable separatrices, each yielding to a cognitive mode (see figure 4.8, plate 9). As a result, OCD dynamics are represented by a $(N+M)$-dimensional transient, which distinguishes itself qualitatively from the other dynamics with a specific instability that leads to uncertainty. The results of this sort of modeling predict that, in OCD, the interaction of sequential cognitive activity (e.g., sequential decision-making) with emotion is characterized by an intermittent dynamical instability. The associated dynamical images and phase portraits are shown in figure 4.8 (plate 9).

The OCD model includes enough parameters to model competition between cognitive processes and the ritual in great detail. It is possible to make the model "noncircular" by arranging the unstable separatrices of the terminal ritual mode. This would, however, require clinical data to specify the return to cognitive function from the ritual (see also McClure, Botvinick, Yeung, Greene, & Cohen, 2007). A very specific object, which we name an "intermittent transient," describes the emotion–cognition interaction during OCD. Along such an intermittent transient, a chain of metastable cognitive modes is interrupted by the ritualistic behavior characteristic of OCD with an unpredictable returning.

4.6   Conclusion

According to the standard definition, a dynamical system is a model of a real system that undergoes a time evolution from the initial moment to infinity. The nervous system, strictly speaking, is not a dynamical system under this definition. However, many brain functions exhibit dynamical features that can be described by appropriate dynamical models over finite intervals of time. Furthermore, the brain is somehow capable of coordinating stable heteroclinic channels and exploiting them in the service of perception and adaptive behavior. See chapter 6 for a discussion of their use as generative models of sequences of sequences commonly encountered in the world. One can hypothesize that, in such cases, neuronal modes must comply with the universal principles that we have discussed in this chapter. To compose these modes hierarchically over space and time, so that they remain sensitive to the external world,

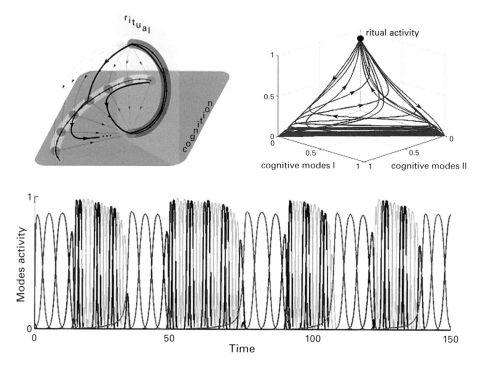

Figure 4.8 (plate 9)
Dynamical representation of obsessive-compulsive disorder (OCD). Top left: A dynamical image of OCD. Here, while the cognitive task evolves on stable transients, the dynamics shift toward a dominant intermittent transient sequence (i.e., the ritual) whose initial mode lies on the unstable manifolds of the cognitive saddles. During this ritual, cognition halts, and upon its completion, the subject returns to a cognitive process, not necessarily through the last cognitive mode visited. Bottom: A simulation of OCD by the proposed model. Here, the individual performs a "normal" cognitive task represented by the five modes colored yellow to red. At certain times, the individual performs a ritual as illustrated by four dark-colored modes in a prescribed ordered. The system can enter this ritual sequence from any cognitive mode, and, upon completion of the ritual, returns back to the cognitive process via an arbitrary mode. Top right: A phase portrait of this dynamical behavior. Adapted from Rabinovich et al. (2010).

may require an additional principle; for example, the free energy principle discussed also in chapter 12.

Acknowledgments

Mikhail I. Rabinovich acknowledges support from ONR grant N00014–07-1-074. Pablo Varona was supported by MICINN BFU2009–08473.

References

Afraimovich, V. S., Zhigulin, V. P., & Rabinovich, M. I. (2004). On the origin of reproducible sequential activity in neural circuits. *Chaos (Woodbury, N.Y.)*, *14*, 1123.

Ashwin, P., Field, M., Rucklidge, A. M., & Sturman, R. (2003). Phase resetting effects for robust cycles between chaotic sets. *Chaos (Woodbury, N.Y.)*, *13*, 973–981.

Baeg, E. H., Kim, Y. B., Huh, K., Mook-Jung, I., Kim, H. T., & Jung, M. W. (2003). Dynamics of population code for working memory in the prefrontal cortex. *Neuron*, *40*(1), 177–188.

Baliki, M. N., Geha, P. Y., Apkarian, A. V., & Chialvo, D. R. (2008). Beyond feeling: chronic pain hurts the brain, disrupting the default-mode network dynamics. *J Neurosci 28*(6), 1398–1403.

Borda, J. C. (1781). Mémoire sur les élections au scrutin. *Histoire de l'Académie Royale des Sciences*. Paris: Académie Royale des Sciences.

Broyd, S. J., Demanuele, C., Debener, S., Helps, S. K., James, C. J., & Sonuga-Barke, E. J. S. (2009.) Default-mode brain dysfunction in mental disorders: a systematic review. *Neurosci Biobehav Rev 33*(3), 279–296.

Buckner, R. L. (2010). Human functional connectivity: new tools, unresolved questions. *Proc Natl Acad Sci USA*, *107*(24), 10769–10770.

Busse, F., & Heikes, K. (1980). Convection in a rotating layer: a simple case of turbulence. *Science*, *208*, 173–175.

Elowitz, M., & Leibler, S. (2000). A synthetic oscillatory network of transcriptional regulators. *Nature*, *403*, 335–338.

Fingelkurts, A. A., & Fingelkurts, A. A. (2006). Timing in cognition and EEG brain dynamics: discreteness versus continuity. *Cogn Process 7*(3), 135–162.

Fornito, A., & Bullmore, E. T. (2010). What can spontaneous fluctuations of the blood oxygenation-level-dependent signal tell us about psychiatric disorders? *Curr Opin Psychiatry*, *23*(3), 239–249.

Friedrich, R. W., & Laurent, G. (2001). Dynamic optimization of odor representations by slow temporal patterning of mitral cell activity. *Science*, *291*(5505), 889–894.

Friston, K. J. (1997). Transients, metastability, and neuronal dynamics. *NeuroImage*, *5*(2), 164–171.

Friston, K. J. (2000). The labile brain. I. Neuronal transients and nonlinear coupling. *Philos Trans R Soc London. Ser B, Biol Sci*, *355*(1394), 215–236.

Friston, K., Phillips, J., Chawla, D., & Buechel, C. (2000). Nonlinear PCA: characterizing interactions between modes of brain activity. *Philos Trans R Soc London. Ser B, Biol Sci*, *355*(1393), 135–146.

Gros, C. (2007). Neural networks with transient state dynamics. *New J Phys*, *9*, 109.

Guckenheimer, J., & Holmes, P. (1988). Structurally stable heteroclinic cycles. *Math Proc Cambridge Philos Soc*, *103*, 189–192.

Hollander, E., Kim, S., Khanna, S., & Pallanti, S. (2007). Obsessive-compulsive disorder and obsessive-compulsive spectrum disorders: diagnostic and dimensional issues. *CNS Spectrums*, *12*(2 Suppl 3), 5–13.

Hopfield, J. J. (1982). Neural networks and physical systems with emergent collective computational abilities. *Proc Natl Acad Sci USA*, *79*(8), 2554–2558.

Huber, M. T., Braun, H. A., & Krieg, J. C. (1999). Consequences of deterministic and random dynamics for the course of affective disorders. *Biol Psychiatry*, *46*(2), 256–262.

Huber, M. T., Braun, H. A., & Krieg, J. C. (2000). Effects of noise on different disease states of recurrent affective disorders. *Biol Psychiatry*, *47*(7), 634–642.

Huerta, R., & Rabinovich, M. (2004). Reproducible sequence generation in random neural ensembles. *Phys Rev Lett*, *93*(23), 238104.

Huppert, J. D, & Franklin, M. E. (2005). Cognitive behavioral therapy for obsessive-compulsive disorder: an update. *Curr Psychiatry Rep*, *7*(4), 268–273.

Ito, J., Nikolaev, A. R., & van Leeuwen, C. (2007). Dynamics of spontaneous transitions between global brain states. *Hum Brain Mapp, 28*(9), 904–913.

Jones, L. M., Fontanini, A., Sadacca, B. F., Miller, P., & Katz, D. B. (2007). Natural stimuli evoke dynamic sequences of states in sensory cortical ensembles. *Proc Natl Acad Sci USA, 104*(47), 18772–18777.

Katerndahl, D., Ferrer, R., Best, R., & Wang, C.-P. (2007). Dynamic patterns in mood among newly diagnosed patients with major depressive episode or panic disorder and normal controls. *Prim Care Companion J Clin Psychiatry*, *9*(3), 183–187.

Kelso, J. A. Scott. 1995. *Dynamic Patterns: The Self-Organization of Brain and Behavior.* The MIT Press.

Koenig, T., Marti-Lopez, F., & Valdes-Sosa, P. (2001). Topographic time-frequency decomposition of the EEG. *NeuroImage*, *14*(2), 383–390.

Krupa, P. (1997). Robust heteroclinic cycles. *J Nonlinear Sci*, *7*, 129.

Kubota, S., & Sakai, K. (2002). Relationship between obsessive-compulsive disorder and chaos. *Med Hypotheses*, *59*(1), 16–23.

Laurent, G., & Davidowitz, H. (1994). Encoding of olfactory information with oscillating neural assemblies. *Science*, *265*(5180), 1872–1875.

Lin, L., Osan, R., Shoham, S., Jin, W., Zuo, W., & Tsien, J. Z. (2005). Identification of network-level coding units for real-time representation of episodic experiences in the hippocampus. *Proc Natl Acad Sci USA*, *102*(17), 6125–6130.

Lörincz, M. L., Geall, F., Bao, Y., Crunelli, V., & Hughes, S. W. (2009). ATP-dependent infra-slow (<0.1 Hz) oscillations in thalamic networks. *PLoS ONE*, *4*(2), e4447.

Lotka, A. J. (1925). *Elements of Physical Biology.* Baltimore, MD: Williams & Wilkins.

Mannell, M. V., Franco, A. R., Calhoun, V. D., Cañive, J. M., Thoma, R. J., & Mayer, A. R. (2010). Resting state and task-induced deactivation: A methodological comparison in patients with schizophrenia and healthy controls. *Hum Brain Mapp, 31*(3), 424–437.

Masterpasqua, F., & Perna, P. A. (Eds.). (1997). *The Psychological Meaning of Chaos.* Washington, DC: American Psychological Association.

Mazor, O., & Laurent, G. (2005). Transient dynamics versus fixed points in odor representations by locust antennal lobe projection neurons. *Neuron*, *48*(4), 661–673.

McClure, S. M., Botvinick, M. M., Yeung, N., Greene, J. D., & Cohen, J. D. (2007). Conflict monitoring in cognition-emotion competition. In *Handbook of Emotion Regulation* (pp. 204–226), edited by J. J. Gross. New York: Guilford.

McKeown, M. J., Makeig, S., Brown, G. G., Jung, T. P., Kindermann, S. S., Bell, A. J., & Sejnowski, T. J. (1998). Analysis of fMRI data by blind separation into independent spatial components. *Hum Brain Mapp*, *6*(3), 160–188.

Muezzinoglu, M. K., Tristan, I., Huerta, R., Afraimovich, V. S., & Rabinovich, M. I. (2010). Transient versus attractors in complex networks. *Int J Bifurcation Chaos Appl Sci Engn*, *20*, 1–23.

Nowotny, T., & Rabinovich, M. I. (2007). Dynamical origin of independent spiking and bursting activity in neural microcircuits. *Phys Rev Lett*, *98*(12), 128106.

Ott, E. (1993). *Chaos in Dynamical Systems*. Cambridge, UK: Cambridge University Press.

Oullier, O., & Scott Kelso, J. A. (2006). Neuroeconomics and the metastable brain. *Trends Cogn Sci*, *10*(8), 353–354.

Postlethwaite, C. M., & Dawes, J. H. P. (2005). Regular and irregular cycling near a heteroclinic network. *Nonlinearity*, *18*, 1477–1509.

Rabinovich, M. I., & Varona, P. (2011). Robust transient dynamics and brain functions. *Front Comput Neurosci*, *5*, 24.

Rabinovich, M. I., Ezersky, A. B., & Weidman, P. D. (2000). *The Dynamics of Patterns*. Singapore: World Scientific.

Rabinovich, M., Huerta, R., & Laurent, G. (2008a). Neuroscience. Transient dynamics for neural processing. *Science*, *321*(5885), 48–50.

Rabinovich, M. I., Huerta, R., Varona, P., & Afraimovich, V. S. (2008b). Transient cognitive dynamics, metastability, and decision making. *PLoS Comput Biol, 4*(5):e1000072.

Rabinovich, M. I., Muezzinoglu, M. K., Strigo, I., & Bystritsky, A. (2010). Dynamical principles of emotion-cognition interaction: mathematical images of mental disorders. *PLoS ONE, 5*(9), e12547.

Rabinovich, M. I., Varona, P., Selverston, A. I., & Abarbanel, H. D. I. (2006). Dynamical principles in neuroscience. *Rev Mod Phys*, *78*(4), 1213–1265.

Rabinovich, M., Volkovskii, A., Lecanda, P., Huerta, R., Abarbanel, H. D., & Laurent, G. (2001). Dynamical encoding by networks of competing neuron groups: winnerless competition. *Phys Rev Lett*, *87*(6), 68102.

Rolls, E. T., Loh, M., & Deco, G. (2008). An attractor hypothesis of obsessive-compulsive disorder. *Eur J Neurosci*, *28*(4), 782–793.

Saari, D. G. (1995). *Basic Geometry of Voting*. Berlin: Springer.

Salvador, R., Suckling, J., Schwarzbauer, C., & Bullmore, E. (2005). Undirected graphs of frequency-dependent functional connectivity in whole brain networks. *Philos Trans R Soc London. Ser B, Biol Sci*, *360*(1457), 937–946.

Scott Kelso, J. A. (1995). *Dynamic Patterns: The Self-Organization of Brain and Behavior*. Cambridge, MA: MIT Press.

Stone, E., & Armbruster, D. (1999). Noise and 0(1) amplitude effects on heteroclinic cycles. *Chaos (Woodbury, N.Y.)*, *9*, 499–505.

Stopfer, M., Jayaraman, V., & Laurent, G. (2003). Intensity versus identity coding in an olfactory system. *Neuron*, *39*(6), 991–1004.

Taylor, K. S., Seminowicz, D. A., & Davis, K. D. (2009). Two systems of resting state connectivity between the insula and cingulate cortex. *Hum Brain Mapp*, *30*(9), 2731–2745.

Tomasi, D., & Volkow, N. D. (2010). Functional connectivity density mapping. *Proc Natl Acad Sci USA*, *107*(21), 9885–9890.

Uchida, N., & Mainen, Z. F. (2003). Speed and accuracy of olfactory discrimination in the rat. *Nat Neurosci*, *6*(11), 1224–1229.

Varona, P., Rabinovich, M. I., Selverston, A. I., & Arshavsky, Y. I. (2002). Winnerless competition between sensory neurons generates chaos: A possible mechanism for molluscan hunting behavior. *Chaos*, *12*(3), 672–677.

Venaille, A., Varona, P., & Rabinovich, M. I. (2005). Synchronization and coordination of sequences in two neural ensembles. *Phys Rev E Stat Nonlin Soft Matter Phys*, *71*(6 Pt 1), 61909.

Zor, R., Hermesh, H., Szechtman, H., & Eilam, D. (2009). Turning order into chaos through repetition and addition of elementary acts in obsessive-compulsive disorder (OCD). *World J Biol Psychiatry*, *10*(4 Pt 2), 480–487.

5   A Dynamic Field Account of Language-Related Brain Potentials

Peter beim Graben and Roland Potthast

Summary

We present a phenomenological modeling account of event-related brain potentials (ERPs) in syntactic language processing. For a paradigmatic ERP experiment on the processing of phrase structure violations using the German language (Hahne & Friederici, 1999), we derive a context-free grammar representation of the stimulus material. We describe the phrase structure violation by a prediction error in an interactive left-corner parser that is mapped onto a dynamic field by means of dynamic cognitive modeling. Our model phenomenologically replicates the experimentally observed P600 ERP component elicited by the violation.

5.1   Introduction

Event-related brain potentials (ERPs) are an important online measure in the cognitive neurosciences (Kutas & van Petten, 1994; Handy, 2005). Conventionally, ERPs are obtained from averaging stimulus-locked electroencephalograms (EEGs) across trials. They exhibit characteristic topographies of positive and negative voltage deflections in comparison with a baseline condition at particular latency times. ERPs are commonly classified according to their polarity and latency, such that "N400" denotes a negative peak 400 ms after stimulus presentation, and "P600" refers to a positive peak 600 ms after stimulus. The conventional ERP averaging analysis presupposes the existence of an invariant "ERP signal" that is concealed by the spontaneous EEG and regarded as stationary and ergodic noise (Regan, 1972; beim Graben, Saddy, Schlesewsky, & Kurths, 2000). However, other interpretations assume stimulus-induced phase resetting (Makeig et al., 2002; Makeig, Debener, Onton, & Delorme, 2004) or stimulus-induced amplitude modulation (Nikulin et al., 2007) (for a critical comparison of these models, see also Becker, Ritter, & Villringer, 2008). From a dynamical system point of view, Başar (1980, 1998) and beim Graben et al. (2000) interpreted single-trial ERP time series as images of phase space trajectories originating from randomly distributed initial conditions under an appropriate observation model. Compatible with this picture is also the suggestion of Hutt, Svensén, Kruggel, and Friedrich (2000) and Hutt (2004) that ERP components correspond to saddle nodes forming (stable) heteroclinic sequences (SHS; Afraimovich, Zhigulin, & Rabinovich, 2004; Rabinovich, Huerta, Varona, & Afraimovich, 2008; see also Chapt. 4). In this interpretation, ERP phase space trajectories would be confined to a stable heteroclinic channel (SHC; Afraimovich et al., 2004; Rabinovich et al., 2008) forming a kind of "bottleneck" (beim Graben et al., 2000).

In the language domain, ERPs found several applications. The so-called mismatch negativity (MMN) reflects phonological and lexical mismatches (Rugg, 1984; Pulvermüller, Lutzenberger, & Birbaumer, 1995; Dehaene-Lambertz, 1997; Näätänen et al., 1997). Whereas the above-mentioned N400 and P600 are sensitive for semantic (Kutas & Hillyard, 1980, 1984; Kolk, Chwilla, van Herten, & Oor, 2003; Herten, Kolk, & Chwilla, 2005), syntactic (Osterhout & Holcomb, 1992; Hagoort, Brown, & Groothusen, 1993), and pragmatic (Noveck & Posada, 2003; Drenhaus, beim Graben, Saddy, & Frisch, 2006; Nieuwland & Kuperberg, 2008) processing problems.

Neurodynamical models of language-related brain potentials have to take one crucial characteristic of language into account: Language is categorical and symbolic. In a recent publication, Kiebel, von Kriegstein, Daunizeau, and Friston (2009; cf. also chapter 6) used SHS dynamics for phonetic speech recognition in order to model the observed mismatch negativity (Dehaene-Lambertz, 1997; Näätänen et al., 1997). The same ERP component observed in word recognition experiments (Rugg, 1984; Pulvermüller et al., 1995) has been tackled by Garagnani, Wennekers, and Pulvermüller (2007, 2008). In the syntactic domain, Hagoort (2003, 2005) described the P600 ERP component through unification costs in the unification model of Vosse and Kempen (2000, 2009). Using different kinds of formal grammars, beim Graben, Gerth, and Vasishth (2008a) and Gerth and beim Graben (2009) made the first attempts toward a dynamical systems model of syntactic reanalysis within the framework of dynamic cognitive modeling (beim Graben & Potthast, 2009).

In this chapter, we demonstrate the basic steps of dynamic cognitive modeling by means of a paradigmatic ERP experiment (Hahne & Friederici, 1999). We use functional representations of complex linguistic data structures (beim Graben, Pinotsis, Saddy, & Potthast, 2008b) to provide a phenomenological account of the observed syntactic ERP components.

5.2   ERP Experiment

In an ERP experiment using the German language, Hahne and Friederici (1999) presented three types of sentences visually word-by-word to their subjects. The conditions are illustrated by means of the following examples.

(1) Die Gans wurde **gebraten**.
The goose was **grilled**.
"The goose was grilled."

(2) *Die Gans wurde im **gebraten**.
The goose was in the **grilled**.
"The goose was grilled in the."

(3) Die Gans wurde im Ofen **gebraten**.
The goose was in the oven **grilled**.
"The goose was grilled in the oven."

Sentences of type (1) are grammatically well-formed. They served as the controlling baseline condition. By contrast, sentences of type (2) exhibit a *phrase structure violation* (indicated by the asterisk) that is illustrated by the filler sentences of type (3): Here, a prepositional phrase *im Ofen* ("in the oven") modifies the main verb *gebraten* ("grilled"). A prepositional phrase is introduced by a preposition, such as *im* ("in the"), which requires an adjacent noun, here *Ofen*. This noun is omitted in type (2), thereby leading to the phrase structure violation that becomes manifest with the concluding, critical word *gebraten*, printed in boldface in the examples above. Measuring event-related brain potentials elicited by the critical word entails a P600 component broadly distributed over parietal recording sites. Figure 5.1 displays the P600 in the grand ERP average.

The P600 ERP is robustly associated with many kinds of ungrammaticalities (Osterhout & Holcomb, 1992; Hagoort et al., 1993), syntactic ambiguities (Osterhout, Holcomb, & Swinney, 1994; beim Graben et al., 2000; Frisch, Schlesewsky, Saddy, & Alpermann, 2002), and syntactic complexity (Kaan, Harris, Gibson, & Holcomb, 2000; Kaan & Swaab, 2003). In the context of the experiment of Hahne and Friederici (1999), it can be related to the violation of a particular expectancy generated by the human language processor: Encountering the preposition *im* predicts

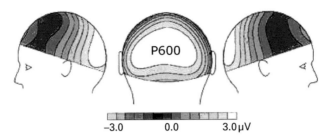

Figure 5.1
The P600 ERP component elicited by phrase structure violation condition (2) in comparison with the correct condition (1) in the experiment by Hahne and Friederici (1999) (20% contrast). Shown are spherical splines of difference waves (2) – (1). Modified reprint with permission of The MIT Press.

the occurrence of a noun, such as *Ofen*, as the next input word. In the next section, we present a computational model for this predictive dynamics.

5.3   Dynamic Cognitive Modeling

According to the "computer metaphor of the mind" (Pylyshyn, 1986), cognition is essentially time-discrete symbol manipulation obeying combinatorial rules. In contrast, the brain as a nonlinear dynamical system operates in continuous time with continuous activation patterns instead of discrete symbolic representations. To bridge the gap between computational psycholinguistics on the one hand and computational neuroscience on the other hand, thereby constituting a new discipline of *computational neurolinguistics*, two different mapping problems have to be solved. First, discrete mental symbolic representations have to be mapped onto continuous activation patterns in neurodynamical systems. This mapping can be achieved through filler/role decompositions and tensor product representations (Mizraji, 1989; Smolensky, 1990; Smolensky, 2006; Smolensky & Legendre, 2006). Second, these activation patterns have to be connected through trajectories in continuous time. This embedding can be straightforwardly established by means of winnerless competition and heteroclinic sequences (Rabinovich et al., 2001; Afraimovich et al., 2004; Rabinovich et al., 2008; chapter 4).

Taken together, tensor product representations and winnerless sequential dynamics constitute dynamic cognitive modeling (DCM; beim Graben & Potthast, 2009) as a three-tier top-down approach comprising the levels of (1) cognitive processes; (2) their state-space representations;

and (3) their neurodynamical realizations. In the following subsections, we illustrate DCM on the basis of the language-processing ERP experiment from section 5.2.

5.3.1   Data Structures and Algorithms

Because DCM is a top-down approach, we first have to find an appropriate linguistic representation of the sentence examples (1)–(3). Sentences such as the filler (3) are hierarchically organized symbolic data structures: A sentence S consists of a subject, realized as a first *noun phrase* NP_1 *die Gans* ("the goose"), and a predicate, called *verbal phrase* VP′. In our example (3), the predicate is headed by an auxiliary Aux *wurde* ("was") complemented by another verbal phrase VP. This phrase in turn consists of the verb V *gebraten* ("grilled") modified by the prepositional phrase PP. Finally, the prepositional phrase is headed by the preposition P *im* ("in the") with noun phrase complement NP_2 *Ofen* ("oven"). A suitable way to display such syntactic dependencies are *phrase structure trees*. Figure 5.2 shows the phrase structure tree of sentence (3) reflecting our hierarchical analysis.

In the next step, we create a context-free grammar (CFG) (Hopcroft & Ullman, 1979) from the tree in figure 5.2 after discarding the particular lexical material because that varied across the different trials in the ERP study. A CFG is a collection of rules $A \to \gamma$ where $A \in N$ is a syntactic category (a nonterminal) and $\gamma \in (T \cup N)^*$ is a string formed of terminal or nonterminal symbols. As terminals, we regard the symbols from the set $T = \{NP_1, NP_2, Aux, V, P\}$, whereas the remaining categories $N = \{S, VP', VP, PP\}$ are considered to be nonterminals. Because every branching in the tree corresponds to a production in the CFG, we obtain the following CFG:

$$
\begin{aligned}
S &\to NP_1 \quad VP' \\
VP' &\to Aux \quad VP \\
VP &\to PP \quad V \\
PP &\to P \quad NP_2.
\end{aligned}
\tag{5.1}
$$

In terms of phrase structure trees and context-free grammars, the human language processor can be most appropriately described as an interactive (Wegner, 1998; beim Graben et al., 2008a) left-corner parser (Aho & Ullman, 1972; Demers, 1977; Hale, 2011). Interactivity refers to the fact that the parser is permanently perturbed by new incoming input words. In a left-corner architecture, the parser takes new input as evi-

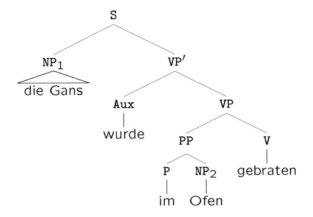

Figure 5.2
Linguistic phrase structure tree of filler sentence (3). Syntactic categories are as follows: S, sentence; NP_1, NP_2, noun phrases; VP′, VP, verbal phrases; Aux, auxiliary; V, verb; PP, prepositional phrase; P, preposition.

dence for making predictions about subsequent words. Then, ungrammatical input leads to prediction failure, which becomes reflected by the P600 ERP observed in experiments such as in our example (Hahne & Friederici, 1999).

For the sake of simplicity, we refrain from elaborating a complete left-corner parser here. Instead, we present the required cognitive architecture as an algebraic representation π (beim Graben et al., 2008a; beim Graben & Potthast, 2009) of the terminal alphabet $\boldsymbol{T}$ on the space of phrase structure trees P; that is, for every input word $w \in \boldsymbol{T}$, $\pi(w){:}P \to P$ maps a tree $p \in P$ to another tree $p' = [\pi(w)](p) \in P$.

To process example sentence (3), we first initialize the parser with a "vacuum state" s_1, the empty tree[1] $\varnothing \in P$. Scanning the first noun phrase NP_1 *die Gans* ("the goose") from the environment in the second step yields the second state $s_2 = [\pi(NP_1)](s_1)$, which is a tree where NP_1 is the confirmed left corner as a result of expanding the first rule $S \to NP_1\ VP'$ of CFG (5.1). In contrast, the right corner is being predicted, indicated by brackets, [VP′] (Hale, 2011).

In the third step, the parser scans the auxiliary Aux *wurde* ("was") from the input, thereby confirming the previous prediction of a verbal phrase VP′, yielding tree $s_3 = [\pi(Aux)](s_2)$. According to the second rule of CFG (5.1), another verbal phrase [VP] then becomes predicted. The processor proceeds with the preposition P *im* ("in the") in the fourth

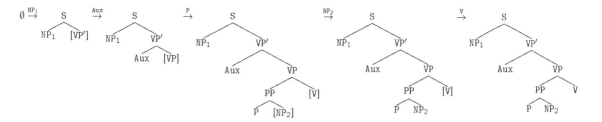

Figure 5.3
Interactive left-corner parse of example sentence (3) according to CFG (5.1).

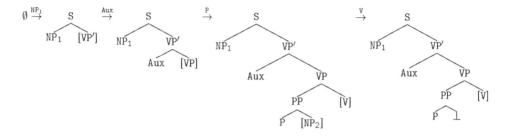

Figure 5.4
Interactive left-corner parse of phrase structure violation (2) according to CFG (5.1). Prediction failure is indicated by ⊥ ("bottom") and reflected by the P600 ERP (figure 5.1).

step, confirming the predicted VP, by making two further predictions of [NP₂] and [V]. Scanning the noun phrase NP₂ *Ofen* ("oven") in the fifth step confirms NP₂. In the final step, the scanned verb V *gebraten* ("grilled") eventually confirms the predicted V, retaining the phrase structure tree of the well-formed sentence from figure 5.2. Figure 5.3 shows the complete parse as a sequence $(s_1, s_2, s_3, s_4, s_5, s_6)$ of six left-corner trees generated by the input (3).

Applying the left-corner algorithm to the phrase structure violation sentence (2) yields another tree sequence $(s_1, s_2, s_3, s_4, s_7)$ of five left-corner trees displayed in figure 5.4.

Obviously, the first four processing steps are the same as in figure 5.3 because the input is interactively fetched from the environment. However, in the fifth step the scanned verb fails to confirm the predicted noun phrase NP₂, indicated by the symbol ⊥ ("bottom") in the respective tree s_7. At this point, the processing breaks down, which is reflected by the ungrammaticality P600 in the ERP (figure 5.1).

5.3.2   State-Space Representations

To solve the first mapping problem mentioned at the beginning of section 5.3, the construction of vector space representations of complex symbolic data structures, we use a filler/role decomposition of the trees in figures 5.3 and 5.4 (Smolensky, 1990; Smolensky, 2006; Smolensky & Legendre, 2006). To this end, we first identify the syntactic categories with a set of *fillers* $F = T \cup N \cup N' \cup \{\bot\} = \{NP_1, NP_2, Aux, V, P, S, VP', VP, PP, [VP'],$ $[VP], [PP], \bot\}$. Note that both basic categories N of the grammar (5.1) and their predicted left-corner counterparts N' become fillers in this step. Moreover, the indicator of prediction failure $\bot$ in tree s_7 also assumes a filler variable. Second, we introduce a set of *roles* $R = \{r_1, r_2, r_3\}$ for the positions in an elementary binary branching tree: r_1 for the mother node, r_2 for the left daughter node, and r_3 for the right daughter node (for details, see beim Graben et al., 2008a, 2008b; beim Graben & Potthast, 2009). A filler/role decomposition for an elementary tree such as s_2 in figure 5.3 is then a set of ordered pairs of fillers *bound* to their respective roles. In our example, we obtain $f_2 = \{(S, r_1), (NP_1, r_2), ([VP'], r_3)\}$, as S occupies the mother node, NP_1 the left daughter, and the predicted $[VP']$ the right daughter node position. The set f_2 itself is a *complex filler* that could bind to another role in a more complex tree. As an example, consider the third step s_3 in the tree sequence in figure 5.3. Here, the complex subtree filler $f_R = \{(VP', r_1), (Aux, r_2), ([VP], r_3)\}$ is bound to the right daughter node of the first-level tree: $f_3 = \{(S, r_1), (NP_1, r_2), (f_R, r_3)\}$, or, after evaluation, $f_3 = \{(S, r_1), (NP_1, r_2), (\{(VP', r_1), (Aux, r_2), ([VP], r_3)\}, r_3)\}$. In general, the set of complex fillers is recursively defined as

$$F_0 = F$$
$$F_{n+1} = \wp(F_n \times R)$$
$$F_\infty = \bigcup_{n=0}^{\infty} F_n,$$

(5.2)

where $\wp(\cdot)$ denotes the power set of an argument (beim Graben et al., 2008b).

After having mapped all trees in figures 5.3 and 5.4 to sets of ordered pairs (of sets of ordered pairs, etc.) by virtue of the filler/role decomposition (5.2), we next carry out tensor product representations (Mizraji, 1989; Smolensky, 1990; Smolensky, 2006; Smolensky & Legendre, 2006) by mapping the fillers F onto a vector space $V_F = \psi(F)$ and by mapping the roles R onto another vector space $V_R = \psi(R)$, where $\psi : F_\infty \to \mathcal{F}$ additionally obeys

$$\psi\left(\{(f,r),(f',r')\}\right) = \psi(f) \otimes \psi(r) \oplus \psi(f') \otimes \psi(r'), \tag{5.3}$$

for fillers $f \in F_n, f' \in F_m$ and roles $r, r' \in R$. Hence, the resulting space $\mathcal{F}$ is the *Fock space*

$$\mathcal{F} = \left(\bigoplus_{n=1}^{\infty} \mathcal{V}_F \otimes \bigotimes_{k=0}^{n} \mathcal{V}_R \right) \oplus \mathcal{V}_R \tag{5.4}$$

well known from quantum field theory (Haag, 1992; Smolensky & Legendre, 2006; Aerts, 2009). Here, we choose a particular Fock space representation, namely a function space over the unit sphere, figuring a compact *feature space* in dynamic field theory (Erlhagen & Schöner, 2002; Schöner & Thelen, 2006).

The unit sphere $S \subset \mathbb{R}^3$ is parameterized through polar coordinates: radius $r \in [0,1]$, polar angle $\vartheta \in [0,\pi]$, and azimuth $\varphi \in [0,2\pi[$. In our model, we use complex radial oscillations

$$f_i(r) = e^{ikr+\phi_i}, \qquad k = \frac{2\pi i}{N_F}, \tag{5.5}$$

for the *i*th filler where $N_F = 10$ is the number of basic categories, including prediction failure $\perp$. The additional phases $\phi_i = 0$ for thus basic categories and $\phi_i = \pi/8$ for left-corner predicted categories render the latter similar to the former (Smolensky & Legendre, 2006). For the tree roles R, we use spherical harmonics

$$Y_{jm}(\vartheta,\varphi) = \sqrt{\frac{2j+1}{4}\frac{(j-m)!}{(j+m)!}}\, P_{jm}(\cos\vartheta)e^{im\varphi} \tag{5.6}$$

with $j = 1$ and $m \in \{-1,0,1\}$ as elaborated in great detail by beim Graben et al. (2008b) and beim Graben and Potthast (2009). Spherical harmonics are particularly well suited for DCM as they exhibit nice recursion properties, expressed by Clebsch–Gordan expansions, in order to represent deeper tree levels by means of higher-order spatial harmonics [the P_{jm} in equation (5.6) are the associated Legendre polynomials]. Then, tensor products (5.3) become point-wise products

$$q_{ijm}(r,\vartheta,\varphi) = (f_i \otimes Y_{jm})(r,\vartheta,\varphi) = f_i(r) Y_{jm}(\vartheta,\varphi) \tag{5.7}$$

in function space. Accordingly, tree s_k in a parser sequence figure 5.3 or figure 5.4 is represented by a linear combination

$$s_k(r,\vartheta,\varphi) = \text{Re}\left[\sum_{ijm} a_{kijm}\, q_{ijm}(r,\vartheta,\varphi) \right] \tag{5.8}$$

of functions, where the a_{kijm} abbreviate the Clebsch–Gordan coefficients, saying that filler i is bound to a superposition of spherical harmonics Y_{jm} in tree k. Additionally, we take real parts in order to obtain real-valued representations.

Furthermore, we introduce an *observation model* (beim Graben et al., 2008a) for visualization purposes by

$$E(\vartheta,\varphi) = \int_0^1 |s(r,\vartheta,\varphi)|\,dr, \tag{5.9}$$

which can be regarded as our model EEG. Figure 5.5 (plate 10) depicts the resulting functional representation of the tree sequence of figure 5.3.

Next, we encounter the second mapping problem, embedding the time-discrete tensor product representations (5.7) into continuous time. This is achieved by regarding the seven different states s_k from both parses figures 5.3 and 5.4 as saddle nodes in an SHS (Rabinovich et al., 2001; Afraimovich et al., 2004; Rabinovich et al., 2008). To this end, we introduce an order parameter expansion (Haken, 1983)

$$u(r,\vartheta,\varphi,t) = \sum_{k=1}^{n} \alpha_k(t) s_k(r,\vartheta,\varphi), \tag{5.10}$$

where n is the total number of representation states, and $\alpha_k(t) \in [0,1]$ is the time-dependent activation of the kth state. These amplitudes are delivered by a winnerless competition in a generalized Lotka–Volterra system of $n = 7$ populations

$$\frac{d\xi_k}{dt} = \xi_k\left(\sigma_k - \sum_{j=1}^{n}\rho_{kj}\xi_j\right) \tag{5.11}$$

$$\alpha_k(t) = \frac{\xi_k}{\sigma_k}$$

with growth rates $\sigma_k > 0$, and interaction weights $\rho_{kj} > 0, \rho_{kk} = 1$, separately trained by the algorithm of Afraimovich et al. (2004) and Rabinovich et al. (2008) for the sequence $(s_1, s_2, s_3, s_4, s_5, s_6)$ of filler states from figure

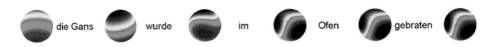

die Gans   wurde   im   Ofen   gebraten

Figure 5.5 (plate 10)
Sequence of functional tensor product representations (5.7) in the observation model (5.9) for the tree sequence of figure 5.3.

5.3 and for the sequence $(s_1, s_2, s_3, s_4, s_7)$ of violation states from figure 5.4. The result of this continuous time embedding is shown in figure 5.6 (plate 11) for the evolution of filler states.

5.3.3 Dynamic Fields

In the third step of DCM, the constructed spatiotemporal dynamics $u_{\text{filler}}(x, t)$, $u_{\text{violation}}(x, t)$ for the parsing of filler sentences (3) and phrase structure violation sentences (2), respectively, can be used as training data for solving the *inverse problem* in dynamic field theory (beim Graben & Potthast, 2009; Potthast & beim Graben, 2009). Starting from the often deployed Amari equation (Amari, 1977) for a neural field $u(x, t)$,

$$\tau \frac{\partial u(x,t)}{\partial t} + u(x,t) = \int_D w(x,y) f(u(y,t)) \, \mathrm{d}y, \tag{5.12}$$

with time constant τ, synaptic weight kernel $w(x, y)$, sigmoidal activation function $f(u)$, and feature space D, the inverse problem is posed by determining the kernel $w(x,y)$ from a prescribed trajectory $u(x, t)$. Here, $x = (r, \vartheta, \varphi) \in D = S$ denotes a point within the unit sphere. Going along the lines of Potthast and beim Graben (2009), we construct a biorthogonal function system $s_j^{\perp}(x)$ from the representational states (5.8), obeying

$$\int_D s_j^{\perp}(x) s_k(x) \, \mathrm{d}x = \delta_{jk}. \tag{5.13}$$

Then, we obtain from (5.10)

$$\int_D s_j^{\perp}(x) u(x,t) \, \mathrm{d}x = \sum_{k=1}^{n} \alpha_k(t) \int_D s_j^{\perp}(x) s_k(x) \, \mathrm{d}x$$

$$\int_D s_j^{\perp}(x) u(x,t) \, \mathrm{d}x = \sum_{k=1}^{n} \alpha_k(t) \delta_{jk}$$

$$\alpha_j(t) = \int_D s_j^{\perp}(x) u(x,t) \, \mathrm{d}x$$

$$\xi_j(t) = \sigma_j \int_D s_j^{\perp}(x) u(x,t) \, \mathrm{d}x. \tag{5.14}$$

Next, we derivate (5.10) with respect to time t, by exploiting (5.11)

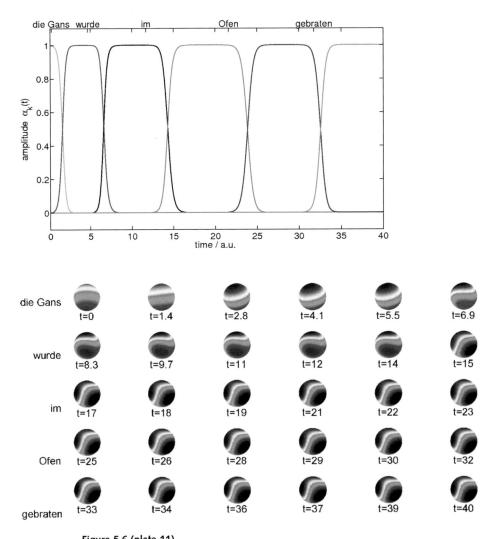

Figure 5.6 (plate 11)
Continuous time embedding of tensor product representations from figure 5.5 through winnerless competition of activation (equation 5.14) amplitudes (equation 5.13). (Top) Sequential amplitude dynamics. (Bottom) Snapshots of EEG model (equation 5.12) dynamics for filler sentence (3) (color-coded amplitude range: −30 to 30).

$$\frac{\partial u(x,t)}{\partial t} = \sum_k \frac{1}{\sigma_k} \frac{d\xi_k}{dt} s_k(x)$$

$$\frac{\partial u(x,t)}{\partial t} = \sum_k \frac{1}{\sigma_k} \left[\xi_k \left(\sigma_k - \sum_j \rho_{kj}\xi_j \right) \right] s_k(x)$$

$$\frac{\partial u(x,t)}{\partial t} = \sum_k \xi_k s_k(x) - \sum_{kj} \frac{\rho_{kj}}{\sigma_k} \xi_k \xi_j s_k(x). \tag{5.15}$$

Multiplying with τ and adding (5.10), we obtain the left-hand side of the Amari equation (5.12):

$$\tau \frac{\partial u(x,t)}{\partial t} + u(x,t) = \sum_k \tau \xi_k s_k(x) - \sum_{kj} \frac{\tau \rho_{kj}}{\sigma_k} \xi_k \xi_j s_k(x) + \sum_k \frac{1}{\sigma_k} \xi_k s_k(x)$$

$$\tau \frac{\partial u(x,t)}{\partial t} + u(x,t) = \sum_k \left(\tau + \frac{1}{\sigma_k} \right) \xi_k s_k(x) - \sum_{kj} \frac{\tau \rho_{kj}}{\sigma_k} \xi_k \xi_j s_k(x). \tag{5.16}$$

Now we can eliminate all occurrences of ξ by means of (5.14), which gives

$$\tau \frac{\partial u(x,t)}{\partial t} + u(x,t) = \sum_k \left(\tau + \frac{1}{\sigma_k} \right) \sigma_k \int_D s_k^\perp(y) u(y,t) s_k(x) \, dy$$

$$- \sum_{kj} \frac{\tau \rho_{kj}}{\sigma_k} \sigma_k \sigma_j \iint_{DD} s_k^\perp(y) u(y,t) s_j^\perp(z) u(z,t) s_k(x) \, dy \, dz$$

$$\tau \frac{\partial u(x,t)}{\partial t} + u(x,t) = \int_D \sum_k (\tau \sigma_k + 1) s_k^\perp(y) s_k(x) u(y,t) \, dy$$

$$- \iint_{DD} \sum_{kj} \tau \rho_{kj} \sigma_j s_k^\perp(y) s_j^\perp(z) s_k(x) u(y,t) u(z,t) \, dy \, dz. \tag{5.17}$$

In the next step, we consider the right-hand side of the Amari equation (5.12), which describes a nonlinear integral transformation in space

$$v_t(x) = \mathcal{J}[u(\cdot,t)](x) = \int_D w(x,y) f(u(y,t)) \, dy, \tag{5.18}$$

when fixing the time point t. The transformation (5.18) can be expressed as a functional Taylor expansion (sometimes called *Volterra series* when applied to the time domain),

$$v_t(x) = w_0(x) + \sum_{m=1}^{\infty} \frac{1}{m!} \int_D \cdots \int_D w_m(x, y_1, y_2, \ldots, y_m) u(y_1, t) u(y_2, t) \ldots$$
$$u(y_m, t) \, dy_1 \, dy_2 \cdots dy_m. \tag{5.19}$$

Taking only the first three terms into account yields

$$\tau \frac{\partial u(x,t)}{\partial t} + u(x,t) \tag{5.20}$$

$$= w_0 + \int_D w_1(x, y) u(y, t) \, dy + \frac{1}{2} \int_D \int_D w_2(x, y, z) u(y, t) u(z, t) \, dy \, dz.$$

Finally, we compare (5.17) and (5.20) to obtain the kernels

$$w_0 = 0 \tag{5.21}$$

$$w_1(x, y) = \sum_k (\tau \sigma_k + 1) s_k^{\perp}(y) s_k(x)$$

$$w_2(x, y, z) = 2\tau \sum_{kj} \rho_{kj} \sigma_j s_k^{\perp}(y) s_j^{\perp}(z) s_k(x).$$

Basically, kernel $w_1(x,y)$ describes a Hebbian synapse between sites y and x that have been trained with pattern sequence s_k. This finding confirms the previous result of Potthast and beim Graben (2009). Besides, the three-point kernel $w_2(x,y,z)$ further generalizes Hebbian learning to interactions between three sites x, y, z in feature space. Hence, we explicitly solved the inverse problem for dynamic field theory with winnerless competition.

5.3.4   Results

First we present the dynamics of the Amari field equation (5.12) with kernels (5.21) constructed for the parse of the filler sentence (3) in figure 5.7 (plate 12).

Comparison with figure 5.6 (plate 11) reveals some slight phase shifts in the amplitude dynamics that are due to the numerical instability of the Lotka–Volterra dynamics (5.11). Nevertheless, the simulated data are in considerably good agreement with the training data.

Finally, we present the EEG observation model of the differences $u_{\text{violation}}(x, t) - u_{\text{filler}}(x, t)$ in figure 5.8 (plate 13). An animation of the parsing dynamics can be found at http://www.beimgraben.info/fockspace.html.

A

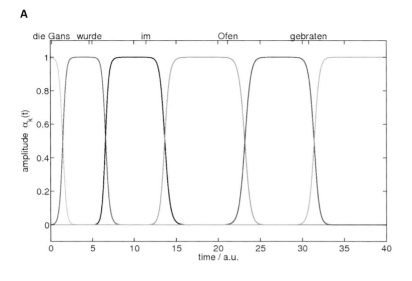

B

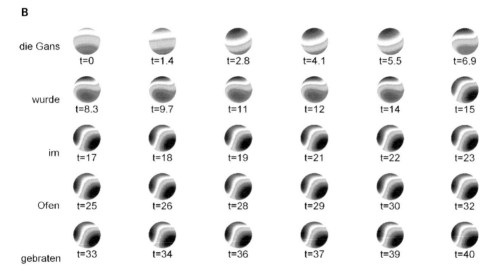

Figure 5.7 (plate 12)
Solutions of the Amari equation (5.15) with kernels (5.24) constructed for the parse of the filler sentence (3). (A) Sequential amplitude dynamics. (B) Snapshots of EEG model (equation 5.12) dynamics for filler sentence (3) (color-coded amplitude range: −30 to 30).

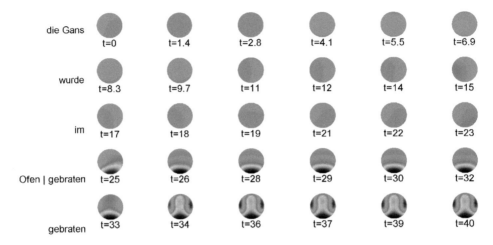

Figure 5.8 (plate 13)
Snapshot of the temporal evolution of the model EEG differences (equation 5.12) between dynamic field patterns $u_{filler}(x,t)$, $u_{violation}(x,t)$. The difference elicited by the prediction failure in condition (2) compared with condition (3) resembles the observed P600 ERP in figure 5.1 (color-coded amplitude range: −5 to 5).

There are no differences between conditions (2) and (3) until *gebraten* ("grilled") was presented to the parser in the violation condition (2) when the parser expects a noun *Ofen* ("oven") immediately after the preposition *im* ("in the"). In fact, this happens in the filler condition (3), whereas the verb *gebraten* in condition (2) leads to a prediction failure, symbolically indicated by ⊥ in figure 5.4. Here, the parse breaks down, eliciting a P600 component in the ERP, shown in figure 5.1. Notably, our dynamic field model replicates this effect, at least phenomenologically, as a positivity with a distinct, parietally focused topography.

5.4 Conclusion

In this contribution, we presented a phenomenological account of dynamic field models for language-related brain potentials. For a paradigmatic ERP experiment on the processing of phrase structure violations using the German language (Hahne & Friederici, 1999), we first derived a context-free grammar representing the stimulus material. Then, we described the phrase structure violation by a prediction error in an interactive left-corner parser. Using filler/role decompositions, tensor product representations, and winnerless competition (Mizraji, 1989; Smolensky, 1990; Rabinovich et al., 2001; Afraimovich et al., 2004; Smolensky,

2006; Smolensky & Legendre, 2006; Rabinovich et al., 2008) in DCM (beim Graben & Potthast, 2009), we constructed dynamic fields over compact feature spaces (Erlhagen & Schöner, 2002; Schöner & Thelen, 2006) to represent the cognitive computations by neurodynamic systems. We solved the inverse problem for synaptic weight kernel construction for the Amari neural field equation (Amari, 1977; beim Graben & Potthast, 2009; Potthast & beim Graben, 2009). Finally, we replicated the experimentally observed P600 ERP component elicited by the phrase structure violation in our phenomenological DCM model. In the current state, DCM establishes a framework to solve neurodynamic inverse problems in a top-down fashion. It does not yet address another inverse problem prevalent in the cognitive neurosciences; namely, the bottom-up reconstruction of neurodynamics from observed physiologic time series, such as EEG or ERP data (Regan, 1972; beim Graben et al., 2000; Makeig et al., 2002, 2004). In particular, it is not related to dynamic causal modeling (David & Friston, 2003; David et al., 2006) addressing the inverse problem of finding neural generators from physiologic data. Certainly, dynamic causal modeling and dynamic cognitive modeling ought to be connected at the intermediate level of neurodynamics. We hope that dynamic cognitive modeling and dynamic causal modeling could eventually be unified.

Note

1. Note that a tree in graph theoretical sense is a set of nodes K connected through edges $E \subset K \times K$. Therefore, the empty tree corresponds to the empty set of nodes $= \varnothing$.

References

Aerts, D. (2009). Quantum structure in cognition. *Journal of Mathematical Psychology*, *53*(5), 314–348.

Afraimovich, V. S., Zhigulin, V. P., & Rabinovich, M. I. (2004). On the origin of reproducible sequential activity in neural circuits. *Chaos*, *14*(4), 1123–1129.

Aho, A. V., & Ullman, J. D. (1972). *The Theory of Parsing, Translation and Compiling* (Vol. I). Englewood Cliffs, NJ: Parsing. Prentice Hall.

Amari, S.-I. (1977). Dynamics of pattern formation in lateral-inhibition type neural fields. *Biological Cybernetics*, *27*, 77–87.

Başar, E. (1980). *EEG-Brain Dynamics. Relations between EEG and Brain Evoked Potentials*. Amsterdam: Elsevier/North Holland Biomedical Press.

Başar, E. (1998). Brain Function and Oscillations. Vol I: Brain Oscillations. Principles and Approaches. Springer Series in Synergetics. Berlin: Springer.

Becker, R., Ritter, P., & Villringer, A. (2008). Influence of ongoing alpha rhythm on the visual evoked potential. *NeuroImage*, *39*(2), 707–716.

beim Graben, P. and Potthast, R. (2009). Inverse problems in dynamic cognitive modeling. *Chaos*, *19*(1), 015103.

beim Graben, P., Gerth, S., and Vasishth, S. (2008a). Towards dynamical system models of language-related brain potentials. *Cognitive Neurodynamics*, *2*(3), 229–255.

beim Graben, P., Pinotsis, D., Saddy, D., and Potthast, R. (2008b). Language processing with dynamic fields. *Cognitive Neurodynamics*, *2*(2), 79–88.

beim Graben, P., Saddy, D., Schlesewsky, M., and Kurths, J. (2000). Symbolic dynamics of event-related brain potentials. *Physical Reviews E*, *62*(4), 5518–5541.

David, O., & Friston, K. J. (2003). A neural mass model for MEG/EEG: coupling and neuronal dynamics. *NeuroImage*, *20*, 1743–1755.

David, O., Kiebel, S. J., Harrison, L., Mattout, J., Kilner, J., & Friston, K. J. (2006). Dynamic causal modelling of evoked responses in EEG and MEG. *NeuroImage*, *30*, 1255–1272.

Dehaene-Lambertz, G. (1997). Electrophysiological correlates of categorical phoneme perception in adults. *Neuroreport*, *8*(4), 919–924.

Demers, A. J. (1977). Generalized left corner parsing. In Proceedings of the 4th ACM SIGACT-SIGPLAN Symposium on Principles of Programming Languages, POPL '77 (pp. 170–182). New York: ACM.

Drenhaus, H., beim Graben, P., Saddy, D., & Frisch, S. (2006). Diagnosis and repair of negative polarity constructions in the light of symbolic resonance analysis. *Brain and Language*, *96*(3), 255–268.

Erlhagen, W., & Schöner, G. (2002). Dynamic field theory of movement preparation. *Psychological Review*, *109*(3), 545–572.

Frisch, S., Schlesewsky, M., Saddy, D., & Alpermann, A. (2002). The P600 as an indicator of syntactic ambiguity. *Cognition*, *85*, B83–B92.

Garagnani, M., Wennekers, T., & Pulvermüller, F. (2007). A neuronal model of the language cortex. *Neurocomputing*, *70*, 1914–1919.

Garagnani, M., Wennekers, T., & Pulvermüller, F. (2008). A neuroanatomically grounded Hebbian-learning model of attention-language interactions in the human brain. *European Journal of Neuroscience*, *27*(2), 492–513.

Gerth, S. and beim Graben, P. (2009). Unifying syntactic theory and sentence processing difficulty through a connectionist minimalist parser. *Cognitive Neurodynamics*, *3*(4), 297–316.

Haag, R. (1992). *Local Quantum Physics: Fields, Particles, Algebras*. Berlin: Springer.

Hagoort, P. (2003). How the brain solves the binding problem for language: a neurocomputational model of syntactic processing. *NeuroImage*, *20*, S18–S29.

Hagoort, P. (2005). On Broca, brain, and binding: a new framework. *Trends in Cognitive Sciences*, *9*(9), 416–423.

Hagoort, P., Brown, C., & Groothusen, J. (1993). The syntactic positive shift (SPS) as an ERP measure of syntactic processing. *Language and Cognitive Processes*, *8*(4), 439–483.

Hahne, A., & Friederici, A. D. (1999). Electrophysiological evidence for two steps in syntactic analysis: early automatic and late controlled processes. *Journal of Cognitive Neuroscience*, *11*(2), 194–205.

Haken, H. (1983). *Synergetics. An Introduction*. Berlin: Springer.

Hale, J. T. (2011). What a rational parser would do. *Cognitive Science*, *35*(3), 399–443.

Handy, T. C. (Ed.). (2005). *Event-Related Potentials. A Methods Handbook*. Cambridge, MA: MIT Press.

Herten, M., Kolk, H. H. J., & Chwilla, D. J. (2005). An ERP study of P600 effects elicited by semantic anomalies. *Brain Research. Cognitive Brain Research*, *22*(2), 241–255.

Hopcroft, J. E., & Ullman, J. D. (1979). *Introduction to Automata Theory, Languages, and Computation*. Menlo Park, California: Addison–Wesley.

Hutt, A. (2004). An analytical framework for modeling evoked and event-related potentials. *International Journal of Bifurcation and Chaos in Applied Sciences and Engineering*, *14*(2), 653–666.

Hutt, A., Svensén, M., Kruggel, F., & Friedrich, R. (2000). Detection of fixed points in spatiotemporal signals by a clustering method. *Physical Review E: Statistical Physics, Plasmas, Fluids, and Related Interdisciplinary Topics*, *61*(5), R4691–R4693.

Kaan, E., & Swaab, T. Y. (2003). Repair, revision, and complexity in syntactic analysis: An electrophysiological differentiation. *Journal of Cognitive Neuroscience*, *15*(1), 98–110.

Kaan, E., Harris, A., Gibson, E., & Holcomb, P. (2000). The P600 as an index of syntactic integration difficulty. *Language and Cognitive Processes*, *15*(2), 159–201.

Kiebel, S. J., von Kriegstein, K., Daunizeau, J., & Friston, K. J. (2009). Recognizing sequences of sequences. *PLoS Computational Biology*, *5*(8), e1000464.

Kolk, H. H. J., Chwilla, D. J., van Herten, M., & Oor, P. J. W. (2003). Structure and limited capacity in verbal working memory: a study with event-related potentials. *Brain and Language*, *85*(1), 1–36.

Kutas, M., & Hillyard, S. A. (1980). Reading senseless sentences: brain potentials reflect semantic incongruity. *Science*, *207*, 203–205.

Kutas, M., & Hillyard, S. A. (1984). Brain potentials during reading reflect word expectancy and semantic association. *Nature*, *307*, 161–163.

Kutas, M., & van Petten, C. K. (1994). Psycholinguistics electrified. event–related brain potential investigations. In M. A. Gernsbacher (Ed.), *Handbook of Psycholinguistics* (pp. 83–133). San Diego: Academic Press.

Makeig, S., Debener, S., Onton, J., & Delorme, A. (2004). Mining event-related brain dynamics. *Trends in Cognitive Sciences*, *8*(5), 204–210.

Makeig, S., Westerfield, M., Jung, T.-P., Enghoff, S., Townsend, J., Courchesne, E., et al. (2002). Dynamic brain sources of visual evoked responses. *Science*, *295*, 690–694.

Mizraji, E. (1989). Context-dependent associations in linear distributed memories. *Bulletin of Mathematical Biology*, *51*(2), 195–205.

Näätänen, R., Lehtokoski, A., Lennes, M., Cheour, M., Huotilainen, M., Iivonen, A., et al. (1997). Language-specific phoneme representations revealed by electric and magnetic brain responses. *Nature*, *385*(6615), 432–434.

Nieuwland, M. S., & Kuperberg, G. R. (2008). When the truth is not too hard to handle: an event-related potential study on the pragmatics of negation. *Psychological Science*, *19*(12), 1213–1218.

Nikulin, V. V., Linkenkaer-Hansen, K., Nolte, G., Lemm, S., Müller, K.-R., Ilmoniemi, R. J., et al. (2007). A novel mechanism for evoked responses in the human brain. *European Journal of Neuroscience*, *25*, 3146–3154.

Noveck, I. A., & Posada, A. (2003). Characterizing the time course of an implicature: an evoked potentials study. *Brain and Language*, *85*, 203–210.

Osterhout, L., & Holcomb, P. J. (1992). Event-related brain potentials elicited by syntactic anomaly. *Journal of Memory and Language*, *31*, 785–806.

Osterhout, L., Holcomb, P. J., & Swinney, D. A. (1994). Brain potentials elicited by garden-path sentences: evidence of the application of verb information during parsing. *Journal of Experimental Psychology. Learning, Memory, and Cognition*, *20*(4), 786–803.

Potthast, R. and beim Graben, P. (2009). Inverse problems in neural field theory. *SIAM Journal on Applied Dynamical Systems*, *8*(4), 1405–1433.

Pulvermüller, F., Lutzenberger, W., & Birbaumer, N. (1995). Electrocortical distinction of vocabulary types. *Electroencephalography and Clinical Neurophysiology*, *94*, 357–370.

Pylyshyn, Z. W. (1986). *Computation and Cognition: Toward a Foundation for Cognitive Science*. Cambrigde, MA: MIT Press.

Rabinovich, M. I., Huerta, R., Varona, P., & Afraimovich, V. S. (2008). Transient cognitive dynamics, metastability, and decision making. *PLoS Computational Biology, 4*(5), e1000072.

Rabinovich, M., Volkovskii, A., Lecanda, P., Huerta, R., Abarbanel, H. D. I., & Laurent, G. (2001). Dynamical encoding by networks of competing neuron groups: winnerless competition. *Physical Review Letters, 87*(6), 068102.

Regan, D. (1972). *Evoked Potentials in Psychology, Sensory, Physiology and Clinical Medicine*. London: Chapman and Hall.

Rugg, M. D. (1984). Event-related potentials and the phonological processing of words and non-words. *Neuropsychologia, 22*(4), 435–443.

Schöner, G., & Thelen, E. (2006). Using dynamic field theory to rethink infant habituation. *Psychological Review, 113*(2), 273–299.

Smolensky, P. (1990). Tensor product variable binding and the representation of symbolic structures in connectionist systems. *Artificial Intelligence, 46*(1–2), 159–216.

Smolensky, P. (2006). Harmony in linguistic cognition. *Cognitive Science, 30*, 779–801.

Smolensky, P., & Legendre, G. (2006). *The Harmonic Mind. From Neural Computation to Optimality-Theoretic Grammar* (Vol. 1). Cambridge, MA: MIT Press.

Vosse, T., & Kempen, G. (2000). Syntactic structure assembly in human parsing: a computational model based on competitive inhibition and a lexicalist grammar. *Cognition, 75*, 105–143.

Vosse, T., & Kempen, G. (2009). The unification space implemented as a localist neural net: predictions and error-tolerance in a constraint-based parser. *Cognitive Neurodynamics, 3*(4), 331–346.

Wegner, P. (1998). Interactive foundations of computing. *Theoretical Computer Science, 192*, 315–351.

6 Recognition of Sequences of Sequences Using Nonlinear Dynamical Systems

Stefan J. Kiebel and Karl J. Friston

Summary

Despite tremendous advances in neuroscience, we cannot yet build machines that recognize the world as effortlessly as we do. One reason might be that there are computational approaches to recognition that have not yet been exploited. Here, we demonstrate that the ability to recognize temporal sequences might play an important part. We show that an artificial agent can extract natural speech sounds from sound waves if speech is generated as dynamic and transient sequences of sequences. In principle, this means that artificial recognition can be implemented robustly and online using dynamic systems theory and Bayesian inference.

6.1 Introduction

We live in a dynamic world. Perhaps the most important source of these dynamics is our own body. We move continually, speaking, walking, and interacting to produce continuous auditory and interoceptive input; that is, internal signals from our body (Craig, 2003). Other organisms, like our conspecifics, also generate dynamics, which we have to register and respond to. We are not aware of much of our visual dynamics because our brain infers a stable and constant world that generates visual signals, even though our eye movements (saccades) are highly dynamic and fleeting (Melcher, 2011).

Not surprisingly, neuroscience is preoccupied by brain dynamics. Theoretical and computational neuroscientists typically model neuronal time series, because this is how they measure brain responses with techniques like two-photon laser microscopy, single-cell and multicell recordings, electroencephalography, functional magnetic resonance imaging, and many other techniques. Computational neuroscience is largely concerned with the modeling of neuronal dynamics and the dynamical mechanics of neurons and networks of neurons (Deco, Jirsa, Robinson, Breakspear, & Friston, 2008). The ensuing nonlinear dynamical systems approach to neuroscience has advanced our understanding of how neurons interact and self-organize, as reviewed in Rabinovich, Varona, Selverston, and Abarbanel (2006) and Cessac and Samuelides (2007). In particular, nonlinear dynamical systems allow one to formalize an understanding of phenomena that are otherwise difficult to grasp (Breakspear et al., 2006).

Although most computational neuroscientists believe that the brain represents events in our environment, there is an explanatory gap between much of computational modeling and the fundamental question: How do our brains represent a dynamic environment? In many models, neuronal dynamics often pertain to responses to sensory input that is delivered as an impulse or stochastically; for example, Poisson spike trains (Ma, Beck, Latham, & Pouget, 2006). This modeling approach is sensible because we yet need to understand how input from our dynamic environment is transformed before it affects the neural system being modeled. However, simply modeling dynamic responses to sensory perturbations like impulses may overlook a fundamental coupling between neuronal dynamics and dynamics in the sensorium. For example, conceptually, one could view the environment and the brain as two coupled nonlinear dynamical systems (Kiebel, Daunizeau, & Friston, 2009a). This coupling may entail some fundamental principles that disclose the function of neuronal dynamics and the mechanisms on which they rest.

In this chapter, we ask how one can model the coupling of continuous brain dynamics and sensory input. The task is to specify a nonlinear dynamical system (called an *agent* in the following), which changes its internal states to represent the hidden causes of dynamic sensory input (Friston, Kilner, & Harrison, 2006). This agenda is pursued by neural network modeling, where specific input patterns affect a network of neurons modeled by rate equations (e.g., Deco & Rolls, 2004). The notion that sensory input changes the internal states of a nonlinear dynamical system can be taken further by exploiting nonlinear phenomena like bifurcations to compute some desired output (Jirsa, Fink, Foo, & Kelso, 2000; Erlhagen & Schoner, 2002; Varona, Rabinovich, Selverston, & Arshavsky, 2002; Sandamirskaya & Schoner, 2010). Similarly, in machine learning, recurrent neural networks have been used for many years, where network and output parameters are learned so that the network maps sensory input to desired outputs (Rumelhart, Hinton, & Williams, 1986; Pearlmuttter, 1989; Williams & Zipser, 1989; Jäger, 2001; Maass,

Natschlager, & Markram, 2002; Verstraeten, Schrauwen, Stroobandt, & Van Campenhout, 2005; Sussillo & Abbott, 2009).

These studies show that one can construct dynamical systems that not only model neuronal responses to sensory input but can also perform brain-like functions; for example, the recognition of what caused sensory input and the retrieval of memories about past input sequences or internal states. However, there are two important issues that are not addressed by these approaches: The first is that our brains must comply with some optimality constraint when representing the environment: Ultimately, nature compares different phenotypes by natural selection (Friston et al., 2006). One may therefore ask what is the optimal agent for representing sensory input from a given econiche? For example, a decisive selection feature may be the time an agent needs to infer that a change in the environment has occurred. This implies there must be a way of comparing different agents using a common optimality criterion. In other words, it should, in principle, be possible to define a single optimality criterion or objective function, which neuronal dynamics optimizes. This may be important when it comes to modeling the brain because it suggests that there is some underlying quantity that neuronal dynamics are trying to optimize. The second issue concerns the design of two coupled nonlinear dynamical systems where one (the agent) is entrained by input from the other (the environment). Most neural network models avoid this issue by not generating sensory input using a nonlinear dynamical system but rather by specifying input as a (deterministic or probabilistic) function of time. This approach precludes deep (hierarchical) dynamical structure in sensory input, which may be a key determinant of optimal neuronal responses. In short, sensory input should mimic the dynamics of our natural world (e.g., speech or kinematics).

In this chapter, we describe how both these issues, adhering to an optimality criterion and the coupling of sensory and agent dynamics, can be addressed in a single approach. To motivate our scheme, we frame the problem as follows: We assume that one of the brain's functions is to decode, in an online fashion, its sensory input. By decoding we mean that the brain receives dynamic sensory input from the environment and represents the hidden causes of that input by its internal states, in an online fashion. This perspective motivates a Bayesian approach, where the brain is a Bayesian observer of the hidden environment generating sensory input (Friston et al., 2006). To pursue this approach, one has to specify a so-called generative model (a nonlinear dynamical system) that describes the mapping from the hidden causes in the environment (e.g., the category of an object producing sensations) to sensory input. The dynamic decoding performed by the brain is the ensuing Bayesian inference that maps (inversely) the sensory input back to (a representation of) its causes. Crucially, in this formulation, Bayesian inference on a nonlinear dynamical system (the environment) calls on another nonlinear dynamical system, the so-called Bayesian update equations (Daunizeau, Friston, & Kiebel, 2009). This means that dynamics in the environment entail dynamics in the brain under (Bayesian) optimality criteria. In other words, deriving Bayesian update equations for the hidden causes (states of the environment) effectively prescribes neuronal dynamics that underlie perception and how they couple to the environment. The only requirement for this optimality modeling is a generic Bayesian online inversion scheme for nonlinear dynamical systems. Fortunately, such schemes exist in the form of extended Kalman filters and more general Bayesian filtering schemes (e.g., Friston, Trujillo-Barreto, & Daunizeau, 2008; Daunizeau et al., 2009). These schemes provide, under certain assumptions, optimal inference. Furthermore, they entail the optimality criteria discussed earlier in terms of the evidence for an agent's model of its world, where the evidence is simply the probability of observing sensory dynamics under the agent's model of how those dynamics were caused. This is because the Bayesian updating or filtering that we associate with neuronal dynamics can always be cast as maximizing model evidence. This theme is developed later in the context of the free-energy principle, where free energy is a mathematical bound on (the log of) model evidence.

We will highlight the potential usefulness of this Bayesian inference approach for modeling perception by using auditory processing to focus on an important feature of sensory input generated by our acoustic environment: Sound-wave modulations during speech are generated on various timescales (Kiebel, von Kriegstein, Daunizeau, & Friston, 2009b). For example, in speech, formants form phonemes and phonemes form syllables. Speech also provides an opportunity to make the nonlinear dynamical system modeling the environment more realistic by endowing it with hierarchical structure. This is motivated easily because sequences, which exist at different timescales, are often structured hierarchically, where sequence elements on one timescale constrain the expression of sequences on a finer timescale. An example here would be the fact that a syllable comprises a specific sequence of phonemes. This hierarchy of timescales may be reflected in the hierarchical organization of the brain's anatomy (Kiebel, Daunizeau, & Friston, 2008). For example, in avian brains, there is anatomic and functional evidence that birdsong is generated and perceived by a hierarchical system, where low levels represent transient acoustic details, and high levels encode song structure at slower timescales (Sen, Theunissen, & Doupe, 2001; Long & Fee, 2008). An equivalent temporal hierarchy might also exist in the human brain for representing auditory information, such as speech (Giraud et al., 2000; Davis & Johnsrude, 2003; Overath, Kumar, von Kriegstein, & Griffiths, 2008; Poeppel, Idsardi, & van Wassenhove, 2008; von Kriegstein, Patterson, & Griffiths, 2008). Here, we show how one can model these hierarchical dynamics and use Bayesian inference to recognize them in an online fashion. This rests on decoding the hidden states of the acoustic environment using a coupled, hierarchical nonlinear dynamical system, of the sort that the brain might use. Both our models of the environment and, therefore, the generative models used by our synthetic agents call upon stable heteroclinic channels (SHCs) as the building block of temporal hierarchies.

6.2 Stable Heteroclinic Channels

As rehearsed in previous chapters, SHCs are attractors that prescribe sequences of transient dynamics (Rabinovich et al., 2006). The key aspect of these dynamical systems is that their equations of motion describe a manifold with a series of saddle points. At each saddle point, trajectories are attracted from nearly all directions but are expelled in the direction of another saddle point. If the saddle points are linked to form a chain, the state follows a trajectory that passes through all these points, thereby forming a sequence. These sequences are exhibited robustly, even in the presence of high levels of noise. In addition, the dynamics of the SHCs are itinerant due to dynamical instability in the equations of motion and noise on the states. This noise also induces a variation in the exact times that sequence elements are visited. This can be exploited during recognition, where the SHC places prior constraints on the sequence in which elements (repelling fixed points) are visited but does not specify precisely when these fixed points are encountered. The combination of these two features, robustness of sequence order but flexibility in sequence timing, makes the SHC a good candidate for the neuronal encoding of trajectories (Friston, 1997; Rabinovich, Huerta, & Laurent, 2008). Rabinovich et al. have used SHCs to explain how spatiotemporal neuronal dynamics observed in odor perception or motor control of a marine mollusc can be expressed in terms of a dynamic system (Varona et al., 2002).

Varona et al. used Lotka–Volterra type dynamics to model a network of six neurons in a marine mollusc (Varona et al., 2002). With a particular sort of lateral inhibition between pairs of neurons and input to each neuron, the network displayed sequences of activity. After a specific order, each neuron became active for a short time and became inactive again, while the next neuron became active, and so on. As noted earlier, stable heteroclinic channels rest on a particular form of attractor manifold that supports itinerant dynamics. This itinerancy can result from deterministic chaos in the absence of noise, which implies the presence of heteroclinic cycles. When noise is added, itinerancy can be ensured, even if the original system has stable fixed points. However, our motivation for considering stochastic dynamics is to construct a probabilistic model, where assumptions about the distribution of noise provide a formal generative model of sensory dynamics.

As reviewed in Rabinovich et al. (2006), Lotka–Volterra dynamics can be derived from simple neural mass models of mean membrane potential and mean firing rate. Here, we use a standard neural mass model, where the state vector $x(t)$ can take positive or negative values:

$$\dot{x} = \kappa\left(-\frac{1}{8}x - \rho S(x,0)\right) + w$$

$$y = S(x,2) + z \qquad (6.1)$$

$$S(x,b) = \frac{1}{1 + \exp(-x-b)},$$

where the motion of the state vector (e.g., depolarization) is a nonlinear function of itself with a scalar rate constant κ and a connectivity matrix ρ (see later). The state vector enters a nonlinear function S to generate outcomes y (e.g., neuronal firing rates). Each element ρ_{ij} determines the strength of lateral inhibition from state j to i. Both the state and observation equations above include additive normally distributed noise vectors w and z with zero mean and some standard deviation (specified later as precision or inverse variance). When choosing a specific connectivity matrix, the states display stereotyped sequences of activity (Afraimovich, Zhigulin, & Rabinovich, 2004b; Rabinovich et al., 2008). If the channel forms a ring, once a state is attracted to any saddle point, it will remain in the SHC.

In this chapter, we use SHCs not as a model for neuronal dynamics per se but as the brain's model of how sensory input is generated. This means that we interpret the states as hidden states in the environment, which generate sensory input. The neuronal responses to sampling sensory input are described by recognition dynamics, which decode or deconvolve the states or causes from that input. These recognition dynamics are described later. This use of equation (6.1) is particularly easy to motivate in this context: Sensory input is usually generated by other neural networks. This means equation (6.1) is appropriate as a generative model of sensory dynamics because it is a model of neuronal dynamics generating sensory data.

6.3   Hierarchies of Stable Heteroclinic Channels

An SHC can generate repetitive, stereotyped sequences. For example, in a system with four saddle points, an SHC forces trajectories through the saddle points in a sequence (e.g., "1–2–3–4–1–2–3–4–1..."). In contrast, an SHC cannot generate "1–2–3–4–3–4–2–1..." because the sequence is not repetitive. However, to model sensory input, for example speech, one must be able to recombine basic sequence elements like phonemes in ever-changing sequences. One solution would be to represent each possible sequence of phonemes (e.g., each syllable) with a specific SHC. A more plausible and parsimonious solution is to construct a hierarchy of SHCs, which can encode sequences generated by SHCs whose attractor topology (e.g., the channels linking the saddle points) is changed by a supraordinate SHC. This can be achieved by making the connectivity matrix at a subordinate level a function of the output states of the supraordinate level. This enables the hierarchy to generate sequences of sequences to any hierarchical depth required.

Following a recent account of how macroscopic cortical anatomy might relate to timescales in our environment (Kiebel et al., 2008), we can construct a hierarchy by setting the rate constant $\kappa^{(j)}$ of the jth level to a rate that is slower than its subordinate level, $\kappa^{(j-1)}$. As a result, the states of subordinate levels change faster than the states of the level above. This means the control parameters $\rho^{(j)}$ at any level change more slowly than the states, $x^{(j)}$, because the slow change in the attractor manifold is controlled by supraordinate states:

$$\dot{x}^{(j)} = \qquad f^{(j)} + w^{(j)}$$
$$v^{(j)} = \qquad g^{(j)} + z^{(j)}$$
$$f^{(j)} = \kappa^{(j)} \left(-\frac{1}{8} x^{(j)} - \rho^{(j)} \left(v^{(j+1)} \right) S\left(x^{(j)}, 0 \right) \right) \qquad (6.2)$$
$$g^{(j)} = \qquad S\left(x^{(j)}, 2 \right).$$

Here, the superscript indexes level j (level 1 being the lowest level), $x^{(j)}$ are "hidden states," and $v^{(j)}$ are outputs to the subordinate level, which we will call hidden causes. As before, at the first level, $y = v^{(1)}$ is the sensory stream. In this chapter, we consider hierarchies with relative timescales $\kappa^{(1)}/\kappa^{(2)}$ of around six. This means that the time spent in the vicinity of a saddle point at a supraordinate level is long enough for the subordinate level to go through several saddle points. As before, all levels are subject to noise on the motion of the hidden states $w^{(j)}$ and causes $z^{(j)}$. At the highest level, the control parameters, $\rho^{(L)}$, are constant over time. At all other levels, the causal states of the supraordinate level, $v^{(j+1)}$, enter the subordinate level by changing the control parameters, the connectivity matrix $\rho^{(j)}$:

$$\rho^{(j)}\left(v^{(j+1)}\right) = \sum_k v_k^{(j+1)} R_k^{(j)}. \tag{6.3}$$

Here, $\rho^{(j)}$ is a linear mixture of "template" control matrices $R^{(j)}$, weighted by the hidden causes at level $j + 1$. Each of these templates is chosen to generate an SHC. Later, we will show examples of how these templates can be constructed to generate sequential phenomena. The key point about this construction is that states from the supraordinate level select which template controls the dynamics of the lower level. By induction, the states at each level follow an SHC because the states at the supraordinate level follow an SHC. This means only one state is active at any time and only one template is selected for the lower level. An exception to this is the transition from one state to another, which leads to a transient superposition of two SHC-inducing templates (see later). Effectively, the transition transient at a specific level gives rise to brief spells of non-SHC dynamics at the subordinate levels (see later). These transition periods are characterized by dissipative dynamics, due to the largely inhibitory connectivity matrices, with inhibition controlled by the saturating nonlinearity S (equation 6.2).

In summary, a hierarchy of SHCs generates the sensory stream $y = v^{(1)}$ at the lowest (fastest) level, which forms a sequence of sequences expressed in terms of first-level states. In these models, the lower level follows an SHC (i.e., the states follow an itinerant trajectory through a sequence of saddle points). This SHC will change whenever the supraordinate level, which itself follows an SHC, moves from one saddle point to another. Effectively, we have constructed a system that can generate a stable pattern of transients like an oscillator or central pattern generator; however, as shown later, the pattern can have deep or hierarchical structure. Next, we describe how the hidden causes $v^{(j)}$ can be recognized or deconvolved from sensory input y.

6.4 Bayesian Recognition Using SHC Hierarchies

We have described how SHCs can, in principle, generate sequences of sequences that, we assume, are observed by an agent as its input y. To recognize the causes of the sensory stream, the agent must infer the hidden states and causes online; that is, the system does not look into the future but recognizes the current state of the environment, at all levels of the hierarchy, by the fusion of current sensory input and internal dynamics elicited by past input. An online recognition scheme can be derived from the *free-energy principle*, which states that an agent will minimize its surprise about its sensory input, under a model it entertains about the environment; or, equivalently maximize the evidence for that model (Friston et al., 2006). This requires the agent to have a dynamic model, which relates environmental states to sensory input. In this context, recognition is the Bayesian inversion of a generative model. This inversion corresponds to mapping sensory input to the posterior or conditional distribution of hidden states. In general, Bayesian accounts of perception rest on a generative model. Given such a model, one can use the ensuing recognition schemes in artificial perception and furthermore compare simulated recognition dynamics (in response to sensory input) with evoked responses in the brain. The generative model in this chapter is dynamical and based on the nonlinear equations (6.1) and (6.2). More precisely, these stochastic differential equations play the role of empirical priors on the dynamics of hidden states causing sensory data.

In the following, we review briefly the Bayesian model inversion described in Friston (2008) for stochastic, hierarchical systems and apply it, in the next section, to hierarchical SHCs. Given some sensory data vector y, the general inference problem is to compute the model evidence or marginal likelihood of y, given a model m:

$$p(y \mid m) = \int p(y, u \mid m)\, du, \tag{6.4}$$

where the generative model $p(y, u|m) = p(y|u, m)p(u|m)$ is defined in terms of a likelihood $p(y|u,m)$ and prior $p(u|m)$ on hidden states. In equation (6.4), the state vector $u = \{x,v\}$ subsumes the hidden causes and states at all levels of a hierarchy (equation 6.2). The model evidence can be estimated by converting this difficult integration problem (equation 6.4) into an easier optimization problem by optimizing a free-energy bound on the log-evidence (Beal, 2003). This bound is constructed using Jensen's inequality and is a function of an arbitrary *recognition* density, $q(u)$:

$$F(q,y) = -\ln p(y\mid m) + D = U - S$$
$$D = \int q(u)\ln\frac{q(u)}{p(u\mid y,m)}\,du \geq 0. \tag{6.5}$$

The free energy comprises an energy term $U = -\langle \ln p(y\mid u) + \ln p(u)\rangle_q$ and an entropy term $S = -\langle \ln q(u)\rangle_q$ and is defined uniquely, given a generative model m. The free energy is an upper bound on the surprise or negative log-evidence, because the Kullback–Leibler divergence D, between the recognition and conditional density, is always positive. Minimizing the free energy minimizes the divergence, rendering the recognition density $q(u)$ an approximate conditional density. When using this approach, one usually employs a parameterized fixed-form recognition density, $q(u\mid\lambda)$ (Friston, 2008). Inference corresponds to optimizing the free energy with respect to the sufficient statistics, λ, of the recognition density:

$$\lambda^* = \arg\min_{\lambda} F(\lambda, y)$$
$$q(u\mid\lambda^*) \approx p(u\mid y,m). \tag{6.6}$$

The optimal statistics λ^* are sufficient to describe the approximate posterior density; that is, the agent's belief about (or representation of) the trajectory of the hidden and causal states. We refer the interested reader to Friston et al. (2008) for technical details about this variational Bayesian treatment of dynamical systems. Intuitively, this scheme can be thought of as augmented gradient descent on a free-energy bound on the model's log-evidence. In other words, the Bayesian update equations underlying equation (6.6) implement a gradient descent on the optimality criterion discussed in the introduction. Crucially, this scheme outperforms conventional Bayesian filtering (e.g., extended Kalman filtering) and eschews the computation of probability transition matrices. This means it can be implemented in a simple and neuronally plausible fashion (Friston, 2008). In addition, one can apply this gradient descent to different models m (equation 6.6) and use their model evidences for model selection among alternatives of how an agent may be constructed. Here, we will not use model (agent) selection because we will assume that the agent knows how the environmental stimuli are generated. In short, this recognition scheme operates online and recognizes current states of the environment by combining current sensory input with internal recognition dynamics, elicited by past input.

A recognition system that minimizes its free energy efficiently will come to represent the environmental dynamics in terms of the sufficient statistics of recognition density; for example, the conditional expectations and variances of $q(u \mid \lambda) = N(\mu, \Sigma) : \lambda = \{\mu, \Sigma\}$. We assume that the conditional moments are encoded by neuronal activity; this means that equation (6.6) prescribes neuronal recognition dynamics. These dynamics implement Bayesian inversion of the generative model, under the approximations entailed by the form of the recognition density. Neuronally, equation (6.6) can be implemented using a message-passing scheme, which, in the context of hierarchical models, involves passing prediction errors up and passing predictions down, from one level to the next. These prediction errors are the difference between the causal states (equation 6.2),

$$\varepsilon^{(j)} = v^{(j)} - g^{(j)}, \tag{6.7}$$

at any level j, and their prediction from the level above, evaluated at the conditional expectations (Friston, 2005; Friston et al., 2006). In addition, there are prediction errors that mediate dynamical priors on the motion of hidden states within each level (equation 6.2):

$$e^{(j)} = \dot{x}^{(j)} - f^{(j)}. \tag{6.8}$$

This means that neuronal populations encode two types of dynamics: the conditional predictions about states of the world and prediction errors. The dynamics of the first are given by equation (6.6), which can be formulated as a function of prediction error. These dynamics effectively suppress or explain away prediction error; see Friston et al. (2008) for details. This inversion scheme is a generic recognition process that receives dynamic sensory input and can, given an appropriate generative model, rapidly identify and track environmental states that are generating input. More precisely, the recognition dynamics resemble the environmental (hidden) states they track (to which they are indirectly coupled) but differ from the latter because they are driven by a gradient descent on free energy (i.e., minimize prediction errors). This is important because we want to use SHCs as a generative model, not as a model of neuronal encoding per se. This means that the neuronal dynamics will only recapitulate the dynamics entitled by SHCs in the environment if the recognition scheme can suppress prediction errors efficiently in the face of sensory noise and prior beliefs about the world.

We are now in a position to formulate hierarchies of SHCs as generative models, use them to generate sensory input, and simulate recognition of hidden causes generating that input. In terms of low-level speech processing, this means that any given phoneme will predict the next phoneme. At the same time, as phonemes are recognized, there is also a prediction about which syllable is the most likely context for generating these phonemes. This prediction arises due to the learned regularities in speech. In turn, the most likely syllable predicts the next phoneme. This means that speech recognition can be described as a dynamic process, on multiple timescales, with recurrently evolving representations and predictions, all driven by the sensory input.

6.5 A Model of Speech Recognition

In the auditory system, higher cortical levels appear to represent features that are expressed at slower temporal scales (Creutzfeldt, Hellweg, & Schreiner, 1980). Wang, Lu, Bendor, and Bartlett (2008) present evidence from single-neuron recordings suggesting that there is a "slowing down" of representational trajectories from human auditory sensory thalamus (a "relay" to the primary auditory cortex), to medial geniculate body (MGB), to primary auditory cortex (AI). In humans, it has been found that the sensory thalamus responds preferentially to faster temporal modulations of sensory signals, whereas primary cortex prefers slower modulations (Giraud et al., 2000). These findings indicate that neuronal populations, at lower levels of the auditory system (e.g., MGB), represent faster trajectories than higher levels (e.g., AI). Specifically, the MGB responds preferentially to temporal modulations of ~20 Hz (~50 ms), whereas AI prefers modulations at ~6 Hz (~150 ms) (Giraud et al., 2000). Such a temporal hierarchy would be optimal for speech recognition, in which information over longer timescales provides predictions for processing at shorter timescales. In accord with this conjecture, optimal encoding of fast (rapidly modulated) dynamics by top-down predictions has been found to be critical for communication (Nahum, Nelken, & Ahissar, 2008; Poeppel et al., 2008; von Kriegstein et al., 2008).

We model this "slowing down" with a hierarchical generative model based on SHCs. This model generates sequences of syllables, where each syllable is a sequence of phonemes. Phonemes are the smallest speech sounds that distinguish meaning, and a syllable is a unit of organization for a sequence of phonemes. Each phoneme prescribes a sequence of sound-wave modulations that correspond to sensory data. We generated data in this fashion and simulated online recognition (see figure 6.1). By recognizing speech-like phoneme sequences, we provide a proof of principle that a hierarchical system can use sensory streams to infer sequences. This not only models the slowing down of representations in the auditory system (Giraud et al., 2000; Nahum et al., 2008; von Kriegstein et al., 2008; Wang et al., 2008) but also may point to computational approaches to speech recognition. In summary, the recognition dynamics following equation (6.6) are coupled to a generative model based on SHCs via sensory input. The systems generating and recognizing states in

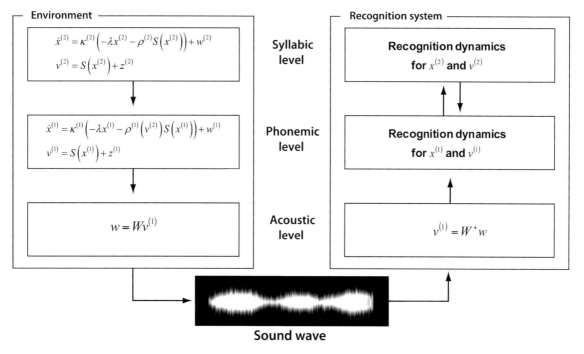

Figure 6.1
Schematic of the generative model and recognition system. This schematic shows the equations that define both the generation of stimuli (left; see equation 6.2) and the recognition scheme based on a generative model. There are three levels; the phonemic and syllabic levels use stable heteroclinic channels, whereas the acoustic level is implemented by a linear transform. W corresponds to sound file extracts, and w is the resulting sound wave. This sound wave is input to the recognition system, with a linear (forward) projection using the pseudo-inverse W^+. The recognition of the phonemic and syllabic level uses bottom-up and top-down message passing between the phonemic and syllabic level, following equation (6.6). Adapted from Kiebel et al. (2009b).

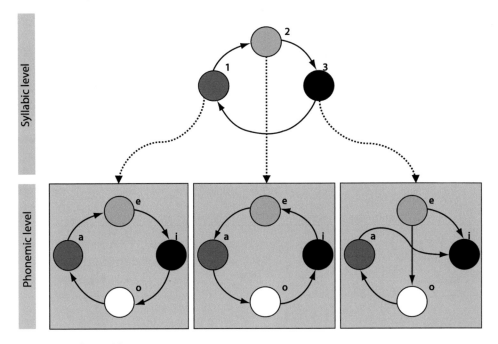

Figure 6.2
Two-level model to generate phoneme sequences. Schematic illustration of the phoneme sequence generation process. At the syllabic level, one of three syllables is active and induces a specific lateral connectivity structure at the phonemic level (equation 6.9). The transition speed at the phonemic level is six times faster than at the syllabic level. The resulting phoneme and syllable dynamics of the model are shown in figure 6.3A (plate 14). Adapted from Kiebel et al. (2009b).

figure 6.1 are both dynamic systems, where a non-autonomous recognition system is coupled to an autonomous system generating speech.

All our simulations use hierarchies with two levels (figure 6.2). The first (phonemic) level produces a sequence of phonemes, and the second (syllabic) level encodes sequences of syllables. We used equation (6.2) to produce phoneme sequences. The template matrices $R^{(j)}$ (equation 6.3) were produced in the following way: We first specified the sequence each template should induce; for example, sequence 1–2–3 for three neuronal populations. We then set elements on the main diagonal to 0.1, the elements (2,1), (3,2), (1,3) to value 0.5, elements (1,2), (2,3), (3,1) to value 1.5, and all other elements to 1 (Afraimovich, Rabinovich, & Varona, 2004a). More generally, the connectivity matrices have the following form:

$$R_{il} = \begin{bmatrix} .1 & 1.5 & 1 & \cdots & .5 \\ .5 & .1 & 1.5 & & 1 \\ 1 & .5 & .1 & & 1 \\ \vdots & & & \ddots & \vdots \\ 1.5 & 1 & 1 & \cdots & .1 \end{bmatrix}. \tag{6.9}$$

Note that SHC hierarchies can be used to create a variety of different behaviors using different connectivity matrices. Here, we explore only a subset of possible sequential dynamics.

When generating sensory data y, we added noise $w^{(j)}$ and $z^{(j)}$ to both the hidden states and causes. At the first and second levels, this was normally distributed zero-mean noise with log-precisions of 12 and 16, respectively. These noise levels were chosen to introduce noisy dynamics but not to the extent that the recognition became difficult to visualize. We repeated all the simulations reported later with higher noise levels and found that the findings remained qualitatively the same (see also second simulation, figure 6.4). Synthetic stimuli were generated by taking a linear mixture of sound waves extracted from sound files, in which a single speaker pronounced each of four vowel-phonemes: [a], [e], [i], [o]. These extracts W were sampled at 22,050 Hz. The mixture was weighted by the causal states of the phonemic level: $w = Wv^{(1)}$. This resulted in a concatenated sound-wave file w. When this sound file is played, one perceives a sequence of vowels with smooth, overlapping transitions; see the supplemental material of Kiebel et al. (2009b) for a sound-file sample. These transitions are driven by the SHCs guiding the expression of the phonemes and syllables at both levels of the generative hierarchy.

For computational simplicity, we circumvented a detailed generative model of the acoustic level. For simulated recognition, the acoustic input (the sound wave) was transformed to phonemic input by inverting the linear mixing described above every 7 ms of simulated time (one time bin). This means that our recognition scheme at the acoustic level assumes forward processing only (figure 6.1). However, in principle, given an appropriate generative model (Sumner, Lopez-Poveda, O'Mard, & Meddis, 2002; Holmberg, Gelbart, & Hemmert, 2007), one could invert a full acoustic model, using forward and backward message-passing between the acoustic and phonemic levels.

6.6   Some Simulated Examples

In this section, we illustrate that the recognition scheme described earlier can reliably decode syllabic and phonemic structure from sensory input online if it has the correct generative model. We will also illustrate that this scheme is robust to observation noise and small deviations in the expected dynamics. Furthermore, we will describe how recognition fails when the generative model deviates from the dynamics predicted. These simulations relate to empirical studies of brain responses evoked by unpredicted linguistic stimuli and show that known experimental phenomena can be modeled by an autonomous system (the environment), which provides rapidly varying input to another (neuronal) system that performs Bayesian decoding.

6.6.1   Recognizing a Sequence of Sequences

To create synthetic stimuli, we generated syllable sequences consisting of four phonemes or states, [a], [e], [i], and [o], over 5.625 seconds (400 time points) using a two-level SHC model (figure 6.2). Using the generative model (equations 6.2 and 6.3), we produced syllable sequences consisting of phonemes (figure 6.3A, top left; plate 14). At the syllabic level, we used three syllables or states to form the second-level sequence $(1–2–3)^{(2)}$; where the numbers denote the sequence, and the superscript indicates the sequence level. The three hidden causes $v^{(2)}$ at the syllabic level entered the phonemic level as control parameters to induce their template matrices as in equation (6.3). This means that each of the three syllable states at the second level causes a phoneme sequence at the first: $(a–e–i–o)^{(1)}$, $(o–i–e–a)^{(1)}$, and $(a–i–e–o)^{(1)}$ (see figure 6.2). In figure 6.3A (plate 14), we show the hidden states and causes, at both levels, generated by this model with $\kappa^{(1)} = 1$ and $\kappa^{(2)} = \frac{1}{6}$. In other words, the rate constant of the syllabic level generates dynamics that are six times slower than at the phonemic level. As expected, the phoneme sequence at the first level changes as a function of the active syllable at the second level. The transients caused by transitions between syllables manifest at the first level as temporary changes in the amplitude or duration of the active phoneme.

We then simulated recognition of these sequences. Figure 6.3B (plate 14) shows that our recognition model successfully tracks the true states at both levels. For recognition, we used prior log-precision of 8 and 12 for the hidden causes and states at the first level and 12 and 10 at the second level. Note the recognition dynamics immediately "lock onto" the hidden causes from the onset of the first phoneme of the first syllable. Note that this was achieved with initial states that were uninformed about the true (but unknown) states of the environment: At both levels, we set all initial states $x_0^{(j)}$ to –4. These results show that the coupling of the agent system to the environment and its internal dynamics are

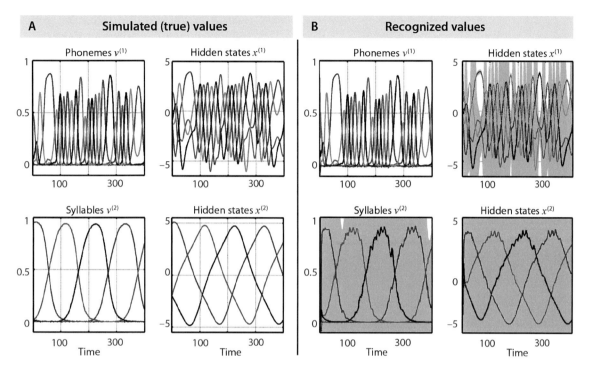

Figure 6.3 (plate 14)
Recognition of a sequence of sequences. (A) Dynamics of generated causal and hidden states at the phonemic and syllabic level using equation (6.2). At the syllabic level (lower row), there are three different syllables (1, blue; 2, green; 3, red), following the syllable sequence 1→2→3. The slowly changing state syllable 1 causes the faster-moving phoneme sequence a→e→i→o (blue→green→red→cyan); syllable 2, o→i→e→a (cyan→red→green→blue); and syllable 3, a→i→e→o (blue→red→green→cyan). See figure 6.2 for a schematic description of these sequences. The four phonemic variables $v^{(1)}$ (upper row) cause sound waves, resolved at 22,050 Hz (see figure 6.1, not shown here). These sound waves are the input to the recognition system. (B) The recognition dynamics after inverting the sound wave. At the phonemic level, the states follow the true states closely. At the syllabic level, the recognized hidden causes $v^{(2)}$ are slightly rougher than the true states but track the true syllable sequence veridically. Note that the hidden states, at both levels, experience high uncertainty whenever a phoneme or syllable is inactive (plotted in gray: confidence intervals of 95% around the mean).

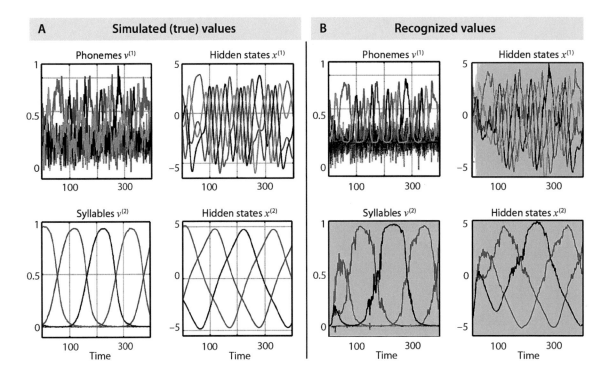

Figure 6.4 (plate 15)
Recognition of a noisy sequence. (A) For these simulations, the parameters and plots are the same as in figure 6.3 (plate 14), but here we increased the observation noise by decreasing the log-precision of the hidden causes at the first level $v^{(1)}$ from 12 to 4. The phoneme sequence $v^{(1)}$ is discernible but very noisy. (B) The recognition dynamics after Bayesian inversion. At the phonemic level, the hidden states $x^{(1)}$ follow the true states, and the hidden causes predicted appear as a de-noised version of the true $v^{(1)}$. At the syllabic level, the recognized causal dynamics $v^{(2)}$ are rougher than the true states but track the true syllable sequence veridically. In addition, there is an initial transient of roughly 50 time points. After this initial period, the recognition starts tracking the true states more closely.

optimal in the sense that the prediction error (equations 6.7 and 6.8) is minimized rapidly.

6.6.2   Robustness against Noise and Small Deviations

Next, we illustrate the robustness of the agent's inference to observation noise and small deviations in the expected sensory input. To increase observation noise, we lowered the log-precision of the causal states at the first level from 12 to 4. Similarly, we lowered the prior log-precision of the causal states at the first level to 4. All other precision parameters and parameters remained identical to the first simulation. In figure 6.4

(plate 15), we show the (noisy) observable and hidden dynamics of the environment and the inference dynamics of the agent. Even though there is a large amount of noise, the agent can still track the underlying slow syllable dynamics at the second level.

In the next simulation, we let the second syllable deviate from the agent's expectation $(o–i–e–a)^{(1)}$ to form the phoneme sequence $(o–i–a–e)^{(1)}$; that is, the two phonemes e and a swap their position within this syllable. The other syllables formed the expected phoneme sequences (see previous simulations). In figure 6.5 (plate 16), we show the recognition dynamics in response to this unexpected input. We inverted the model twice with a subtle but important change in the log-precisions. In the first inversion (figure 6.5B), we used a prior log-precision of the hidden causes at the first level of 4, whereas in the second inversion, we increased this log-precision to 6. All other log-precision remained the same as in the first simulation (figure 6.3B). When using a log-precision of 4, the agent exploited the prediction error at the first level to adjust its dynamics to the unexpected input. When we used an increased log-precision of 6, the agent resolved the situation by switching to a different syllable at the second level (around time point 100), in this case to the first because this syllable contains the unexpected phoneme sequence $a–e$. This syllable switching enables the agent to explain away the prediction error at the first level. Note that the agent's switching between syllables (figure 6.5C, lower row) is fast compared with the timescale of the syllables in the environment (see later). This means that the agent's internal representation of the environment can adjust rapidly to unexpected dynamics using minimization of prediction error. The difference between the decoding or inversion shown in figure 6.5B and 6.5C is explained by the "higher cost" of using prediction error at the first level in the second inversion (figure 6.5C): The higher prior precision at the first level practically disabled the use of prediction error at the first level. Therefore, the agent had to explain away deviations from the expected input by switching between syllables at the second level. Although it may seem undesirable that the Bayesian inference is sensitive to a small change in the prior precision parameters, this may be an important feature for modeling brain function. Generally, neuronal responses and behavior may depend in a very sensitive way on the precision ascribed to predictions at different cognitive or sensory levels (Friston, 2010). For example, in an aroused state, humans tend to neglect small details to avoid subverting high-level predictions (figure 6.5B) (Coull, 1998). Conversely, when details are perceived clearly (attended

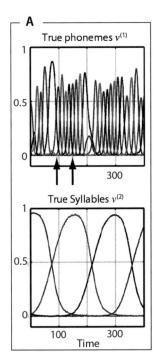

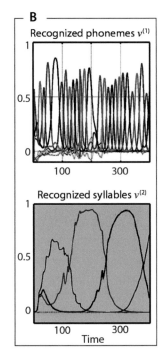

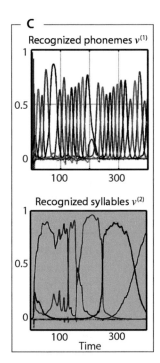

Figure 6.5 (plate 16)
Recognition of a deviating sequence. (A) For these simulations, the parameters
are the same as in figure 6.3 (plate 14), but we used a phonemic sequence of the
second syllable that deviated from the agent's expectation. The agent had expected for
syllable 2 o→i→e→a (cyan→red→green→blue), but the environment played o→i→a→e
(cyan→red→blue→green); that is, we switched the location of the phonemes e and a. Here,
we show only the hidden causes $v^{(1)}$ and $v^{(2)}$ at both levels. The deviations at the phoneme
levels during the presence of syllable 2 are indicated by two red arrows. (B) The recognition
dynamics after Bayesian inversion (conditional expectations or predictions of hidden
causes $v^{(1)}$ and $v^{(2)}$). For inversion, we used a log-precision of 4 for the hidden causes at the
first level and a log-precision of 10 for the hidden states at the second level. At the phoneme
level, there are some small differences between the true and reconstructed causes up to
time point 250. At the syllable level, there are some deviations from the true causes, but
the reconstruction of syllable identity is veridical. (C) Same as in panel B, but for inversion
we used a log-precision of 6 for the hidden causes at the first level and a log-precision
of 10 for the hidden states at the second level. In contrast to the inversion under panel B,
the phonemic level is reconstructed accurately. However, there are deviations from the
true syllabic dynamics between time points 90 to 180. See the text for further description
of the significance of the differences of both reconstructions (B and C) to the true causal
states (A).

to), an unexpected detail may easily switch the percept at a higher level (figure 6.5C).

6.6.3   Robustness to Speed of Speech

Here, we demonstrate that representation or inference is robust in the face of a moderate change in the timescale of the dynamics of the environment. Notably, human speech recognition is robust to the speed of speech (Foulke & Sticht, 1969; Versfeld & Dreschler, 2002). How do our brains recognize speech at different rates? There are two possible mechanisms in our model that can deal with "speaker speed" parameters online. First, one could make the rate constants $\kappa^{(1)}$ and $\kappa^{(2)}$ free parameters and optimize them during inversion. Adjusting to different speaker parameters is probably an essential faculty, because people speak at different speeds (Pisoni, 1993). The second mechanism is that the recognition itself might be robust to deviations from the expected rate of phonemic transitions: In other words, even though recognition uses the rate parameters appropriate for canonical speech, it still can recognize fast speech. This might explain why human listeners can understand speech at rates that they have never experienced previously, at two or three times of the typical speech rate (Foulke & Sticht, 1969). In the following, we show that our scheme exhibits the same robustness.

To simulate speed differences, we used the same two-level model as in the simulations above but with $\kappa^{(1)} = 1.5$ for the generation of phonemes and with $\kappa^{(1)} = 1.0$ for recognition, so that the stimulus stream was 50% faster than expected by the agent. As can be seen in figure 6.6A (plate 17), recognition can successfully track the syllables (and phonemes, not plotted). This was because the second level adapted to the fast sensory input by changing its recognition dynamics in responses to prediction error (see figure 6.6B, plate 17; note the differences in figure 6.6A between the true and recognized $v^{(2)}$). The prediction errors at both levels, $e^{(1)}$ and $e^{(2)}$, are shown in figure 6.6C (plate 17). At the first level, the agent uses mostly positive prediction error to speed up the internal dynamics to match the faster than expected input phoneme sequence. At the second level, the agent uses prediction error mostly during the transitions between syllables. These results show that the system can track true syllables veridically, where the prediction error accommodates the effects caused by speed differences. This robustness to variations in the speed of phoneme transitions might be a feature shared with the auditory system (Vaughan, Storzbach, & Furukawa, 2006).

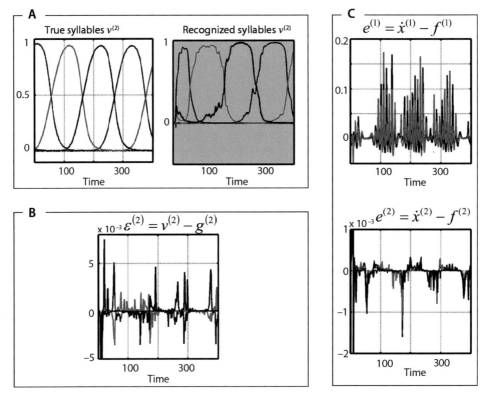

Figure 6.6 (plate 17)
Recognition of unexpectedly fast phoneme sequences. (A) True and recognized syllable dynamics of a two-level model when the phoneme sequence is generated with a rate constant of $\kappa^{(1)} = 1.5$ but recognized with a rate constant of $\kappa^{(1)} = 1.0$ (i.e., for the agent, speech was 50% faster than expected). Left: True dynamics of $v^{(2)}$. Right: Recognition dynamics for $v^{(2)}$, which is mostly veridical. (B) Prediction error $\varepsilon^{(2)}$ (on hidden causes) at syllabic level, see equation (6.7). (C) Top: Prediction error $e^{(1)}$ (on hidden states) at phonemic level, see equation (6.8). Bottom: Prediction error $e^{(2)}$ (on hidden states) at syllabic level.

6.7   Discussion

We have presented a model of how perception may be implemented by a dynamic agent: Sensory input is generated by a hierarchy of dynamic systems in the environment (Friston et al., 2006; Kiebel et al., 2008; Kiebel et al., 2009b). We couple this dynamic system, via sensory sampling, to our recognition system implementing the inversion dynamics (figure 6.1). The recognition system minimizes a proxy for surprise or model evidence; the negative free energy (equation 6.6). To do this, the states of the recognition system move on manifolds, defined through the free energy by the generative model. Here, we used a hierarchy of SHCs as a generative model, so that the manifold changes continuously at various timescales. The inferred SHC states never reach a fixed point but are perpetually following a trajectory through state space, in the attempt to mirror the generative dynamics of the environment. When sensory input is unexpected (see third and fourth simulation, figures 6.5 and 6.6, plates 16 and 17), the system uses the prediction error to change its representation rapidly, at all levels, such that it best explains the sensory stream.

We have shown that SHCs can be used as generative models for online recognition of sensory dynamics. In particular, we have provided proof-of-concept that sensory input generated by these hierarchies can be filtered (in a Bayesian sense) or deconvolved to disclose the hidden states causing that input. This is a nontrivial observation because nonlinear, hierarchical, and stochastic dynamical systems are difficult to invert online (Judd & Smith, 2004; Budhiraja, Chen, & Lee, 2007). However, we found that the inversion of models based on SHCs is relatively simple. Furthermore, the implicit recognition scheme appears robust to noise and deviations from true model parameters. This suggests that SHCs may be a candidate for neuronal models that contend with the same problem of deconvolving causes from sensory consequences. Moreover, hierarchical SHCs seem, in principle, an appropriate description of natural sequential input, which is usually generated by our own body or other agents, and can be described as a mixture of transients and discrete events.

In general, appropriate dynamic models of the environment may be requisite to make strong predictions about observed neuronal dynamics. Given the complexity and detail of neuronal dynamics, one might argue that the identification of appropriate environmental models is a daunting task. However, the "dual-system" approach of modeling both the environment and brain as two coupled nonlinear dynamical systems would essentially recast the question "How does the brain work?" to "What is a good model of the environment that discloses how the brain works?" (see, e.g., Chiel & Beer, 1997; Proekt et al., 2008). This approach has the advantage that environmental models, which cannot be inverted, disqualify themselves and are unlikely to be used as generative models by the brain. The main advantage of this approach, given invertible generative models, is that it results in optimal (under some assumptions) Bayesian update equations, which can be used to predict observed neuronal dynamics. Here, we assume that the brain uses the same optimal inference for a given inference problem as we find with optimal Bayesian inference. This approach has been used successfully for functional magnetic resonance imaging (fMRI) (called "computational fMRI"; O'Doherty, Dayan, Friston, Critchley, & Dolan, 2003; Friston & Dolan, 2010), and may also apply to observations of brain dynamics at different spatiotemporal scales.

In this chapter, we used a generative model that was formally identical to the process actually generating sensory input. We did this for simplicity; however, any generative model that could predict sensory input would be sufficient. In one sense, there is no true model because it is impossible to disambiguate between models that have different forms but make the same predictions. This is a common issue in ill-posed inverse problems, where there are an infinite number of models that could explain the same data. In this context, the best model is usually identified as the most parsimonious. The advantage of using Bayesian inference is that the approximated model evidence can also be used for comparison between different models (agents), when they are embedded in an otherwise identical environment (and receive the same sensory input). We did not use this selection technique in this chapter because we would have found that the model we used was the best (given that it recapitulated the causal structure of the environment). However, for unknown environments, the use of the model evidence (approximated by the negative free energy) may provide a way of comparing (and selecting) among alternative models.

The dual-system approach offers also an interesting perspective for machine learning: Typically, recurrent neural networks (RNNs), either in their continuous or discrete formulation, are used as a coarse-grained model of real brain networks in classification applications (e.g., Schrauwen & Büsing, 2009). For example, equation (6.1) is nothing more than a continuous RNN with specifically chosen connectivity weights to construct SHCs. In RNNs, as they are typically used in machine learning, the internal states, after some computation time, provide input to some classifier. With the dual-system approach, we go a little further: Rather than using equation (6.1) directly, we use dynamic Bayesian filtering, where the generative model is an RNN. As we have seen in our simulations, the agent's dynamics, which result from the inversion of the RNN equations (equation 6.1), show phenomena (fast adjustment to changes in environment, prediction, prediction error, robustness to speed changes) that are reminiscent of real neuronal phenomena and are probably more difficult to achieve by using equation (6.1) directly. In particular, the rapid adjustment of the agent dynamics in case of an unexpected deviation is probably very hard if not impossible to obtain with conventional RNN dynamics. This is because RNN dynamics have their intrinsic timescale (rate constant κ in equation 6.1), which prescribes the speed of their dynamics. Fast changes in their hidden states can only be induced by fast changes to their input. We have shown cases when hidden state dynamics are much faster than the timescale of the input (e.g., figure 6.5C, lower row; plate 16). These fast agent dynamics were caused by the mismatch between relatively slow input dynamics and internal prediction dynamics at the same timescale. Although using Bayesian update equations for RNNs requires more computation, we believe that the potential of this approach outweighs this disadvantage by far. Of course, for this approach to work, one cannot invert any RNN model: One must carefully select the generative model (or learn the network parameterization from input observed in nature like speech or kinematics). In our case, we showed that SHCs, which are a specific parameterization of an RNN, ordered in hierarchies, are a promising starting point for a generative model of sequences of sequences observed in nature.

References

Afraimovich, V. S., Rabinovich, M. I., & Varona, P. (2004a). Heteroclinic contours in neural ensembles and the winnerless competition principle. *International Journal of Bifurcation and Chaos in Applied Sciences and Engineering, 14*, 1195–1208.

Afraimovich, V. S., Zhigulin, V. P., & Rabinovich, M. I. (2004b). On the origin of reproducible sequential activity in neural circuits. *Chaos (Woodbury, N.Y.), 14*, 1123–1129.

Beal, M. J. (2003) Variational algorithms for approximate Bayesian inference. PhD. Thesis, Gatsby Computational Neuroscience Unit, University College London.

Breakspear, M., Roberts, J. A., Terry, J. R., Rodrigues, S., Mahant, N., & Robinson, P. A. (2006). A unifying explanation of primary generalized seizures through nonlinear brain modeling and bifurcation analysis. *Cerebral Cortex, 16*, 1296–1313.

Budhiraja, A., Chen, L. J., & Lee, C. (2007). A survey of numerical methods for nonlinear filtering problems. *Physica D. Nonlinear Phenomena, 230*, 27–36.

Cessac, B., & Samuelides, M. (2007). From neuron to neural networks dynamics. *European Physical Journal. Special Topics, 142*, 7–88.

Chiel, H. J., & Beer, R. D. (1997). The brain has a body: adaptive behavior emerges from interactions of nervous system, body and environment. *Trends in Neurosciences, 20*, 553–557.

Coull, J. T. (1998). Neural correlates of attention and arousal: insights from electrophysiology, functional neuroimaging and psychopharmacology. *Progress in Neurobiology, 55*, 343–361.

Craig, A. D. (2003). Interoception: the sense of the physiological condition of the body. *Current Opinion in Neurobiology, 13*, 500–505.

Creutzfeldt, O., Hellweg, F. C., & Schreiner, C. (1980). Thalamocortical transformation of responses to complex auditory-stimuli. *Experimental Brain Research, 39*, 87–104.

Daunizeau, J., Friston, K. J., & Kiebel, S. J. (2009). Variational Bayesian identification and prediction of stochastic nonlinear dynamic causal models. *Physica D. Nonlinear Phenomena, 238*, 2089–2118.

Davis, M. H., & Johnsrude, I. S. (2003). Hierarchical processing in spoken language comprehension. *Journal of Neuroscience, 23*, 3423–3431.

Deco, G., & Rolls, E. T. (2004). A neurodynamical cortical model of visual attention and invariant object recognition. *Vision Research, 44*, 621–642.

Deco, G., Jirsa, V. K., Robinson, P. A., Breakspear, M., & Friston, K. (2008). The dynamic brain: from spiking neurons to neural masses and cortical fields. *PLoS Computational Biology, 4*, e1000092.

Erlhagen, W., & Schoner, G. (2002). Dynamic field theory of movement preparation. *Psychological Review, 109*, 545–572.

Foulke, E., & Sticht, T. G. (1969). Review of research on intelligibility and comprehension of accelerated speech. *Psychological Bulletin, 72*, 50.

Friston, K. J. (1997). Transients, metastability, and neuronal dynamics. *NeuroImage, 5*, 164–171.

Friston, K. (2005). A theory of cortical responses. *Philosophical Transactions of the Royal Society B-Biological Sciences, 360*, 815–836.

Friston, K. (2008). Hierarchical models in the brain. *PLoS Computational Biology, 4*, e1000211.

Friston, K. (2010). The free-energy principle: a unified brain theory? *Nature Reviews. Neuroscience, 11*, 127–138.

Friston, K. J., & Dolan, R. J. (2010). Computational and dynamic models in neuroimaging. *NeuroImage, 52*, 752–765.

Friston, K., Kilner, J., & Harrison, L. (2006). A free energy principle for the brain. *Journal of Physiology, Paris, 100*, 70–87.

Friston, K. J., Trujillo-Barreto, N., & Daunizeau, J. (2008). DEM: a variational treatment of dynamic systems. *NeuroImage, 41*, 849–885.

Giraud, A. L., Lorenzi, C., Ashburner, J., Wable, J., Johnsrude, I., Frackowiak, R., et al. (2000). Representation of the temporal envelope of sounds in the human brain. *Journal of Neurophysiology, 84*, 1588–1598.

Holmberg, M., Gelbart, D., & Hemmert, W. (2007). Speech encoding in a model of peripheral auditory processing: quantitative assessment by means of automatic speech recognition. *Speech Communication, 49*, 917–932.

Jäger, H. (2001). The "Echo State" Approach to Analysing and Training Recurrent Neural Networks. Technical Report. German National Research Center for Information Technology.

Jirsa, V. K., Fink, P., Foo, P., & Kelso, J. A. S. (2000). Parametric stabilization of biological coordination: a theoretical model. *Journal of Biological Physics, 26*, 85–112.

Judd, K., & Smith, L. A. (2004). Indistinguishable states II—the imperfect model scenario. *Physica D. Nonlinear Phenomena, 196*, 224–242.

Kiebel, S. J., Daunizeau, J., & Friston, K. J. (2008). A hierarchy of time-scales and the brain. *PLoS Computational Biology, 4*, e1000209.

Kiebel, S. J., Daunizeau, J., & Friston, K. J. (2009a). Perception and hierarchical dynamics. *Frontiers in Neuroinformatics, 3*, 20.

Kiebel, S. J., von Kriegstein, K., Daunizeau, J., & Friston, K. J. (2009b). Recognizing sequences of sequences. *PLoS Computational Biology, 5*, e1000464.

Long, M. A., & Fee, M. S. (2008). Using temperature to analyse temporal dynamics in the songbird motor pathway. *Nature, 456*, 189–194.

Ma, W. J., Beck, J. M., Latham, P. E., & Pouget, A. (2006). Bayesian inference with probabilistic population codes. *Nature Neuroscience, 9*, 1432–1438.

Maass, W., Natschlager, T., & Markram, H. (2002). Real-time computing without stable states: a new framework for neural computation based on perturbations. *Neural Computation*, *14*, 2531–2560.

Melcher, D. (2011). Visual stability introduction. *Philosophical Transactions of the Royal Society B-Biological Sciences*, *366*, 468–475.

Nahum, M., Nelken, I., & Ahissar, M. (2008). Low-level information and high-level perception: the case of speech in noise. *PLoS Biology*, *6*, 978–991.

O'Doherty, J. P., Dayan, P., Friston, K., Critchley, H., & Dolan, R. J. (2003). Temporal difference models and reward-related learning in the human brain. *Neuron*, *38*, 329–337.

Overath, T., Kumar, S., von Kriegstein, K., & Griffiths, T. D. (2008). Encoding of spectral correlation over time in auditory cortex. *Journal of Neuroscience*, *28*, 13268–13273.

Pearlmuttter, B. A. (1989). Learning state space trajectories in recurrent neural networks. *Neural Computation*, *1*, 263–269.

Pisoni, D. B. (1993). Long-term-memory in speech-perception—some new findings on talker variability, speaking rate and perceptual-learning. *Speech Communication*, *13*, 109–125.

Poeppel D., Idsardi W.J., van Wassenhove, V. (2008). Speech perception at the interface of neurobiology and linguistics. *Philosophical Transactions of the Royal Society of London. Series B, Biological Sciences*, *363*, 1071–1086.

Proekt, A., Wong, J., Zhurov, Y., Kozlova, N., Weiss, K. R., & Brezina, V. (2008). Predicting adaptive behavior in the environment from central nervous system dynamics. *PLoS ONE*, *3*, e3678.

Rabinovich, M., Huerta, R., & Laurent, G. (2008). Neuroscience—transient dynamics for neural processing. *Science*, *321*, 48–50.

Rabinovich, M. I., Varona, P., Selverston, A. I., & Abarbanel, H. D. I. (2006). Dynamical principles in neuroscience. *Reviews of Modern Physics*, *78*, 1213–1265.

Rumelhart, D. E., Hinton, G. E., & Williams, R. J. (1986). Learning representations by back-propagating errors. *Nature*, *323*, 533–536.

Sandamirskaya, Y., & Schoner, G. (2010). An embodied account of serial order: how instabilities drive sequence generation. *Neural Networks*, *23*, 1164–1179.

Schrauwen, B., & Büsing, L. (2009) A hierarchy of recurrent networks for speech recognition. In Proceedings of 23nd Annual Conference on Neural Information Processing Systems (NIPS 2009).

Sen, K., Theunissen, F. E., & Doupe, A. J. (2001). Feature analysis of natural sounds in the songbird auditory forebrain. *Journal of Neurophysiology*, *86*, 1445–1458.

Sumner, C. J., Lopez-Poveda, E. A., O'Mard, L. P., & Meddis, R. (2002). A revised model of the inner-hair cell and auditory-nerve complex. *Journal of the Acoustical Society of America*, *111*, 2178–2188.

Sussillo, D., & Abbott, L. F. (2009). Generating coherent patterns of activity from chaotic neural networks. *Neuron*, *63*, 544–557.

Varona, P., Rabinovich, M. I., Selverston, A. I., & Arshavsky, Y. I. (2002). Winnerless competition between sensory neurons generates chaos: a possible mechanism for molluscan hunting behavior. *Chaos (Woodbury, N.Y.)*, *12*, 672–677.

Vaughan, N., Storzbach, D., & Furukawa, I. (2006). Sequencing versus nonsequencing working memory in understanding of rapid speech by older listeners. *Journal of the American Academy of Audiology*, *17*, 506–518.

Versfeld, N. J., & Dreschler, W. A. (2002). The relationship between the intelligibility of time-compressed speech and speech in noise in young and elderly listeners. *Journal of the Acoustical Society of America*, *111*, 401–408.

Verstraeten, D., Schrauwen, B., Stroobandt, D., & Van Campenhout, J. (2005). Isolated word recognition with the liquid state machine: a case study. *Information Processing Letters*, *95*, 521–528.

von Kriegstein, K., Patterson, R. D., & Griffiths, T. D. (2008). Task-dependent modulation of medial geniculate body is behaviorally relevant for speech recognition. *Current Biology*, *18*, 1855–1859.

Wang, X., Lu, T., Bendor, D., & Bartlett, E. (2008). Neural coding of temporal information in auditory thalamus and cortex. *Neuroscience*, *154*, 294–303.

Williams, R. J., & Zipser, D. (1989). A learning algorithm for continually running fully recurrent neural networks. *Neural Computation*, *1*, 270–280.

7   The Stability of Information Flows in the Brain

Mikhail I. Rabinovich, Christian Bick, and Pablo Varona

Summary

In this chapter, we introduce a novel concept and its corresponding dynamical object to analyze brain activity: the informational flow in phase space (IFPS). This concept is directly related to the sequential dynamics of metastable states that are activated by inputs that do not destroy the origin of a competitive process. For the successful execution of a cognitive function, an IFPS as a function of time has to be a laminar (non-chaotic); that is, a stable flow. Such stability guarantees the reproducibility and robustness of the cognitive activity. Based on the requirement of IFPS stability, we analyze here the stability of sequential working memory and discuss the dynamical origin of the finite working memory capacity. We also build a dynamical model of information binding for transients that describes, for example, the interaction of different sensory information flows that are generated in parallel and discuss the stability limit of sequential language processing. Finally, we consider the role of noise on the temporal dynamics of sequential decision making.

7.1   How to Define an Information Flow in the Brain?

When we try to understand brain activity from the point of view of information processing, we face two essential questions: (1) In which space do we have to consider such processing? (2) How is it related to the traditional probabilistic description of information? Let us discuss these issues.

The brain's hierarchical organization (Hawkings & Blakeslee, 2004), that is, from the perception levels to the complex subcore and cortex structures, supports the idea of an also hierarchical organization of its information flows. In fact, the popular view of the existence of one-directional flows of sensory information (which are transferred through centers of preliminary processing to the cortex decision-making centers and behavior generation) does look very attractive. However, the reality is more challenging. The brain is characterized by a huge amount of informational feedback. This is a mechanism to control sensory input: By concentrating attention, the brain chooses what sensory information is critical for executing cognitive functions to survive in extreme conditions. The idea of a hierarchical organization of brain informational flows is very practical and promising (Yamashita & Tani, 2008), not only referring to space but also to time, as we will discuss later.

Regarding the second question, the functional role of information (content and meaning) in cognitive processes cannot be directly measured with a traditional statistical approach. Although Shannon information (Shannon, 1948) has made many valuable contributions and has many very important uses in neuroscience, it is somehow restricted to assess several functional properties of information, in particular the stability of the processes of information transmission and creation. Because the generation of, for example, a motor program or speech requires a sequence of signals, the information flow has to be organized in a specific temporal order that must be kept. In fact, such an idea can be traced back to Wiener, who recognized the importance of temporal ordering in the inference of causal relations (Wiener, 1956). Granger formalized Wiener's idea in terms of autoregressive models of time series (Granger, 1969), and the technique now bears his name. However, we cannot directly use this idea because we first need to find an instrument for the qualitative analysis of dynamical informational flows.

Now we are ready for a definition: let us name *cognitive (mental) information flow* to a specific sequence of items. Note that this concept does not refer to the number of items or events, but to a particular relationship between specific items ordered in time. In contrast to the traditional view, it is our suggestion to consider the informational flows in the phase space of a corresponding dynamical model as an alternative to the physical space of the brain. In other words, an informational flow is a flow along a chain of metastable states. The end of the chain is a state corresponding to a final or intermittent decision or action. One of the critically important features of such an informational sequence is its stability for recalling, which guarantees the usefulness of the sequential information (behavioral or cognitive). The information flow that we have just defined naturally satisfies the causal-answer relationship and is the basis for solving problems that are related to overcoming uncertainty and to generating a decision—the new information. For cognitive processing, a flow in a phase space—a spatiotemporal representation of information—is a natural method that provides the continuality of the processing.

It is important to recall that the brain is not a classical dynamical system (see chapter 4), but in some sense it is a set of dynamical systems that work hierarchically in different timescales and time windows (Hasson, Yang, Vallines, Heeger, & Rubin, 2008), each of them representing a dynamical execution of different perceptional, emotional, or cognitive functions. Thus, several parallel informational flows can coexist but in different phase subspaces. In this view, the information prepared by low levels of the hierarchy are presented to the upper levels as excitatory inputs that can select the building blocks of the heteroclinic channel— the active metastable states. The quantitative description of information flow in phase space can be done by computing the sequence of mutual information along the heteroclinic channel. Another quantitative characteristic of information flow along a heteroclinic channel is the information flow capacity (C_{IF}), which we introduce at the end of section 7.4.

7.2   Working Memory Capacity

The stability conditions of the models that we have discussed in chapter 4 provide us with a very powerful tool to address and predict several dynamical aspects of brain activity. In particular, we can calculate how long a typical heteroclinic channel can be (i.e., how many steps the sequential switching can have). Let us consider here the example of how to use this approach to find the origin of the limited capacity of working memory (Bick & Rabinovich, 2009b).

Working memory (WM) is the ability transiently to hold in mind and manipulate several items that are involved in a given information processing or in actions such as thinking, planning, or producing a motor output. Tasks involving WM include, for example, remembering a sequence of statements that we recently heard in a speech or following directions to an unknown place. Language, as a sequential activity, is also based on WM. However, the capacity of WM is limited, and this is one of the reasons why the metaphorical term "blackboard of the mind" has become popular to describe WM.

The capacity of sequential WM is defined as the number of items that can be recalled correctly after a WM task and varies among different individuals, depending also on age and health conditions. Numerous studies have led to the generally accepted view that the effective capacity for healthy subjects ranges between three and seven items (Swanson,

1999; Oberauer & Kliegl, 2006; Rouder et al., 2008; Edin et al., 2009). This limit has led to coining of the term "magical number seven" (Miller, 1956) in conjunction with WM. In fact, this number is not strictly seven, but something in the range three to seven depending on the subject.

Information processing related to WM activity can be represented in an abstract space (the phase space of the network that implements the working memory) as a continuous flow of "liquid phase": The incoming information encoded in a spatiotemporal manner excites the specific network with a functional reverberate loop that sustains the corresponding information item for a finite time (based on a transient attractor). The item networks are coupled through inhibitory interconnections with each other and build a macroscopic network that keeps the whole sequence of items. The cooperative dynamics of this macro-network can be based on the winnerless competition (WLC) principle (see chapter 4) and guarantee that the sequential items are recalled in the right order. Thus all three processes—storing, maintaining, and retrieving of sequential information—in fact can be thought of as continuous transient dynamical activity of hierarchically organized functional neuronal networks (Rabinovich & Varona, 2011). This perspective has also been discussed in another model based on an echo state network (Pascanu & Jaeger, 2011).

As many experiments show (for a review, see Jensen & Mazaheri, 2010), functional inhibition is reflected in oscillatory activity in the brain at the frequency band of 8–13 Hz (alpha rhythm). The alpha activity can facilitate sequential inhibition by reducing the activity of a given network. There are several models of WM based on the idea that all steps of WM information processing in the engaged distributed networks are reflected by neuronal synchronization in the gamma band (30–80 Hz) accompanied by a theta (5–8 Hz) or an alpha band (Lisman & Idiart, 1995; Roopun et al., 2008; Tort et al., 2008; Schroeder & Lakatos, 2009). It is reasonable to hypothesize that such synchronization leads to a temporal coordination between the fast one-item processing and the slow sequential-item interaction. One can expect that this coordination supports the robustness of information processing and contributes to a larger WM capacity (Palva, Monto, Kulashekhar, & Palva, 2010). Now we show that sequential WM capacity in the context of our model is limited by conditions of the retrieval process stability (Bick & Rabinovich, 2009a, 2009b). The dynamical model for sequential WM that we would like to discuss here is based on WLC between informational items (Bick & Rabinovich, 2009b). These items are represented in the phase space by saddle fixed points and the mnemonic recall by a trajectory in a stable heteroclinic channel (SHC) (Rabinovich et al., 2008a; Rabinovich et al., 2008b) (see chapters 4 and 14). In contrast to attractor dynamics, the transient itself reflects the sequential memory. Under certain simplifying assumptions, there is an upper bound on the number of items that can be stored in this sequential WM model when implemented by inhibitory-coupled neuronal clusters. Dynamics of such information items can be described by a generalized Lotka–Volterra model

$$\tau_i \frac{dx_i^m}{dt} = x_i^m \left[\sigma_i^m - \sum_{j=1}^{N} \rho_{ij}^m x_j^m - \sum_{k=1}^{M} \sum_{j=1}^{N} \xi_{ij}^{mk} x_j^k \right]$$

$$i, j = 1 \dots N \qquad m, k = 1 \dots M$$

(7.1)

where $x_i^m \geq 0$ represents the instantaneous amplitude of the (i^m)-mode, τ_i is the time constant that for working memory is around 1–5 s, $\sigma_i^m \geq 0$ is the growth rate for the mode depending on an external stimulus, and $\rho_{ij}^m \geq 0$ and $\xi_{ij}^{mk} \geq 0$ are the interaction strengths between the modes. Here, m, k indicate different brain activity modalities (for simplicity, in our example on working memory we will use $M = 1$) and i, j indicate different modes within the same modality. The parameters ρ_{ij}^m and ξ_{ij}^{mk} can depend on the stimuli. In the case of a single family modality (i.e., $M = 1$), we have the traditional Lotka–Volterra model. One of the remarkable features of this model is the existence in the phase space (for a wide range of control parameters) of a stable heteroclinic channel that corresponds to robust sequential switching from one metastable state to other (Afraimovich et al., 2004; Bick & Rabinovich, 2009a; Rabinovich, Afraimovich, & Varona, 2010; Rabinovich et al., 2008).

Bick and Rabinovich (2009b) assumed that the relative connection strengths are sampled from uniform distributions and cannot exceed an order of magnitude. They found that the bound for the number of items is about seven. This is remarkable because the model dynamics exhibit the very same inherent bound for sequential WM capacity as given by the "magical number." Let us briefly explain this result. Sequential WM dynamics is separated into two stages: the storage of sensory information and its retrieval. Storage means initiation of a specific pattern in the phase space of the corresponding dynamical system by both sensory input and the contents of WM. Based on the hypothesis that WLC between different informational items is the main mechanism for the correct retrieval in sequential WM, Bick and Rabinovich (2009b) analyzed the structural stability of sequential switching; that is, the correct reproducibility of the sequence of the informational items (which is the key property for memory performance). The stability conditions require a strong enough inhibition in the WM random network, and, what is a key point, the level of the inhibition increases exponentially with the WM capacity. If we suppose that the ratio between the level of external inhibition and the self-inhibition ρ_{ij}/ρ_{ii} is about 20 (large enough from the neurobiological point of view), the number of successfully recalled informational items, according to the exponential law, has to be between seven and eight (see figure 7.1). Recently, a functional magnetic resonance imaging (fMRI) study (Edin et al., 2009) has provided experimental evidence for the dependence of the capacity limitation for visual WM on the level of inhibition.

WM capacity depends on both the environment and the individual itself. In our case, this is reflected in the model's architecture through subject- and environment-dependent parameters (i.e., connection strengths that represent lateral inhibition). In particular, the dependence on the individual has to be emphasized, as it modulates how an external stimulus actually changes the parameters themselves. For example, "cognitive control" plays a role in the individual perception of a painful stimulus because it determines how the external stimulus is translated into parameter changes. Therefore, individual traits can modulate the subjective experience, leading to a subject-dependent experience of the same stimulus. If we assume a relationship between the level of

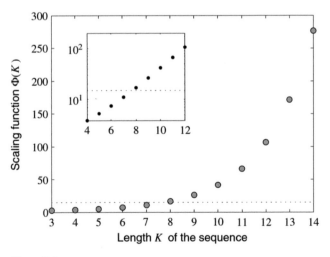

Figure 7.1
Dependence of sequential memory capacity on the normalized level of network inhibition $\Phi(K) = \rho_{ij}/\rho_{ii}$. Adapted from Bick and Rabinovich (2009b).

pain and inhibition, the suggested model can be used to predict the dependence of working memory capacity in the presence of pain. More specifically, assume that a painful stimulus $P > 0$ will result in the modulation of lateral inhibition $\rho_{ij} = \rho_{ij}(P)$. For P small, we can write

$$\rho_{ij}(P) = \rho_{ij}(0) + \frac{d\rho_{ij}(P)}{dP}\bigg|_{P=0} P + O(P^2). \tag{7.2}$$

Ignoring higher-order terms, the parameter

$$h := \frac{d\rho_{ij}(P)}{dP}\bigg|_{P=0}$$

determines how the painful stimulus influences the dynamics.

To get a dynamical bound on the capacity of sequential working memory, we can consider the bounds on the elements of the connection matrix: ρ_u denoting the upper bound for the off-diagonal elements and ρ_l the lower bound for the remaining non-diagonal matrix elements. We have $\rho_l > \rho_u$, and their ratio is of crucial importance (Bick & Rabinovich, 2009a; Bick & Rabinovich, 2009b). Analyzing the influence of pain on these bounds gives functions $\rho_x(P) = \rho_x + hP$ for $x \in \{u, l\}$. Hence,

$$\frac{\rho_l(P)}{\rho_u(P)} - \frac{\rho_l(0)}{\rho_u(0)} = \frac{hP(\rho_u - \rho_l)}{\rho_u(\rho_u + hP)}. \tag{7.3}$$

For $h > 0$, increasing P lowers the bound on relative connection strength in our neural interpretation. Therefore, sequential WM capacity is increased. Conversely for h negative, a nonzero value of P separates the bounds further, resulting in decreased sequential WM capacity.

7.3   Limits of Sequential Language Processing

"Language, like a beaver's dam, is a collectively constructed transgenerational phenomenon. But human language, unlike the beaver's dam, provides our species with a distinctive, general purpose cognitive niche: a persisting, though never stationary, symbolic edifice whose critical role in promoting thought and reason remains surprisingly ill-understood" (Clark, 2005). At the same time, processing language is a neural feature that dominates our everyday lives. How does language processing work? Here, we want to consider the problem of message transduction from a speaker to a listener from a dynamical point of view. It is well known that in a real-world context, language contains much more information than just a formal message, such as information about the speaker; for example, about his social background, his emotional state of mind, and other things. Within this section, however, we want to assume that only the formal message plays a role. How is such a message transmitted to the listener?

Usually, language is organized hierarchically. Words, which are themselves collections of phonemes, make up sentences, which again make up paragraphs or other larger collections of information. In this hierarchy, sequential ordering plays a prominent role as it is an essential part of the semantic and syntactic structure. Rather than talking about words in a classical sense, we should consider *informational units*. A sequentially ordered sequence of these informational units then constitutes an *informational sentence* (i.e., the shortest form of a message). Messages usually consist of several such sentences. How can these informational units—we will also refer to them as *linguistic modes*—be interpreted? In our context, they can be seen as entities that carry semantic information, such as things like "red apple" or "table" and relations thereof "on the," which can relate two or more objects. These informational units combined give the informational sentence "red apple on the table." Although intermediate levels of combining information are present in natural language (e.g., "chunking," phrases, relative clauses), we want to restrict ourselves here to two levels in the hierarchy, one to describe informational units and a second for informational sentences as sequences of informational units.

We want to formalize this intuition. Suppose the speaker wants to convey a message. He then has to decompose the message into informational sentences, which themselves consist of informational units. A sequence of informational units is uttered as a sequence of phonetic words to the listener. The listener now has to interpret this sequence of phonetic words to extract the message. His brain has to be capable of interpreting the (language-dependent) phonetic words to recover the informational units while doing an online integration to reconstruct the informational sentences and finally the message itself. The dynamical model that we propose consists of two unidirectionally coupled dynamical systems, one for the speaker and one for the listener. Each of these systems consists of coupled dynamical systems with distinct timescales representing the different levels in the hierarchy. Informational units and informational sentences are represented by saddle sets in the phase space of the system corresponding to the level in the hierarchy (see figure 7.2). Temporal relations in the form of sequential ordering can be realized as heteroclinic connections between these saddle sets (SHCs; cf. chapter 4).

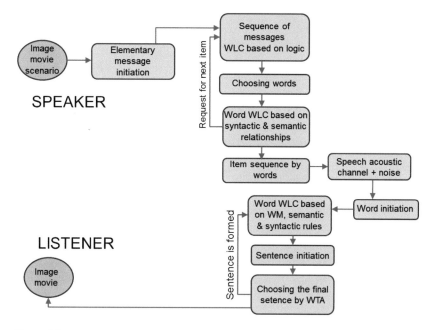

Figure 7.2
Schematic of message transduction. Here for simplicity, we name the informational units as words.

Through the hierarchy, sequences of informational units will be identified with an informational sentence.

This dynamical system can be described by the following set of differential equations. Let Q denote the message to be transmitted. The speaker's dynamics are given by

$$\tau_R \frac{dR_j}{dt} = R_j \left(\alpha_j(Q,V) - \sum_{k=1}^{M} \beta_{jk}(Q,V)R_j \right)$$

$$\tau_V \frac{dV_i}{dt} = V_i \left(\gamma_i(R) - \sum_{k=0}^{N} \delta_{ik}(R)V_i \right), \tag{7.4}$$

where $j = 1,\ldots, M$ and $i = 0,\ldots, N$. Here, R corresponds to the activity of the speaker's informational units and V to the activity of the informational sentences. The dependency of the parameters on the dynamical variables will be described below. With $\tilde{V}$ being the distorted sequence of words uttered by the speaker, the listener's dynamics are described by

$$\tau_W \frac{dW_i}{dt} = W_i \left(\theta_i(\tilde{V}, S) - \sum_{k=0}^{N'} \iota_{ik}(\tilde{V}, S) W_j \right)$$

$$\tau_S \frac{dS_j}{dt} = S_j \left(\kappa_j(W) - \sum_{k=1}^{M'} \lambda_{jk}(W) S_k \right),$$

(7.5)

where $i = 0, \ldots, N'$ and $j = 1, \ldots, M'$. Correspondingly, W and S stand for the activity of the listener's informational units and sentences. All parameters denoted by lowercase Greek letters have positive, real values, and $\tau_V < \tau_R$, $\tau_W < \tau_S$ denote the timescales.

The speaker's dynamics are closely related to the concept of hierarchically coupled heteroclinic channels as proposed by Kiebel, Daunizeau, and Friston (2008) (cf. chapter 6). When the speaker initiates the transduction of a message, the formation of informational sentences corresponds to the formation of a stable heteroclinic channel in the topmost level of the speaker's dynamical system. Because of the nature of the channel, the dynamics will follow the heteroclinic sequence, leading to sequential activity of the nodes corresponding to the informational sentences. While an informational sentence is active, it imposes a stable heteroclinic sequence on the lower level, which corresponds to the corresponding temporally ordered sequence of informational units. The result is a sequence of sequences of informational units that is uttered to the listener in the form of a sequence of phonetic words in a specific language. It is important to emphasize the difference between a sequence of informational units and a sequence of phonetic words in a language: A sequence of informational units is a temporal, logically sound sequence of semantic units, whereas a sequence of phonetic words is a grammatical sentence in a language. Furthermore, some of the information in the sequence of informational units will not necessarily be contained in the sequence of phonetic words but might result in a change of prosody (e.g., different stress patterns) or other mechanisms that carry semantic information.

The uttered words will reach the listener through a noisy channel. The listener has to use his own lexicon of informational units and sentences to recover the message. Note that such a lexicon is different and complimentary to a lexicon of phonetic words. We suggest that the mechanism for this reconstruction is competitive interaction in a non-autonomous dynamical system that is driven by the input provided by the speaker. This is in contrast to probabilistic models that have been proposed before, and it is important to emphasize here the principal differences of a dynamic approach versus the traditional structured probabilistic approaches to semantic cognition (see, e.g., McClelland et al., 2010). The task of the listener is not just to discriminate between predefined structures, but learning should ideally also enable the addition of new, previously unknown items through a dynamical process. Input by a speaker's informational unit will activate a subset of the listener's informational units; namely, the units that are "similar." Here, *similar* means for example that it could be a synonym (semantically similar unit) or it could be an informational unit corresponding to a phonetically similar word (but a potential mismatch in semantic information). Each case corresponds to a match in the corresponding lexicon, the first in the lexicon of informational units, the second in the phonetic lexicon. At the same time, the upper level tries to infer the informational sentence from the temporal sequence of informational units through bottom-up interaction, possibly similar to the activation pattern in the TRACE model (e.g., McClelland & Elman, 1986), where initially equivalent items are activated simultaneously. Ideally, this level could provide feedback to the lower level, resulting in anticipation of upcoming words (Stephens, Silbert, & Hasson, 2010). The resulting sequence of informational sentences then corresponds to the message that was received by the listener.

Let us illustrate the above by giving an example. Imagine we want to tell the fairy tale *Three Little Pigs* (Halliwell, 1842) to our grandson. The first step of telling the story is to sequence it into sentences; for example,

The three little pigs built their new houses.
The first pig built his house out of straw.
The second pig built his house out of sticks.
The third pig built his house out of bricks.
The wolf huffed and puffed and blew the straw house down.
The wolf huffed and puffed and blew the stick house down.
The wolf huffed and puffed but couldn't blow the third house down.
The wolf ran to the woods and never came back again.

Every one of these sentences now contains various informational units. The second sentence, for example, contains the items "first pig," "house," and "straw," and the verb "built" relates those three items. Note that informational units are difficult to define, and our suggestion in this example depends on intuition. The result of the sequencing process is a sequence of sequences of informational units.

It is important to note the similarities between the model of message transduction and working memory. In fact, it is well accepted that working memory plays a key role in language processing. For our model, working memory can be seen as a key ingredient; an informational sentence imposes a stable heteroclinic channel on the word level. This can be interpreted as a sequence of items being loaded into working memory. Correspondingly, the message itself is such a sequence of informational sentences that are active in working memory. A restriction on the number of items that can be held in working memory, which comes from the conditions on the existence of a stable heteroclinic channel (cf. earlier), now corresponds to a restriction of the number of informational units that a message can consist of in our language model. In other words, our model predicts a maximum number of informational units and informational sentences that a message will be split up into by the speaker.

The situation is a bit more subtle for the listener's dynamics. If we assume that the input by the speaker not only activates the corresponding informational units and sentences but also leads to an active formation of a stable heteroclinic sequence in the phase space of the listener's dynamical system, then the results for working memory also carry over to the listener's dynamics. In fact, such an assumption is not unreasonable, because if such a structure in the phase space is not built up, a recall of the information that was just processed would be impossible. Being able to recall, however, should be one feature of "understanding the message."

The limit of informational units, which is induced by limited working memory capacity, is a limit on abstraction representations of information. How can such a limitation be quantified in the context of natural language processing? It is wrong to assume that such a limit will just translate to a limit of the number of words in a sentence, as words and informational units are usually not in a directly corresponding one-to-one relationship. If one had a (language-dependent) estimation of the average number of words per informational unit, this would result in an average limit of the number of words, depending on the language. Thus, the question that we have to address is more general: How can one quantify the number of informational units that are present in a sentence in natural language? Semantic complexity measures (Pollard & Biermann, 2000) could provide a way to measure the amount of information that is present in natural language. Moreover, there are approaches that relate language and working memory through cognitive load theory (Sweller, van Merrienboer, & Paas, 1998), which has mostly been used for instructional purposes. Based on this theory, bounds for the length of an optimally understandable sentence were investigated (Mikk, 2008).

The model we proposed above gives rise to additional mathematical challenges. The restrictions that working memory imposes for the speaker carry over only when there is a unidirectional coupling. For the listener, a feedback connection leads to the desirable feature of anticipation, but also the speaker's dynamics feedback could lead to the accommodation of sentences of different lengths. Recurrently interacting heteroclinic dynamics, however, are still poorly studied. Moreover, the learning rule to generate the input-dependent heteroclinic channel in the phase space of the listener's dynamical system has yet to be formulated, a necessity for the applicability of the results. We hope that future work will give further insight to the underlying dynamical mechanisms of language processing.

7.4   Interaction of Heteroclinic Channels: Binding Problem

Suppose we are tasting a fine wine. Although its flavor is typically perceived as a unitary perceptual experience, this perception reflects processing of inputs from multiple sensory systems: from gestation (through the stimulation of receptors on the tongue and in the mouth), smell (through the stimulation of receptors in the olfactory mucosa), and oral somato-sensation (through the stimulation of diverse receptors in the oral cavity, providing information about viscosity, temperature, pungency, and spiciness). Even though they derive from signals transmitted over several nerves, flavors often appear remarkably coherent in phenomenal perception. Integrating information across the senses enhances our ability to detect and classify objects in the environment. For example, to find flowers, honeybees use the same multimodality approach—their sensory and central systems process in an integrative way at least three flows of sensory information (i.e., the color, odor, and taste of flowers). How does the brain do it?

Multi-electrode recordings from different areas of sensory systems in different animals have shown that sensory information on the first level of processing is encoded as spatiotemporal patterns by neural networks that implement a WLC interaction of different dynamical modes (variables). In the phase space, such dynamics is represented by a heteroclinic channel. Motivated by the multisensory dynamics observed in neural systems, Rabinovich et al. (2010) built a model that describes the heteroclinic integration of channels representing different modalities (binding dynamics). This model is described by model (7.1) with $M > 1$.

Our interest aims to describe the neural dynamics associated with the binding problem in terms of a sequence of metastable states in the phase space. Each metastable state marked by the index i is represented in neuronal space by a distributed set of excited neurons participating in a given brain mode. We denote the ith mode as $x_i(t)U_i(k)$, where $U_i(k)$ is the normalized ratio of activity of the kth member of the ith set averaged in time, and $x_i(t) \geq 0$ represents the level of the activity of the ith mode. Such a set is the result of the temporal self-organization in a complex neuronal system. Metastable states on the x_i axes, $x_i = $ const $\neq 0$, are saddles. We suppose that the interaction between different modalities is weak. By keeping just the simplest nonlinearities, we can suggest a phenomenological model of heteroclinic binding in the form of kinetic equations, in particular, as the generalized Lotka–Volterra model (7.1).

The main results of theoretical and computational analyses in Rabinovich et al. (2010) can be summarized as follows: (i) for a wide range of control parameters (i.e., the levels of excitation and inhibition) in the phase space of model (7.1), there exists an object that the authors named a multimodality heteroclinic channel (see figure 7.3), and the trajectories in the vicinity/inside of this dynamical object represent an integrated (binded) information flow of different modalities (see figure 7.4); (ii) the time series and spectrum of these multimodality trajectories demonstrate new features—mutual modulation and regularization of the different modality and, correspondingly, the appearance of new components in the power spectrum. The properties displayed by the model can be key features for the next step of multimodality information processing, such as object recognition, speech generation, and so forth. The proposed dynamical mechanism for binding accounts for different levels of temporal hierarchy, from milliseconds to minutes.

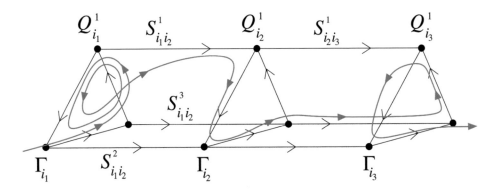

Figure 7.3
Illustration of a multimodality heteroclinic sequence and a trajectory corresponding to the binding activity. Adapted from Rabinovich et al. (2010).

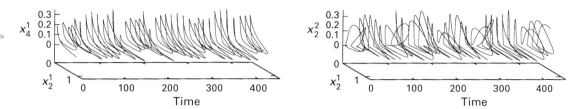

Figure 7.4
Mutual modulation due to the heteroclinic binding of three coupled modalities built with three 6-neuron networks. The modulation is illustrated by the joint time evolution of x_2^1 and x_4^1 (neurons 2 and 4 in modality 1; left panel) and the joint time evolution of x_2^1 and x_2^2 (corresponding neurons in two modalities; right panel). Adapted from Rabinovich et al. (2010).

In fact, the heteroclinic binding is a method for transient self-organization of perceptual spatiotemporal modes. The information about the recognizable image coding by such modes is transferred to the cognitive and behavioral modes for the next processing. This phenomenon can be analyzed based on fMRI data (for a review, see Raizada & Krieges-korte, 2010).

To characterize quantitatively the effectiveness of the heteroclinic binding, let us introduce a new function called information flow capacity (C_{IF}) (Rabinovich et al. 2011),

$$C_{IF}(L) = \sum_{l}^{L} [\Delta C_{IF}(l)], \tag{7.6}$$

where

$$\Delta C_{IF}(l) = J_l + \sum_{j=1}^{J_l} \frac{\operatorname{Re}\lambda_j^l}{|\lambda_{J_l+1}^l|} \tag{7.7}$$

Here, l is the index of the metastable state (saddle) along a channel, L is the number of saddles that the system passes until time t_L, λ_j^l are the eigenvalues of the Jacobian of the l saddle, and the integer J satisfies the following conditions ($\operatorname{Re}\lambda_1 > \ldots \geq \operatorname{Re}\lambda_m > 0 > \operatorname{Re}\lambda_{m+1} \geq \ldots \geq \operatorname{Re}\lambda_n$):

$$\sum_{j=1}^{J}\operatorname{Re}\lambda_j > 0, \quad \sum_{j=1}^{J+1}\operatorname{Re}\lambda_j < 0$$

In other words, J is the number of eigenvalues at which the cumulative sum over real parts becomes negative. If the unstable separatrices of all saddles along the heteroclinic channel are one-dimensional, such that $J_l=1$, we have

$$C_{IF}(L) = \sum_{l}^{L}\left(1+\frac{1}{\nu_l}\right).$$

(7.8)

In this case, the the ratio between positive and negative eigenvalues is equal to the saddle value ν_l in degree -1 (see chapter 4; we wish to recall here that for the channel stability, the product of all saddle values has to be larger than one).

Now we will illustrate the usefulness of the C_{IF} for a quantitative description of the example of heteroclinic binding problem. As one can see in figure 7.3, each saddle along a "binding heteroclinic channel" has two unstable separatrices. That means all $J_l = 2$. Thus, the estimation of the C_{IF} described earlier tells us that the flow capacity for a binding channel is at least two times larger than the C_{IF} of three independent channels. We can interpret this result in the following way: The information flow capacity characterizes the complexity level of the trajectories within a network of heteroclinic channels. We can hypothesize that such complexity supports fast and rich information encoding mechanisms about a subject.

It would be very interesting to connect the function C_{IF} with Shannon information and the capacity dimension of chaotic sets (see Baker & Gollub, 1996). However, there are two principal steps that have to be done to build a bridge between the description of transient trajectories in heteroclinic channels and asymptotic dynamics on chaotic attractors: (1) it is necessary to introduce a specific (non-invariant measure) and (2) to consider not continuous flows but maps. We are sure that this is doable in the near future.

7.5   Sequential Decision Making

Decisions need to be reproducible to allow for memory and learning. In contrast, a decision making (DM) system also has to be sensitive to new information from the environment. These requirements are fundamentally contradictory, and current approaches (Briggman, Abarbanel, & Kristan, 2005; Brown et al., 2005; Loh & Deco, 2005; Wong & Wang, 2006) are not sufficient to explain the use of sequential activity for DM. Here, we describe a new class of models suitable for analyzing sequential decision making (SDM) based on the SHC concept (Rabinovich et al., 2008b).

A key finding in decision theory (Kahneman & Tversky, 1979) is that the behavior of an individual shifts from risk aversion (when possible gains are predicted) to risk seeking (when possible losses are predicted). In particular, Kahneman and Tversky (1982) conducted several experiments to test decision making under uncertainty. They showed that when potential profits are concerned, decision makers are risk averse, but when potential losses are concerned, subjects become risk seeking.

To illustrate how the SHC concept can be applied to the execution of a risk-seeking decision making, we can consider a simple fixed time (T^*) game: a player takes sequential actions in a changing environment so as to maximize the reward. The success of the game depends on the decision strategy. Formally, the SDM model can consist of (1) a set of environment states $\sigma(I)$; (2) a set of dynamical variables $A_j \geq 0$ characterizing the level of activity of the cognitive modes that correspond to the execution of the decision strategy; and (3) a scalar representing the cumulative reward that depends on the number of achieved steps in the available time T^* and on the values of the instantaneous reward at the steps along different transients (i.e., different choices) (Rabinovich et al., 2008b). Depending on the environment conditions, the game can end at step ($k + 1$) or it can continue using one or many different alternatives based on the different choices. It is clear that to get the maximum cumulative reward, the player has to pass as many steps within the game's time T^*. Thus, the strategy that will make the game successful has to be based on two conditions: (1) the game does not have to end in an attractor (stable fixed point) at time $t < T^*$, and (2) the player has to encounter as many metastable states as possible during the time T^*.

It is difficult to estimate analytically which strategy is the best to solve the first problem. This can be done in a computer simulation, but we can make a prediction for the second problem. Let us assume that we have a successful game and, for the sake of simplicity, that the reward on each state is identical (as our computer simulations indicate, the results do not qualitatively change if the rewards for each step are different). Thus, the game dynamics in the phase space can be described by the system

$$\dot{A}_j = A_j(t)\left[\sigma_j(I_k) - \left(A_j - \sum_{i \neq 1}^{N} \rho_{ji} A_i\right)\right] + A_j(t)\eta_j(t) \tag{7.9}$$

$$\sigma_j(I_k) \in [\sigma_j^0 + S_i^m(I_k)], \quad m \in \{1, ..., m_k\}, \tag{7.10}$$

where $A_j \geq 0$, m_k is the number of admissible values of σ_j at the decision step t_k, S_i^m represents the stimulus determined by the environment information I_k at the step t_k, and η_j is a multiplicative noise (Rabinovich et al., 2008b). We can think that the game is a continued process that is represented by a trajectory arranged in a heteroclinic channel. The saddle vicinities correspond to the decision steps. Evidently, the number of such steps increases with the speed of the game, which depends on the time that the system spends in the vicinity of the saddle (metastable state) as given by $t_k = 1/\lambda_k \ln(1/|\eta|)$, where $|\eta|$ is the level of perturbation (average distance between the game trajectory and the saddle at decision step t_k), and λ_k is a maximal increment that corresponds to the unstable separatrices of this saddle. From this estimate, we can make a clear prediction. If the system does not stop in the middle of the game, to get the best reward a player has to choose the $\sigma(I_k)$ that corresponds to the maximal λ_k (risk seeking) and to have an optimal level of the noise (not too much to avoid leaving the heteroclinic channel). Suppose that we have noise in the input I that controls the next step of the decision making. Since

$$A_j \{\sigma[\xi = I + \eta(t)]\} \approx A_j \sigma(I) + A_j \left. \frac{d\sigma}{d\xi} \right|_I \eta(t), \tag{7.11}$$

such additive informational noise appears on the right side of the dynamical model as a multiplicative noise.

The parameters of the model that we will review here were selected according to a uniform distribution in the range $\sigma_j^0 \in [5,10]$ (Rabinovich et al., 2008b). As a proof of concept, the specific order of the sequence is not important. Therefore, the sequence order is set from saddle 0 to N, which is obtained by setting a connectivity matrix so that $\rho_{i-1\,i} = \sigma_{i-1}^0 / \sigma_i^0 + 0.51$ for $i = 2,\ldots,N$, $\rho_{i+1\,i} = \sigma_{i+1}^0 / \sigma_i^0 - 0.5$ for $i = 1,\ldots,N-1$, and $\rho_{ij} = \rho_{j-1\,j} + (\sigma_i^0 - \sigma_{j-1}^0) / \sigma_j^0 + 2$ for $i \notin \{j-1, j, j+1\}$. Note that there are infinite matrices that will produce the same sequence. All the rest of the parameters that form the basis of all possible perturbations or stimulations at each of the saddles or decision steps were taken from a uniform distribution $S_i^m \in [-4,9]$. The specific selection of these parameters does not have any major impact on the results that are described here. For the sake of simplicity, we assume that the external perturbations at each of the decision steps are uncorrelated. See Rabinovich et al. (2008b) for simulation details.

When the trajectory reaches the vicinity of a saddle point within some radius $\varepsilon = 0.1$, then the decision-making function is applied. The rule applied in this case is the high-risk rule, which is implemented as follows.

At each saddle, the increments $\lambda_{j(q)i} = \sigma_{j(q)} - \rho_{j(q)i}\sigma_{j(q)}$ can be calculated such that a specific q is chosen to obtain a maximal $\lambda_{j(q)i}$ at each saddle. In other words, we choose the maximal increment, which corresponds to the fastest motion away from the saddle S_i, and therefore, the shortest time for reaching the next saddle.

To evaluate the model, the effect of the strength of uncorrelated multiplicative noise $\langle\eta_j(t)\eta_j(t')\rangle = \mu\delta(t-t')$ can be analyzed. The results shown in figure 7.5 show that there exists an optimal level of noise. For low noise, the system travels through most of the saddles in a slower manner as $t_k = 1/\lambda_k\ln(1/|\eta|)$, whereas for increasing values of the noise, the number of metastable states involved in the game are reduced. The top panel in figure 7.5 shows the cumulative reward for different noise levels. Two interesting cases can be pointed out. As we can see from the figure, the optimal cumulative reward is obtained for a particular noise

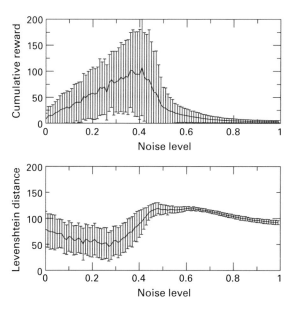

Figure 7.5
Estimation of the cumulative reward for different noise levels using multiplicative noise. (Top) Cumulative reward calculated as the number of cognitive states that the system travels through until the final time of the game T^*, which is 100 in this case. For each level of noise, 1000 different sequences are generated (for $N = 15$ and a total of 15 choices). (Bottom) Reproducibility index of the sequence calculated with the average Levenshtein distance across all generated sequences. The lower the distance, the more similar the sequences are for 1000 different runs. The pair distances are calculated and averaged to obtain the mean and the standard deviation, which is represented by the error bars. Adapted from Rabinovich et al. (2008b).

level. For levels of moderate noise, the system enters partially repeated sequences, because the two or more unstable directions allow the system to move to two or more different places in a random fashion. The reproducibility measure of the obtained sequences is shown in the bottom panel of figure 7.5. We can see that the most reproducible sequences are generated for a slightly smaller level of noise than the one that corresponds to the maximum cumulative reward. To estimate the reproducibility across sequences, we used the Levenshtein distance, which basically finds the easiest way to transform one sequence into another (Levenshtein, 1966). This distance is appropriate to identify the repetitiveness of the sequence, and it is used in multiple applications. Sometimes it happens that the sequence becomes repetitive, and in other cases it just dies. The error bars in this figure denote the standard deviation. While the Levenshtein distance does not have large error bars, the cumulative reward does, because for that level of noise, it is common to enter limit cycles that reach the maximum time. It is more likely to find two extremes: (1) ending quickly and (2) reaching a limit cycle.

Concerning the formation of a habit, it is important to note that the memorized sequence is subjected to the external stimulation, which can change the direction at any given time. This fact is reflected in the results shown in figure 7.5 where the Levenshtein distance does not go exactly to zero. The heteroclinic skeleton that forms the SHC can be broken and can even repeat itself to produce limit cycles for a given set of external stimulus. So the model does have alternatives that are induced by the set of external perturbations under the risk-taking decision-making rule.

The simple game that we have described here illustrates a type of transient cognitive dynamics with multiple metastable states. We suggest that other types of sequential decision making could be represented by similar dynamical mechanisms.

7.6   Future Directions

To analyze information flows in phase space, we have focused our attention on the interaction of metastable states that represent brain modes ignoring their fast intrinsic temporal structure. In reality, the temporal hierarchy is a key principle that is characterized by both the environment and the brain intrinsic dynamics (Kiebel et al., 2008). In particular, the lowest level of the hierarchy corresponds to fast (~100 ms) sensory processing, whereas the highest levels encode slow (minutes, hours, and longer) cognitive and emotional dynamics. The hierarchical activation approach to connect functional brain modes helps us to understand the dynamical mechanisms of fast information flows from perception to emotion, cognition, and between different stages of execution of complex functions like speech generation, correction, and pronunciation. In spite of the fact that the mathematical formalism of such approach is not developed yet, we wish to discuss here a couple of ideas that can be useful for this goal.

One idea is related to the temporal receptive window (TRW). Lerner, Honey, Silbert, and Hasson (2011) reported the results of mapped TRWs in auditory and language areas by measuring fMRI activity in subjects listening to a real-life story scrambled at the timescales of words, sentences, and paragraphs. Their results revealed a hierarchical architecture of TRWs. In particular, in early auditory cortices, brain responses were driven by the momentary incoming input. In areas with an intermediate TRW, coherent information at the sentence timescale or longer was necessary to evoke reliable responses. At the apex of the TRW hierarchy, the authors found areas that responded reliably only when intact paragraphs were heard in a meaningful sequence. These results suggest that the timescale of processing is a functional property that may provide an organizing principle for the activation of different brain modes and for the sequential temporal stages of information flow in a unified phase space that integrates the subspaces with different timescales.

In this chapter, we have concentrated on stable information flows in the brain. However, it is widely accepted that the brain is often working on the edge of instability (Jirsa & Ghosh, 2010). What can we expect on the other side of the stability boundary? It depends on the kind of instability. It is reasonable to separate all instabilities into intrinsic and external. Intrinsic instabilities mean that new dynamics appear between modes of the same family (i.e., the activity is based on the same repertoire). In contrast, external instabilities mean that modes of new families appear (i.e., the repertoire is changing itself). The development of intrinsic instabilities has been considered by Tristan and Rabinovich (2012). In this paper, the authors analyzed the corresponding phenomena in a heteroclinic network with active elements whose equilibria have multidimensional unstable manifolds. They introduced a new characteristic of sequential transient dynamics—an uncertainty function that measures the level of nonreproducibility of generalized heteroclinic channels. It has been shown that the probability to get a heteroclinic channel with fixed uncertainty depends on both the number of saddles along the heteroclinic chain and the number of elements in the network. These results indicate that in complex networks, in spite of the multidimensionality of the unstable manifold of saddles, some amount of order along transients remains feasible: Many trajectories follow a strongly unstable direction, and the probability to keep a generalized heteroclinic sequence is high enough.

The scenario of external perturbation development can be much more dramatic. New transients—new heteroclinic channels—can appear. Such changes can represent behavioral or cognitive patterns that did not exist before (Abraham, 1996). This generation or creation of information is the result of the instability. Departing from the approach that we described in this chapter, it is very appealing to analyze self-organization bifurcations leading to novel channels (i.e., novel informational flows).

Acknowledgments

Mikhail I. Rabinovich acknowledges support from ONR grant N00014-07-1-074. Valentin S. Afraimovich was partially supported by PROMEP grant UASLP-CA21. Chris Bick was partially supported by the German Academic Exchange Service through a DAAD Doktorandenstipendium. Pablo Varona was supported by MICINNBFU2009-08473.

References

Abraham, F. D. (1996). The dynamics of creativity and the courage to be. In W. Sulis & A. Combs (Eds.), *Nonlinear Dynamics in Human Behavior. Studies of Nonlinear Phenomena in Life Science* (Vol. 5, pp. 364–400). Singapore: World Scientific.

Afraimovich, V. S., Zhigulin, V. P., & Rabinovich, M. I. (2004). On the origin of reproducible sequential activity in neural circuits. *Chaos (Woodbury, N.Y.)*, *14*, 1123.

Baker, G. L., & Gollub, J. B. (1996). *Chaotic Dynamics: An Introduction*. Cambridge, UK: Cambridge University Press.

Bick, C., & Rabinovich, M. I. (2009a). On the occurrence of stable heteroclinic channels in Lotka–Volterra models. *Dynamical Systems: An International Journal*, *25*, 1–14.

Bick, C., & Rabinovich, M. I. (2009b). Dynamical origin of the effective storage capacity in the brain's working memory. *Physical Review Letters*, *103*(21), 218101.

Briggman, K. L., Abarbanel, H. D. I., & Kristan, W. B. (2005). Optical imaging of neuronal populations during decision-making. *Science*, *307*(5711), 896–901.

Brown, E., Gao, J., Holmes, P., Bogacz, R., Gilzenrat, M., & Cohen, J. D. (2005). Simple neural networks that optimize decisions. *International Journal of Bifurcation and Chaos in Applied Sciences and Engineering*, *15*, 803–826.

Clark, A. (2005). Word, niche and super-niche: how language makes minds matter more. *Theoria*, *54*, 255–268.

Edin, F., Klingberg, T., Johansson, P., McNab, F., Tegnér, J., & Compte, A. (2009). Mechanism for top-down control of working memory capacity. *Proceedings of the National Academy of Sciences of the United States of America*, *106*(16), 6802–6807.

Granger, C. W. J. (1969). Investigating causal relations by economic models and cross-spectral methods. *Econometrica, 37*, 424–438.

Halliwell, J. O. (1842). *The Nursery Rhymes of England*. London: F. Warne and Co.

Hasson, U., Yang, E., Vallines, I., Heeger, D. J., & Rubin, N. (2008). A hierarchy of temporal receptive windows in human cortex. *Journal of Neuroscience, 28*(10), 2539–2550.

Hawkings, J., & Blakeslee, S. (2004). *On Intelligence*. New York: Times Books.

Jensen, O., & Mazaheri, A. (2010). Shaping functional architecture by oscillatory alpha activity: gating by inhibition. *Frontiers in Human Neuroscience, 4*, 186.

Jirsa, V. K., & Ghosh, A. (2010). Spontaneous brain dynamics emerges at the edge of instability. In D. A. Steyn-Ross & M. Steyn-Ross (Eds.), *Modeling Phase Transitions in the Brain* (Vol. 4, pp. 81–98). New York: Springer.

Kahneman, D., & Tversky, A. (1979). Prospect theory: an analysis of decision under risk. *Econometrica, 47*, 263–291.

Kahneman, D., & Tversky, A. (1982). Judgement under Uncertainty: Heuristics and Biases In D. Kahneman, P. Slovic, & A. Tversky (Eds.), *Judgement under Uncertainty: Heuristics and Biases* (pp. 3–23). Cambridge, UK: Cambridge University Press.

Kiebel, S. J., Daunizeau, J., & Friston, K. J. (2008). A hierarchy of time-scales and the brain. *PLoS Computational Biology, 4*(11), e1000209.

Lerner, Y., Honey, C. J., Silbert, L. J., & Hasson, U. (2011). Topographic mapping of a hierarchy of temporal receptive windows using a narrated story. *Journal of Neuroscience, 31*(8), 2906–2915.

Levenshtein, V. I. (1966). Binary codes capable of correcting deletions, insertions, and reversals. *Soviet Physics, Doklady, 10*, 707–710.

Lisman, J. E., & Idiart, M. A. (1995). Storage of 7 +/- 2 short-term memories in oscillatory subcycles. *Science, 267*(5203), 1512–1515.

Loh, M., & Deco, G. (2005). Cognitive flexibility and decision-making in a model of conditional visuomotor associations. *European Journal of Neuroscience, 22*(11), 2927–2936.

McClelland, J. L., & Elman, J. L. (1986). The TRACE model of speech perception. *Cognitive Psychology, 18*(1), 1–86.

McClelland, J. L., Botvinick, M. M., Noelle, D. C., Plaut, D. C., Rogers, T. T., Seidenberg, M. S., & Smith, L. B. (2010). Letting structure emerge: connectionist and dynamical systems approaches to cognition. *Trends in Cognitive Sciences, 14*(8), 348–356.

Mikk, J. (2008). Sentence length for revealing the cognitive load reversal effect in text comprehension. *Educational Studies, 34*(2), 119–127.

Miller, G. A. (1956). The magical number seven plus or minus two: some limits on our capacity for processing information. *Psychological Review, 63*(2), 81–97.

Oberauer, K., & Kliegl, R. (2006). A formal model of capacity limits in working memory. *Journal of Memory and Language, 55*(4), 601–626.

Palva, J. M., Monto, S., Kulashekhar, S., & Palva, S. (2010). Neuronal synchrony reveals working memory networks and predicts individual memory capacity. *Proceedings of the National Academy of Sciences of the United States of America, 107*(16), 7580–7585.

Pascanu, R., & Jaeger, H. (2011). A neurodynamical model for working memory. *Neural Networks, 24*(2), 199–207.

Pollard, S., & Biermann, A. W. (2000). A measure of semantic complexity for natural language systems. In NAACL-ANLP 2000 Workshop: Syntactic and Semantic Complexity in Natural Language Processing Systems (pp. 42–46). Stroudsburg, PA: Association for Computational Linguistics.

Rabinovich, M. I., & Varona, P. (2011). Robust transient dynamics and brain functions. *Frontiers in Computational Neuroscience, 5*, 24.

Rabinovich, M. I., Afraimovich, V. S., & Varona, P. (2010). Heteroclinic binding. *Dynamical Systems: An International Journal, 25*(3), 433–442.

Rabinovich, M., Huerta, R., & Laurent, G. (2008a). Neuroscience. Transient dynamics for neural processing. *Science, 321*(5885), 48–50.

Rabinovich, M. I., Huerta, R., Varona, P., & Afraimovich, V. S. (2008b). Transient cognitive dynamics, metastability, and decision making. *PLoS Computational Biology, 4*(5), e1000072.

Rabinovich, M. I., Afraimovich, V. S., Bick, C., & Varona, P. (2012). Information flow dynamics in the brain. *Physics of Life Reviews, 9,* 51–73.

Rabinovich, M., Huerta, R., & Laurent, G. (2008). Neuroscience. Transient dynamics for neural processing. *Science, 321*(5885), 48–50.

Raizada, R. D. S., & Kriegeskorte, N. (2010). Pattern-information fMRI: new questions which it opens up and challenges which face it. *International Journal of Imaging Systems and Technology, 20,* 31–41.

Roopun, A. K., Kramer, M. A., Carracedo, L. M., Kaiser, M., Davies, C. H., Traub, R. D., et al. (2008). Temporal interactions between cortical rhythms. *Frontiers in Neuroscience, 2*(2), 145–154.

Rouder, J. N., Morey, R. D., Cowan, N., Zwilling, C. E., Morey, C. C., & Pratte, M. S. (2008). An assessment of fixed-capacity models of visual working memory. *Proceedings of the National Academy of Sciences of the United States of America, 105*(16), 5975–5979.

Schroeder, C. E., & Lakatos, P. (2009). Low-frequency neuronal oscillations as instruments of sensory selection. *Trends in Neurosciences, 32*(1), 9–18.

Shannon, C. E. (1948). A mathematical theory of communication. *Bell System Technical Journal, 27,* 379–423.

Stephens, G. J., Silbert, L. J., & Hasson, U. (2010). Speaker-listener neural coupling underlies successful communication. *Proceedings of the National Academy of Sciences of the United States of America, 107*(32), 14425–14430.

Swanson, H. L. (1999). What develops in working memory? A life span perspective. *Developmental Psychology, 35*(4), 986–1000.

Sweller, J., van Merrienboer, J., & Paas, F. (1998). Cognitive architecture and instructional design. *Educational Psychology Review, 10*(3), 251–296.

Tort, A. B. L., Kramer, M. A., Thorn, C., Gibson, D. J., Kubota, Y., Graybiel, A. M., et al. (2008). Dynamic cross-frequency couplings of local field potential oscillations in rat striatum and hippocampus during performance of a T-maze task. *Proceedings of the National Academy of Sciences of the United States of America, 105*(51), 20517–20522.

Tristan, I., & Rabinovich, M. I. (2012). Transient dynamics on the edge of stability. In G. Liu (Ed.), *Nonlinear Dynamics: New Directions.* New York: Springer.

Wiener, N. (1956). The theory of prediction. In E. F. Beckenbach (Ed.), *Modern mathematics for the engineer* (pp. 165–190). New York: McGraw-Hill.

Wong, K.-F., & Wang, X.-J. (2006). A recurrent network mechanism of time integration in perceptual decisions. *Journal of Neuroscience, 26*(4), 1314–1328.

Yamashita, Y., & Tani, J. (2008). Emergence of functional hierarchy in a multiple timescale neural network model: a humanoid robot experiment. *PLoS Computational Biology, 4*(11), e1000220.

8   Multiscale Electroencephalographic Dynamics and Brain Function

Maxim Bazhenov and Scott Makeig

Summary

How the large-scale brain activities represented by electroencephalogram (EEG) and local field potential (LFP) signals recorded at a range of spatial scales emerge from multiscale electrical dynamics in mammalian brain neuropile remains an open question. Even less is known as to what extent electrical fields generated by the partially synchronous collective activity of neural populations influence the dynamics of the individual neurons and the network activities they participate in. Here, we discuss some recent results related to multiscale brain dynamics that emphasize the relative weakness of current neuroscientific understanding of how complex feedback interactions across different spatial scales of brain activity, from the level of individual neurons to spatiotemporally coordinated EEG source activity networks that include separated cortical areas, support coordinated brain/behavioral function.

8.1   Neuronal Correlates of Electroencephalographic and Local Field Potential Rhythms

The term *electroencephalogram* (EEG) refers to electrical signals generated by brain activity and recorded from electrodes placed on the scalp. Cortical electrical activity may also be recorded invasively (in humans during preoperative monitoring) using somewhat smaller electrodes placed directly on the brain surface, giving the so-called electrocorticogram (ECoG), or by still much smaller electrodes inserted into brain tissue, recording local field potential (LFP) signals. Understanding how the EEG, ECoG, and LFP patterns relate to the activities of contributing neurons and neuropile interactions remains an important and largely open problem (Makeig et al., 2002).

Clearly, scalp EEG signals sum volume-conducted changes in electrical activity of multiple cortical sources and ultimately represent weighted mixtures of the net electrical activity patterns of portions of cortical neuropile that each exhibit some degree of LFP synchrony. In some cases, these sources can be well localized to near-synchronous activity occurring across square-centimeter–sized or smaller cortical areas; for example, EEG patterns during waking cognitive processes or during focal seizures as indicated by results of independent component analysis (ICA) applied to high-density scalp EEG recordings (Makeig, Bell, Jung, & Sejnowski, 1996; Makeig et al., 2002; Delorme, Palmer, Onton, Oostenveld, & Makeig, submitted). In other circumstances, EEG signals may largely originate in more or less synchronous LFP activity across larger brain areas; for example, during slow-wave sleep or epileptic seizures (Massamini, Huber, Ferrarelli, Hill, & Tononi, 2004; Milton, Chkcencheli, & Towle, 2007).

In contrast, fine-wire electrode LFP recordings provide (relatively) microscopic measures of brain activity summarizing net electrical activities around up to a few thousand neurons (Niedermeyer & Lopes da Silva, 2005; Katzner et al., 2009). In large part, these activities arise from partial synchrony among membrane voltage gradients between different portions of individual cells, understood or assumed to be largely produced by synaptic activations mediated by action potentials. Excitatory synaptic activation within one neuronal compartment will create a flow of positive ions inside the cell (an active current sink), depolarizing the intracellular space and creating negative potential in surrounding space. These gradients lead to current flows between compartments within the neuron membranes, the extracellular space, and the interdigitated glial syncytium, producing hyperpolarization of the membrane at sites where positive ions leave the cell, thus constituting passive current sources. Active current sources may also arise from inhibitory synaptic currents that produce corresponding passive current sinks.

These distributions of current sinks and sources within and around pyramidal cells oriented perpendicular to the cerebral cortical surface (with somas in the deep layers and dendrites in superficial layers) create electrical fields whose summed, locally partly spatially coherent contributions to potentials measured at larger cortical surface electrodes are major contributors to LFP signals (Creutzfeldt, Watanabe, & Lux, 1966a, 1966b; Klee & Rall, 1977; Lopes da Silva & Van Rotterdam, 2005), with recent evidence pointing to a particularly strong impact of inhibitory processes (Trevelyan, 2009; Bazelot, Dinocourt, Cohen, & Miles, 2010; Oren, Hajos, & Paulsen, 2010).

The unique configuration of large, locally similarly oriented pyramidal neurons in cerebral cortex provide strong contributions to the quasi-dipolar "far-field" potentials that are major contributors to scalp EEG signals—though only when and if there exists enough LFP synchrony at spatial scales well beyond 1000 adjacent neurons. Only such an emergent partial field synchrony across a wider area can avoid the otherwise inevitable phase cancellation of summed incoherent signals from smaller local domains of synchrony at the electrically distant scalp electrodes and so produce a net positive or negative far-field potential ECoG or EEG contribution.

The strength of the electric field produced by an equivalent dipole (i.e., a dipole producing a far-field equivalent to that produced by coherent LFP across a cortical patch) depends both on the degree of spatial synchrony of the cellular generators as well as the distance between their current sinks and sources (Nunez & Srinivasan, 2005); this should make locally synchronous field activities associated with large layer-V and layer-VI pyramidal neurons main contributors to recorded LFP and EEG signals.

In principle, both slower synaptic currents and fast intrinsic currents generated during action potential propagation contribute to LFP and EEG signals. However, in part because of the low-pass filtering properties of the extracellular media (Bedard, Kroger, & Destexhe, 2004), very-high-frequency electric fields associated with action potentials steeply attenuate with distance, so only nearby neurons can produce significant extracellular spike signals in a recording electrode. Therefore, models of LFP and EEG assuming uniform electrical properties in the extracellular medium may overestimate the contribution of fast intrinsic currents and underestimate the effects of slow synaptic and intrinsic currents and conductances. As a result, such models may generate electric signals that decay quickly after offset of cellular spike activity and produce almost no signal during any periods of reduced neuronal firing activity, no matter how brief. They also may discount the effects of areal synchronization by focusing on very narrow spike potentials that rarely synchronize precisely.

8.2   Measuring Multiscale Field Dynamics

The spatiotemporal dynamics of partial local synchrony across slower local field processes in adjacent cortical (or other brain structure) territories are still largely unknown. In particular, until very recently there have been few attempts to measure it using fine electrode grids (Freeman, 1975). Instead, the field of brain electrophysiology may be said to have long ago split into two camps: psychologists and neurologists who study scalp EEG or near square-centimeter–scale cortical LFP activities, and neurobiologists who have for at least 50 years focused near exclusively on the temporal dynamics of spike processes within individual neurons. The former have rarely explored in depth how smaller-scale field activities converge to produce the measured far-field potentials, and the latter long tended to dismiss the importance of field activities, famously referring to them as only the epiphenomenal "roar of the [neuronal] crowd" (see Kirkland, 2002).

Both technical limitations and (perhaps) lack of imagination have prevented serious attempts at concurrently recording local field synchronies multiple spatial scales. For this reason, for example, recent reports that theta band LFP activity in hippocampus takes the form of a traveling wave (Lubenov & Siapas, 2009) and that beta band ECoG activity in motor areas also has a coherent local traveling wave structure (Rubino, Robbins, & Hatsopoulos, 2006) are suggestive of hitherto unappreciated dynamic structure encompassing brain activity at smaller and larger spatial scales. NASA time-lapse movies of hydrogen density across the solar surface clearly exhibit multiscale spatiotemporal dynamic structure spontaneously emerging within the nonlinear solar plasma. To date, no comparable multiscale recording of cortical field density has been recorded—a technological recording challenge that current wireless microelectronic technology would seem to make possible, even in volunteer preoperative human subjects and perhaps involving less discomfort and no greater risk than current wired ECoG recording methods.

8.3 Spatiotemporal Field Dynamics in Sleep

A better-known and modeled example of rhythmic brain activity that leads to large-amplitude EEG oscillations is slow oscillations in sleep. The signature characteristic of slow-wave sleep (SWS) in the EEG is large-amplitude fluctuations of field potential (Blake & Gerard, 1937) that reflect slow alternating periods of relative activity and silence in underlying cortical networks (Steriade, Nuñez, & Amzica, 1993a, 1993b; Contreras & Steriade, 1995; Steriade, Timofeev, & Grenier, 2001; Timofeev, Grenier, & Steriade, 2001; Petersen, Hahn, Mehta, Grinvald, & Sakmann, 2003). Similar patterns were recorded from neostriatal neurons by Wilson and Kawaguchi (1996), who introduced the now widely used terms "Up state" (for the cortical surface depolarized phase) and "Down state" (for the hyperpolarized phase) (Mahon et al., 2006). Each slow oscillation cycle starts in a particular cerebral cortical location

and rapidly propagates to other regions (Massimini et al., 2004; Volgushev, Chauvette, Mukovski, & Timofeev, 2006). In cats, cortical depth
profiles of LFP activity measured *in vivo* during active ("Up") SWS
states include current sources in superficial layers and sinks in deep
layers, and the inverse of this during silent ("Down") SWS states
(Chauvette, Volgushev, & Timofeev, 2010).

It has been recently shown (Bazhenov et al., 2011) that to generate
model LFP profiles in agreement with experimental data requires taking
into account the filtering properties of extracellular media by including
its inhomogeneous electrical properties (Bedard et al., 2004; Bedard &
Destexhe, 2009). By including these properties in the model, the propagation of fast currents is diminished, leaving slow intrinsic and synaptic
currents to provide the major contribution to LFP signals recorded
farther from the source neurons. This generates slow changes in the LFP
(figure 8.1, plate 18), even between active states (i.e., during silent states),

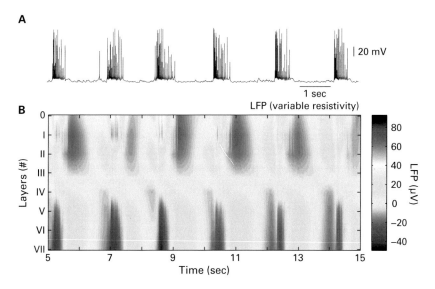

Figure 8.1 (plate 18)
Local field potentials during sleep slow oscillations simulated using a variable media resistivity model. (A) Membrane voltage of a model layer IV pyramidal cell. (B) Depth LFP
profile of the network. Here, for clarity the LFP was low-pass–filtered at 50 Hz. These LFP
profiles include a relatively low-amplitude phase just before active state onset that can be
explained by the relatively long (typically around 1 s) duration of the silent states produced
by the model that were in this respect more *in vitro*–like (Sanchez-Vives & McCormick,
2000) compared with the shorter (typically less than 0.5 s) silent states observed in vivo
(Steriade et al., 1993b). Modified from Bazhenov et al. (2011).

in agreement with experimental observations (Chauvette et al., 2010; Csercsa et al., 2010). In contrast, a conventional constant conductivity model assuming that LFP is generated by current sources embedded in a uniform resistive medium (Nunez & Srinivasan, 2005) may explain *in vivo* distribution of LFP during active phases of slow oscillations. However, it failed to explain the profound LFP structure during silent states of slow oscillation (Chauvette et al., 2010; Csercsa et al., 2010).

The LFP signal model, incorporating a non-homogeneous conductivity by including spatial variations (or inhomogeneities) of both conductivity and permittivity (Bazhenov et al., 2011), also reproduced critical features of the current source density (CSD) profiles between superficial and deep cortical layers including the observed CSD distribution during the silent (Down) states of the slow oscillation (figure 8.2, plate 19). This feature is not reproduced by traditional LFP models assuming uniform resistivity, which may mean that the traditional models are insufficient or alternatively that current Up and Down state network models are too simple.

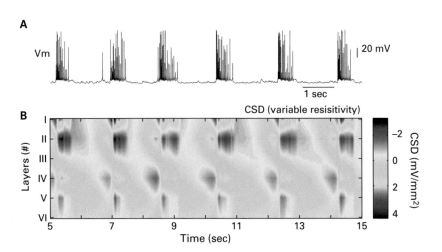

Figure 8.2 (plate 19)
Current source density analysis of the simulated sleep slow oscillations. (A) Membrane voltage of a pyramidal cell from layer IV. (B) Depth CSD profile in the middle of the network arising within the variable (non-homogeneous) media resistivity model. The CSD profile during active (Up) states is similar to that estimated from constant resistivity models. But, in contrast to constant resistivity models, the CSD is also nonzero and non-uniform during silent (Down) states. Modified from Bazhenov et al. (2011).

8.4   Mechanisms of Neuronal Synchronization

Far-field EEG and LFP patterns reflect spatially and temporally synchronized activity within neuronal, intercellular, and interleaved glial neuropile. Neuronal synchronization is usually understood in cellular neurophysiology to refer to a temporal coincidence of two or more discrete neural electrical events (e.g., the near coincidence of two neuronal action potentials or bursts of action potential). Near-synchronous activities of many neurons also lead to coordinated ions flow in extracellular space that can be detected as changes in the LFP. If, for example, a population of neurons fires action potentials periodically in a manner partially synchronous across many cells, periodic LFP oscillations will be produced. Finally, if long-range synchronization takes place between neuronal and extraneuronal field activities in adjacent (and sometimes nonadjacent) brain areas, the resulting broader scale changes in electrical activity may be recorded as scalp EEG rhythms.

Different neuronal mechanisms can be responsible for neuronal synchronization. These include synaptic interactions (both chemical and electrical), ephaptic interactions, and changes in extracellular ionic concentrations (reviewed in Timofeev, Bazhenov, Seigneur, & Sejnowski, 2011).

8.4.1   Synaptic Interactions

Synaptic interaction is a common mechanism of communication between neurons. Transmitter release at a presynaptic terminal leads to receptor activation in the postsynaptic cell and inward or outward currents that depolarize or hyperpolarize the cell. Generally, both excitatory and inhibitory synaptic interactions may contribute to synchronization of neuronal activities. Imagine, for example, two neurons connected by an excitatory synapse. Action potential in one cell may then trigger an excitatory postsynaptic potential (EPSP) in another cell. If this EPSP is large enough, or if the second cell receives near-simultaneous spike-related inputs from several of its connected neurons, these events can trigger an action potential in the postsynaptic cell. Both axonal and conductance delays, however, lead to delay in the generation of action potential in the postsynaptic cell, this delay possibly varying between different cells, potentially leading to progressive decay of synchrony in later EPSP phases.

An efficient way to synchronize a population of excitatory cells involves inhibition. Imagine a group of excitatory neurons generating action potentials in an asynchronous manner. Imagine now that these neurons simultaneously receive inhibitory input from the same inhibitory interneuron arising from an action potential in the inhibitory cell. This will provoke synchronous inhibitory postsynaptic potentials (IPSPs) in all the postsynaptic neurons. When these IPSPs end, all the postsynaptic excitatory neurons may spike near synchronously. If some of these excitatory cells project back to the inhibitory interneuron, the near-synchronous spiking of the excitatory cells might trigger a new spike in the inhibitory interneuron, beginning a new cycle that, repeated, produces an observed field oscillation at a nearby LFP or ECoG electrode (figure 8.3, plate 20). This mechanism of synchronization, commonly referred as *feedback inhibition* (Bazhenov & Stopfer, 2010), is involved in the generation of many brain rhythms including, for example, some types of gamma oscillations, thalamic spindles, and so forth. It is dynamically similar to the *partial phase resetting* of ongoing alpha band (near 10 Hz) scalp EEG activity sometimes observed after sudden visual stimulus onsets (Makeig et al., 2002).

In large-scale network models, synaptic interactions between excitatory and inhibitory neurons may lead to a variety of complex patterns including regimes with spiral wave dynamics (high degree of long-range

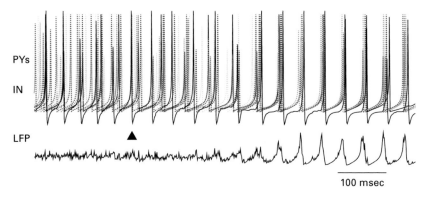

100 msec

Figure 8.3 (plate 20)
The effect of feedback inhibition on spike synchronization. Top: With no inhibitory feedback, eight pyramidal neurons (PYs; dashed lines) oscillate asynchronously in the 20- to 25-Hz frequency range. About 200 ms after an inhibitory GABAergic synapse from the interneuron (IN; black line) to PYs is activated (arrowhead), spikes in the pyramidal neurons became synchronized by IN-mediated IPSPs. Bottom: Increase of PY synchronization is reflected in the emergence of large-amplitude LFP oscillations. Modified from Timofeev et al., (2011).

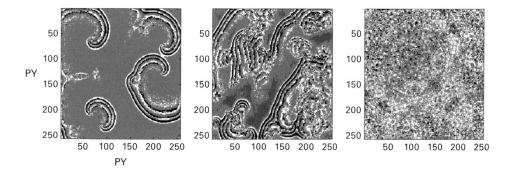

Figure 8.4 (plate 21)
Spatiotemporal dynamics mediated by synaptic coupling. Snapshots of activity in a two-dimensional network of 65,536 excitatory (PY) and 16,384 inhibitory neurons. Changing the balance of excitation and inhibition transformed the network state from only a few isolated spiral waves (left) to a state with multiple spirals (middle) and finally to an asynchronous state with many local spots of correlated firing (right). Synaptic connectivity included 200 presynaptic neurons for excitatory (AMPA) synapses and 12 presynaptic neurons for inhibitory (GABA$_A$) synapses. Modified from Rulkov et al. (2004).

synchrony) and quasi-asynchronous firing (low degree of long-range synchrony) (figure 8.4, plate 21) (Rulkov, Timofeev, & Bazhenov, 2004).

8.4.2   Gap Junction Interactions

The presence of direct electrical synapses between neurons allows a direct flux of ions between connected cells constituting a communication mechanism that is action potential independent. If a few cells are connected by electrical synapses, any change in membrane voltage in one neuron triggers current flow between this and its electrically coupled neighbor neurons leading to a corresponding change of membrane voltage in the other cells, also providing a synchronizing effect. Electrical coupling has high efficacy for the short-range synchronization (Galarreta & Hestrin, 2001), and it can be enhanced by low $[Ca^{2+}]_o$ (Thimm, Mechler, Lin, Rhee, & Lal, 2005) when efficiency of synaptic transmission is reduced. This may play an important role in synchronizing paroxysmal activities during seizures (Seigneur & Timofeev, 2011). Because of the relatively high resistance of electrical synapses, they are much more efficient in transmitting slow membrane voltage changes such as those following bursts of action potentials rather than individual action potentials. The effects of gap junction–mediated neural interactions are similar to effects of coupling present in a variety of systems incorporating diffusion and can be described using a similar mathematical formalism. The

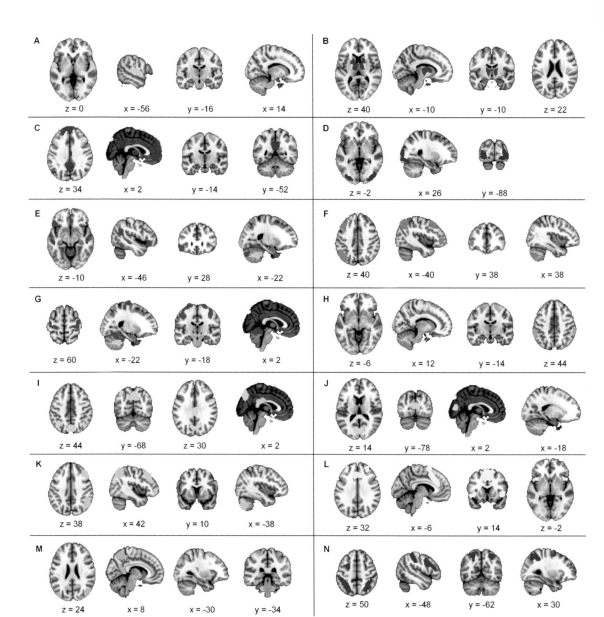

A

z = 0   x = -56   y = -16   x = 14

B

z = 40   x = -10   y = -10   z = 22

C

z = 34   x = 2   y = -14   y = -52

D

z = -2   x = 26   y = -88

E

z = -10   x = -46   y = 28   x = -22

F

z = 40   x = -40   y = 38   x = 38

G

z = 60   x = -22   y = -18   x = 2

H

z = -6   x = 12   y = -14   z = 44

I

z = 44   y = -68   z = 30   x = 2

J

z = 14   y = -78   x = 2   x = -18

K

z = 38   x = 42   y = 10   x = -38

L

z = 32   x = -6   y = 14   z = -2

M

z = 24   x = 8   x = -30   y = -34

N

z = 50   x = -48   y = -62   x = 30

Plate 1 (figure 2.1)

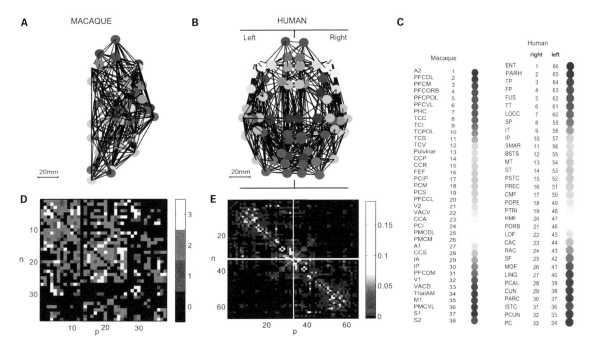

A MACAQUE

B HUMAN
Left   Right

C

	Macaque			Human		
					right	left
A2	1		ENT		1	66
PFCDL	2		PARH		2	65
PFCM	3		TP		3	64
PFCORB	4		FP		4	63
PFCPOL	5		FUS		5	62
PFCVL	6		TT		6	61
PHC	7		LOCC		7	60
TCC	8		SP		8	59
TCI	9		IT		9	58
TCPOL	10		IP		10	57
TCS	11		SMAR		11	56
TCV	12		BSTS		12	55
Pulvinar	13		MT		13	54
CCP	14		ST		14	53
CCR	15		PSTC		15	52
FEF	16		PREC		16	51
PCIP	17		CMF		17	50
PCM	18		POPE		18	49
PCS	19		PTRI		19	48
PFCCL	20		RMF		20	47
V2	21		PORB		21	46
VACV	22		LOF		22	45
CCA	23		CAC		23	44
PCI	24		RAC		24	43
PMCDL	25		SF		25	42
PMCM	26		MOF		26	41
A1	27		LING		27	40
CCS	28		PCAL		28	39
IA	29		CUN		29	38
IP	30		PARC		30	37
PFCDM	31		ISTC		31	36
V1	32		PCUN		32	35
VACD	33		PC		33	34
ThalAM	34					
M1	35					
PMCVL	36					
S1	37					
S2	38					

D

E

Plate 2 (figure 1.2)

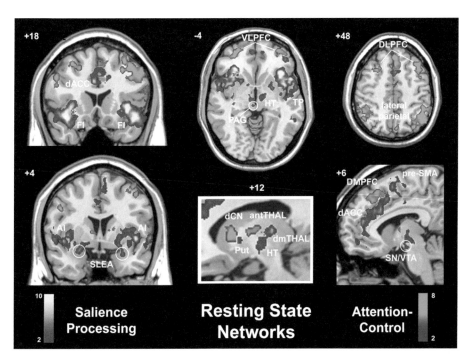

+18 dACC FI FI

-4 VLPFC HT TP PAG

+48 DLPFC lateral parietal

+4 AI AI SLEA

+12 dCN antTHAL dmTHAL Put HT

+6 DMPFC pre-SMA dACC SN/VTA

Salience Processing

Resting State Networks

Attention-Control

Plate 3 (figure 2.2)

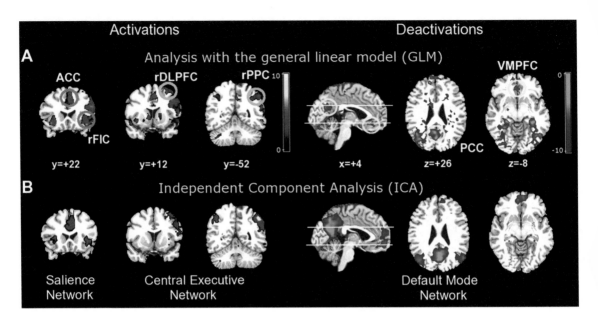

Plate 4 (figure 2.3)

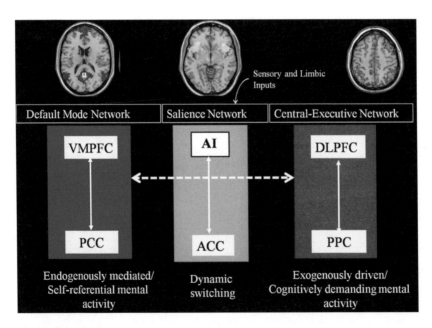

Plate 5 (figure 2.6)

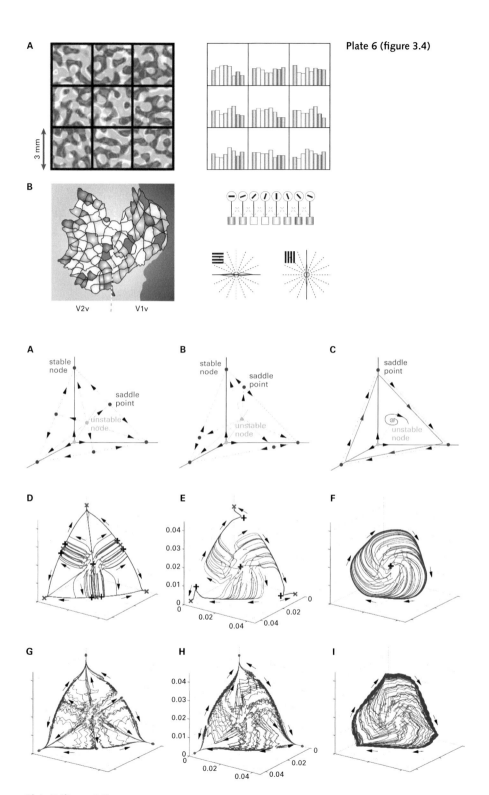

Plate 6 (figure 3.4)

A

3 mm

B

V2v   V1v

A

stable
node

saddle
point

unstable
node

B

stable
node

saddle
point

unstable
node

C

saddle
point

unstable
node

D

E

0.04
0.03
0.02
0.01
0
0   0.02   0.04   0.02

F

G

H

0.04
0.03
0.02
0.01
0
0   0.02   0.04   0.02

I

Plate 7 (figure 4.6)

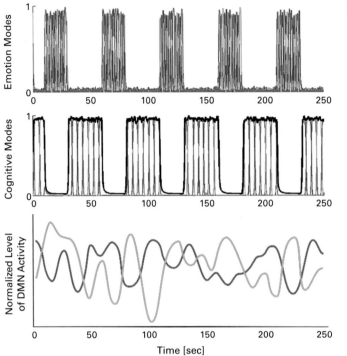

Plate 8 (figure 4.7)

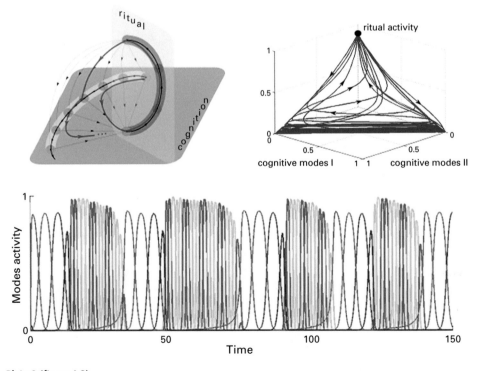

Plate 9 (figure 4.8)

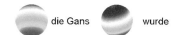 die Gans wurde im Ofen 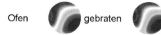 gebraten

Plate 10 (figure 5.5)

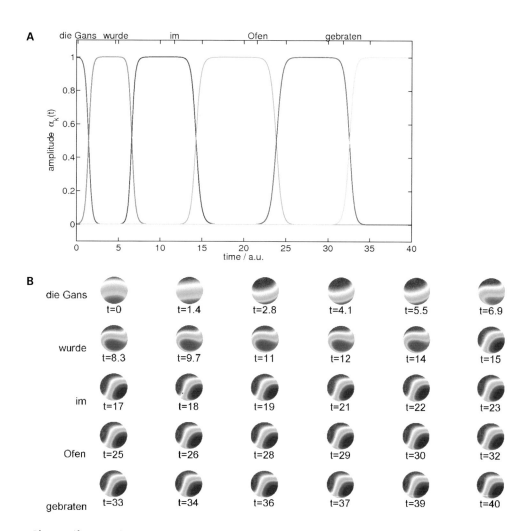

Plate 11 (figure 5.6)

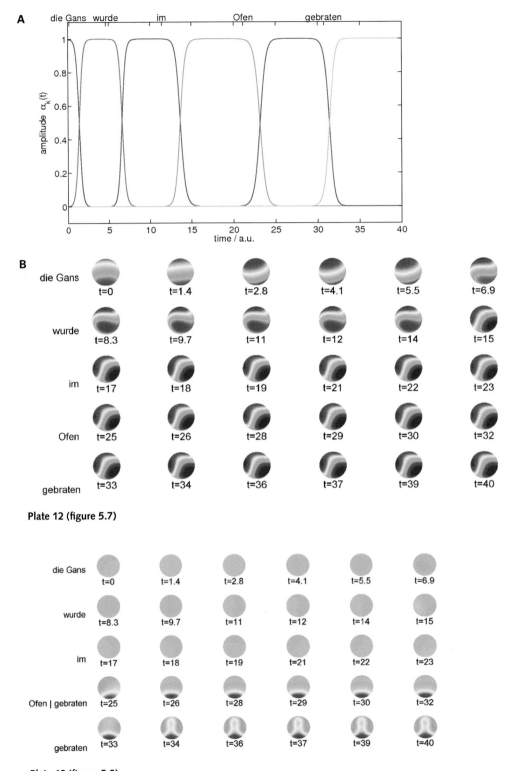

A die Gans wurde im Ofen gebraten

B

die Gans t=0 t=1.4 t=2.8 t=4.1 t=5.5 t=6.9

wurde t=8.3 t=9.7 t=11 t=12 t=14 t=15

im t=17 t=18 t=19 t=21 t=22 t=23

Ofen t=25 t=26 t=28 t=29 t=30 t=32

gebraten t=33 t=34 t=36 t=37 t=39 t=40

Plate 12 (figure 5.7)

die Gans t=0 t=1.4 t=2.8 t=4.1 t=5.5 t=6.9

wurde t=8.3 t=9.7 t=11 t=12 t=14 t=15

im t=17 t=18 t=19 t=21 t=22 t=23

Ofen | gebraten t=25 t=26 t=28 t=29 t=30 t=32

gebraten t=33 t=34 t=36 t=37 t=39 t=40

Plate 13 (figure 5.8)

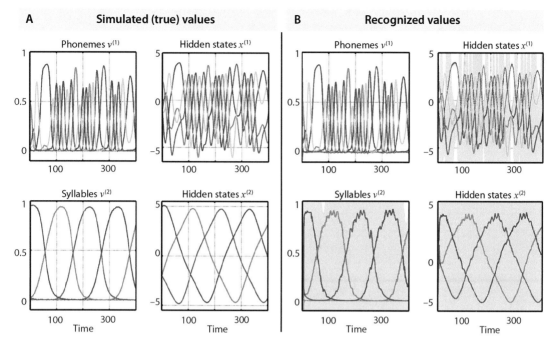

Plate 14 (figure 6.3)

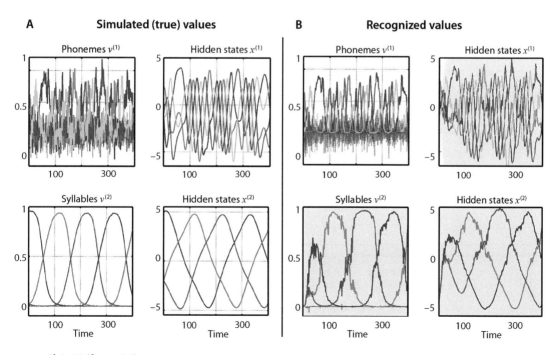

Plate 15 (figure 6.4)

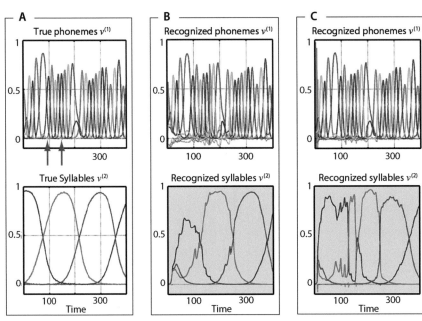

Plate 16 (figure 6.5)

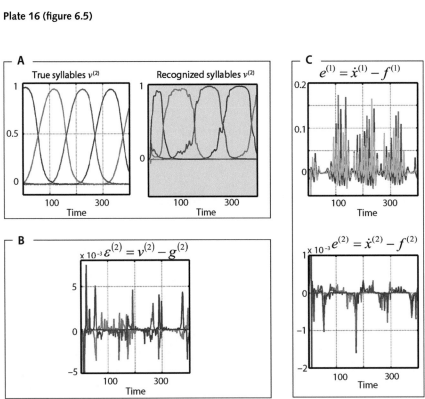

Plate 17 (figure 6.6)

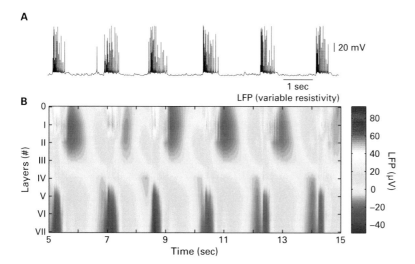

Plate 18 (figure 8.1)

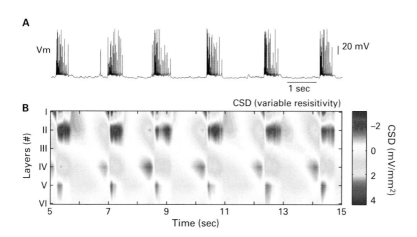

Plate 19 (figure 8.2)

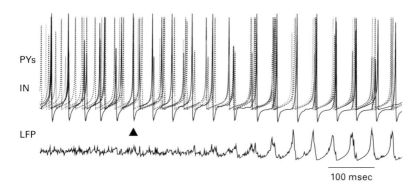

Plate 20 (figure 8.3)

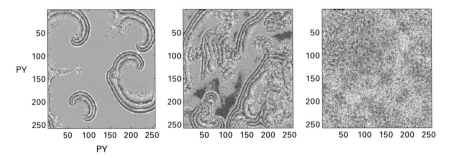

Plate 21 (figure 8.4)

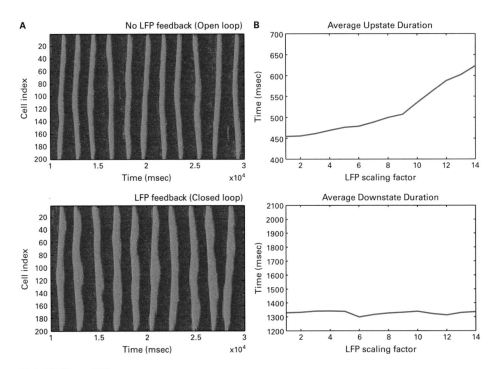

Plate 22 (figure 8.5)

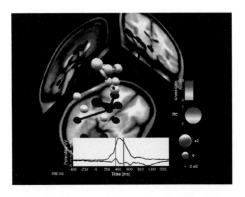

Plate 23 (figure 8.6)

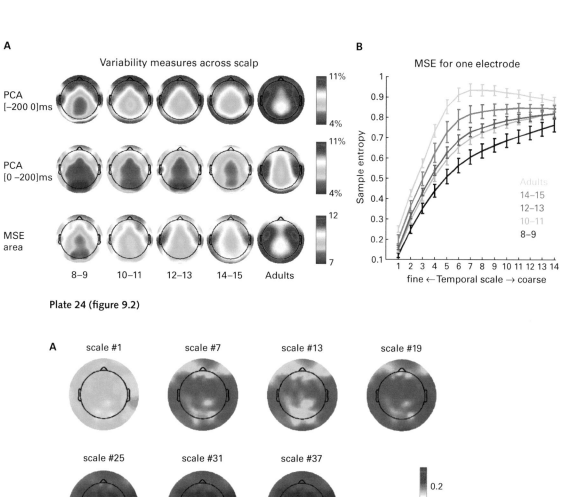

A Variability measures across scalp

PCA
[−200 0]ms

PCA
[0 −200]ms

MSE
area

8–9   10–11   12–13   14–15   Adults

B MSE for one electrode

Sample entropy

fine ← Temporal scale → coarse

Adults
14–15
12–13
10–11
8–9

Plate 24 (figure 9.2)

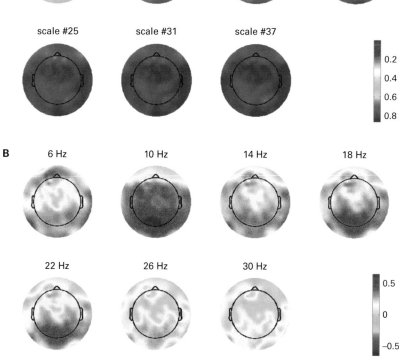

A

scale #1   scale #7   scale #13   scale #19

scale #25   scale #31   scale #37

0.2
0.4
0.6
0.8

B

6 Hz   10 Hz   14 Hz   18 Hz

22 Hz   26 Hz   30 Hz

0.5
0
−0.5

Plate 25 (figure 9.5)

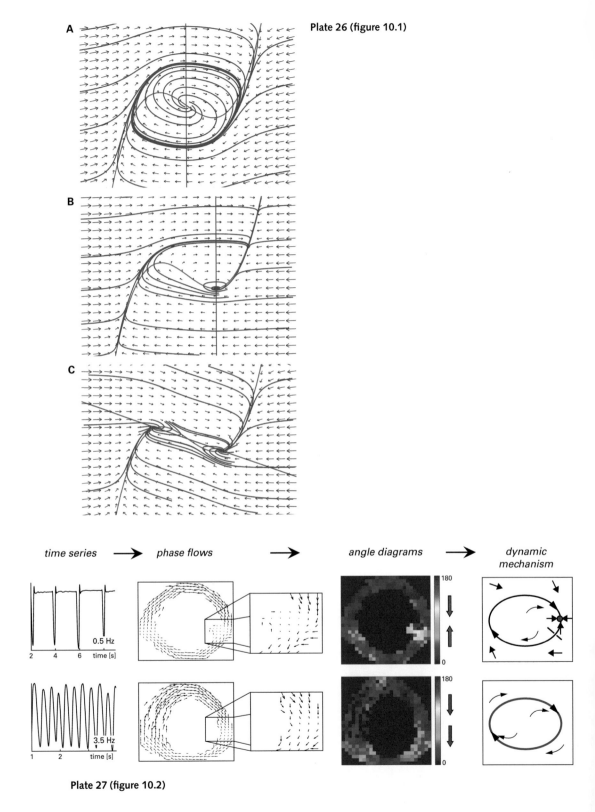

A

B

C

Plate 26 (figure 10.1)

time series ⟶ phase flows ⟶ angle diagrams ⟶ dynamic mechanism

0.5 Hz

2   4   6   time [s]

3.5 Hz

1   2   time [s]

180

0

180

0

Plate 27 (figure 10.2)

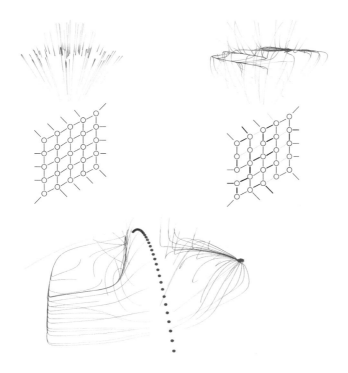

Plate 28 (figure 10.3)

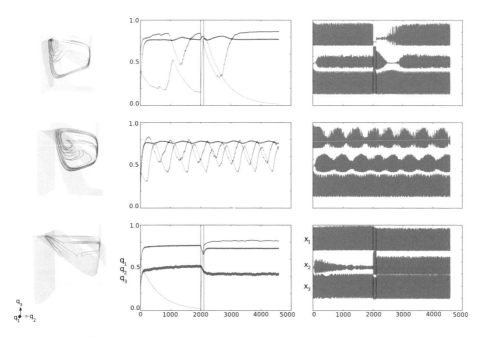

Plate 29 (figure 10.5)

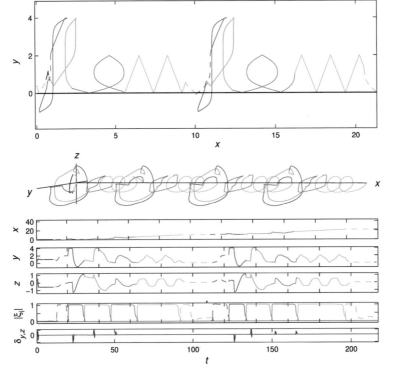

Plate 30 (figure 10.6)

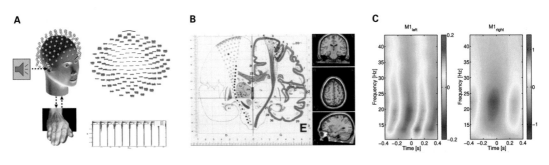

A **B** **C**

Plate 31 (figure 11.3)

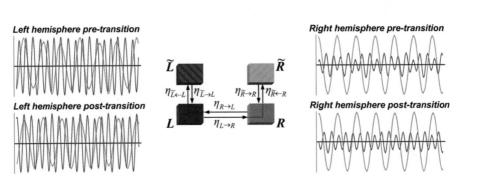

Left hemisphere pre-transition

Left hemisphere post-transition

Right hemisphere pre-transition

Right hemisphere post-transition

Plate 32 (figure 11.6)

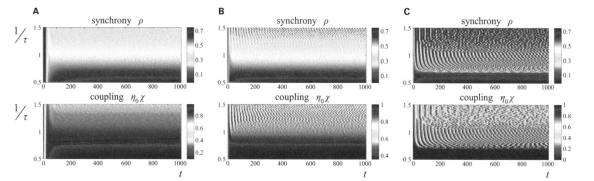

Plate 33 (figure 11.7)

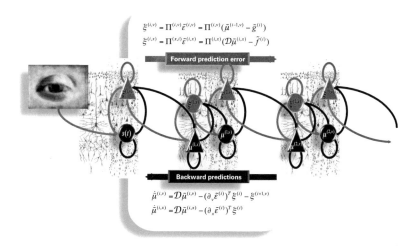

Plate 34 (figure 12.3)

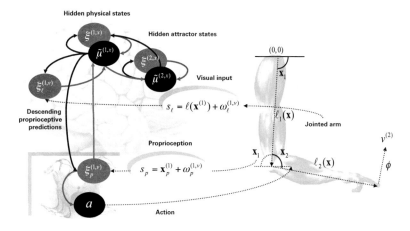

Plate 35 (figure 12.6)

association of gap junctions with inhibitory neurons further intensifies the role of these cells in producing oscillatory patterns in cortical neuropile. In the thalamic reticular formation, for example, gap junctions between inhibitory neurons may produce traveling waves of electrical activity (Fuentealba et al., 2004).

8.4.3 Ephaptic Interactions

Extracellular currents produced by electrical activity of neurons constituting local extracellular field potentials may directly influence the intrinsic electrical properties of neighboring neurons. These effects may include depolarization or hyperpolarization of cell membranes that vary the excitability or synchronous co-excitability of nearby cells. Although relatively weak, these ephaptic effects (Krnjevic, Dalkara, & Yim, 1986) have a global scope that may produce significant impact, particularly when neuronal activity is already partially synchronized by other mechanisms. Examples include sleep slow oscillations and epileptic activity, cases in which a certain degree of synchrony in electrical activity across neurons is already present from chemical or electrical interactions. In that case, a weak but global effect of ephaptic interaction may further augment (or not) the emergent synchrony.

8.4.4 Changes in Extracellular Ionic Concentrations

The electrical activity of neurons is associated with opening and closing of different ionic channels leading to changes in extracellular ion concentrations. These effects are strongest for low-concentration ions such as K^+ and Ca^{2+}. Opening of K^+ channels (such as the delayed and rectified voltage-gated channels involved in action potential generation) or Ca^{2+} channels may increase extracellular K^+ and decrease extracellular Ca^{2+} concentrations. Although these local changes are normally compensated by effects of ionic pumps and interactions with the (always) nearby glial syncytium, significant alternations in ion concentrations triggered by electrical activity in one cell may propagate to neighboring neurons leading to changes in their excitability, therefore contributing to synchronization of electrical activity between neighboring cells. Specifically, this mechanism likely contributes to the spread and synchronization of neuronal activity during epileptic seizures when high activity in groups of neurons leads to a large increase in extracellular potassium concentration whose diffusion increases the excitability of a larger pool of neurons surrounding epileptic focus (Frohlich, Sejnowski, & Bazhenov, 2010). This mechanism may contribute to synchronizing slow electrical activity patterns but is less likely to play a role in synchronizing fast oscillations.

8.5   Effects of Electrical Fields on Neuronal Activity during Sleep

Electric (ephaptic) interactions (Krnjevic, Dalkara, & Yim, 1986) may be particularly relevant during slow-wave sleep activities because of the large-amplitude LFP and EEG oscillations generated by thalamocortical ensembles during transitions between active (Up) and silent (Down) states. In principle, even weak electrical fields generated by neuronal activity might significantly affect overall activity patterns in neuronal networks because of the positive feedback loop they create. That is, extraneuronal electrical fields may act to increase synchronization of neuronal activities, in turn leading to even stronger extraneuronal field, and so on.

The effect of ephaptic interactions during sleep slow activity was recently explored (Frohlich & McCormick, 2010). This study revealed that external electrical field activity applied to cortical slices at strengths comparable with those produced during sleep *in vivo* can change the strength, frequency, and synchronization pattern of sleep-like oscillations in the slice. Applying external sine-wave field patterns triggered more rapid periodic transitions between Up and Down states than those in the same slice preparation without applied electrical fields. In a computer model, simulated electrical field activity generated by network neurons increased the duration of active states when electrical field was applied back to neurons producing it; this effect depended on the strength of ephaptic interactions in the model (figure 8.5, plate 22).

8.5.1   Large-Scale Network Activity Patterns

The primary function of the brain is to organize behavior or, more particularly, to optimize the results of behavior. Approximately 10^{15} synaptic molecular events occur in the human brain every second. From this vast dynamic complexity emerges organized behavior that continuously attempts to maximize rewards and minimize their opposites. This requires that many brain areas function together within tight time constraints. However, observation of brain dynamics has been dominated until recently by single-neuron recording studies at the neurophysiologic level and by single-channel and single-location event-related and task-related activation measures in EEG and hemodynamic imaging.

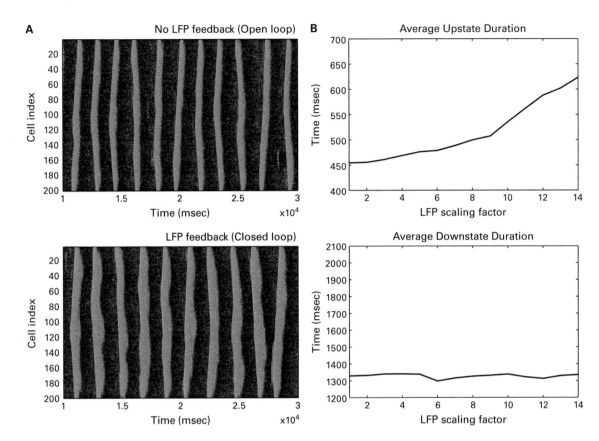

Figure 8.5 (plate 22)
Effect of electrical field feedback on simulated slow-wave sleep oscillations. (A) Raster plots of network activity without (top) and with (bottom) electrical field feedback. (B) Increasing the strength of the electrical field feedback in the model increased the duration of active (but not silent) states (P. Longers, S. Skorheim & M. Bazhenov, unpublished observations).

Attempts to look for network and network-like interactions in human functional magnetic resonance imaging (fMRI) data have given intriguing results including the common reappearance of so-called default-mode activation in the set of cortical and subcortical sites involved in the circuit of Papez (Jones, Mateen, Lucchinetti, Jack, & Welker, 2011) when subjects are told to "rest" while remaining awake in the scanner (J-R. Duann, S. Makeig, et al., unpublished observations). Concurrent and lagged correlations between activity levels in brain areas are observed in fMRI data recorded during watching complex dramatic movie scenes, and so forth (see Rogers, Morgan, Newton, & Gore, 2007). However, co-occurrence of activations at the multisecond scale, available via hemodynamic

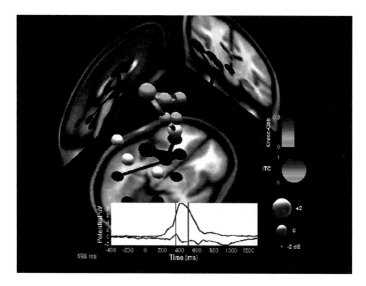

Figure 8.6 (plate 23)
Post-motor theta dynamics. Frame of an animation representing grand mean patterns of
event-related dynamics in the theta band. Black traces in the lower panel show the envelope of the grand mean event-related potential (ERP) time locked to the subject button
press (vertical line) median time of stimulus onset. Theta dynamics computed in a window
(center frequency 4.9 Hz, 3-cycle Hanning taper) centered (second vertical line) 150 ms
after the button press (first vertical line). Each sphere in the upper panel represents the
location of the equivalent dipole for a component cluster grouping maximally independent
EEG components from 15 subjects. Approximate projections of the equivalent-dipole locations are shown in shadow on three planes from an average MR image (Montreal Neuro-
logical Institute). Log spectral power changes (relative to prestimulus baseline) are
indicated by the sizes of the spheres (see key, bottom right). Non-gray sphere colors indicate consistent intertrial coherence (phase locking; ITC). Colored cylinders joining spheres
indicate significant event-related phase coherence (ERC) between cluster components.
From Makeig et al. (2004).

imaging, do not approach the speed of coordination of behavior and
thought (with timescales of tens of milliseconds or shorter). Study of
cortical dynamic interactions across cortical areas is only possible using
high-density EEG data, including noninvasively recorded scalp EEG.

Figure 8.6 (plate 23) shows a result from an animation of a brief
dynamic event involving the temporally coherent appearance of a tripha-
sic theta (ca. 5 Hz) complex in several maximally independent source
clusters surrounding a rapid thumb button press in a visual spatial selective attention task (Makeig et al., 2004). Similar transient theta complex
events may be more robust after manual responses immediately known
by the subject to be in error or after unexpected error (or bonus reward)
feedback. The role of theta band (in humans, 3–8 Hz; in animals, somewhat wider) dynamics in memory and other (here, reward-related) cogni-

tive processes is an attractive target for generative modeling. However, most current efforts to build generative models of cortical field dynamics either do not attempt to fit model behavior to actual field data at all or attempt to fit only a mean event-related response time series or mean channel power spectrum.

The application of ICA to scalp EEG (Makeig et al., 1996) or ECoG data (Whitmer, Worrell, Stead, Lee, & Makeig, 2009) has proved powerful to isolate electrical source processes completely compatible with generation by synchronous local field activity across a single cortical patch (Delorme et al., submitted). For ECoG data, Akalin Acar and colleagues (Acar, Worrell, & Makeig, 2009; Akalin Acar, Palmer, Worrell, & Makeig, 2011) have recently shown that at least in some cases, it is possible to estimate the actual cortical patch generator using a high-resolution model of cortex and a forward electrical head model derived from a magnetic resonance (MR) head image.

The prospect of electrocortical imaging of activity generated near an implanted ECoG array (including source areas located in cortical sulci and therefore projecting perpendicular to the grid) allows imagination of a procedure in which dynamic electrocortical imaging data could be used to train a generative model network to repeat and generalize recorded cortical EEG/ECoG dynamics. The now-being documented ephaptic effects of local field activity on neural spiking (and likely on spike-timing dependent plasticity and long-term potentiation) might be used to train the neural model. If successful, such models might be valuable for both basic and clinical neuroscience. They might constitute the first true multiscale models of electrophysiologic brain dynamics, both revealing new facts about brain dynamics supporting behavior and cognition and usable as test beds for building monitoring systems (e.g., for epilepsy) and for modeling and predicting consequences of drug, surgical, or other therapies for many pathologies.

8.6   Conclusion

Despite decades of studies, the questions how single-neuron activity leads to observed LFP, ECoG, and EEG patterns and how electrical fields in the brain at all spatial scales influence neuronal dynamics remain largely unanswered. Recent advances in both multiresolution data recordings and large-scale computer modeling bring, however, a hope that combining these powerful approaches may shed light on the genesis and functions of the large-scale activity patterns generated by the brain. As these spatiotemporal patterns form the basis of all perception, memory, and action, understanding their dynamics may, therefore, reveal a long mysterious link between neuronal activities and high-level brain functions.

Acknowledgments

This study was supported by NIH-NINDS (grant 1R01NS060870 to M.B.) and by a gift from The Swartz Foundation (Old Field, New York) (to S.M.).

References

Acar, A. Z, Worrell, G., & Makeig, S. (2009). Patch basis electrocortical source imaging in epilepsy. Proc IEEE Engin Med Biol Soc, Minneapolis, MN.

Akalin Acar, Z., Palmer, J., Worrell, G., & Makeig, S. (2011). Adaptive mixture independent component analysis and source localization in epilepsy. Proc IEEE Engin Med Biol Soc, Boston, MA.

Bazelot, M., Dinocourt, C., Cohen, I., & Miles, R. (2010). Unitary inhibitory field potentials in the CA3 region of rat hippocampus. *Journal of Physiology, 588*, 2077–2090.

Bazhenov, M., & Stopfer, M. (2010). Forward and back: motifs of inhibition in olfactory processing. *Neuron, 67*, 357–358.

Bazhenov, M., Lonjers, P., Skorheim, S., Bedard, C., & Destexhe, A. (2011). Non-homogeneous extracellular resistivity affects the current-source density profiles of Up/Down state oscillations. *Philosophical Transactions A, 369*(1952), 3802–3819.

Bedard, C., & Destexhe, A. (2009). Macroscopic models of local field potentials and the apparent 1/f noise in brain activity. *Biophysical Journal, 96*, 2589–2603.

Bedard, C., Kroger, H., & Destexhe, A. (2004). Modeling extracellular field potentials and the frequency-filtering properties of extracellular space. *Biophysical Journal, 86*, 1829–1842.

Blake, H., & Gerard, R. W. (1937). Brain potentials during sleep. *American Journal of Physiology, 119*, 692–703.

Chauvette, S., Volgushev, M., & Timofeev, I. (2010). Origin of active states in local neocortical networks during slow sleep oscillation. *Cerebral Cortex, 20*, 2660–2674.

Contreras, D., & Steriade, M. (1995). Cellular basis of EEG slow rhythms: a study of dynamic corticothalamic relationships. *Journal of Neuroscience, 15*, 604–622.

Creutzfeldt, O. D., Watanabe, S., & Lux, H. D. (1966a). Relations between EEG phenomena and potentials of single cortical cells. I. Evoked responses after thalamic and erpicortical stimulation. *Electroencephalography and Clinical Neurophysiology, 20*, 1–18.

Creutzfeldt, O. D., Watanabe, S., & Lux, H. D. (1966b). Relations between EEG phenomena and potentials of single cortical cells. II. Spontaneous and convulsoid activity. *Electroencephalography and Clinical Neurophysiology, 20*, 19–37.

Csercsa, R., Dombovari, B., Fabo, D., Wittner, L., Eross, L., Entz, L., et al. (2010). Laminar analysis of slow wave activity in humans. *Brain, 133*, 2814–2829.

Delorme, A., Palmer, J., Onton, J., Oostenveld, R., & Makeig, S. (submitted). Independent components of electroencephalographic signals are dipolar.

Freeman, W. (1975). *Mass Action in the Nervous System: Examination of the Neurophysiological Basis of Adaptive Behavior through the EEG.* New York: Academic Press.

Frohlich, F., & McCormick, D. A. (2010). Endogenous electric fields may guide neocortical network activity. *Neuron, 67,* 129–143.

Frohlich, F., Sejnowski, T. J., & Bazhenov, M. (2010). Network bistability mediates spontaneous transitions between normal and pathological brain states. *Journal of Neuroscience, 30,* 10734–10743.

Fuentealba, P., Crochet, S., Timofeev, I., Bazhenov, M., Sejnowski, T. J., & Steriade, M. (2004). Experimental evidence and modeling studies support a synchronizing role for electrical coupling in the cat thalamic reticular neurons in vivo. *European Journal of Neuroscience, 20,* 111–119.

Galarreta, M., & Hestrin, S. (2001). Electrical synapses between GABA-releasing interneurons. *Nature Reviews. Neuroscience, 2,* 425–433.

Jones, D. T., Mateen, F. J., Lucchinetti, C. F., Jack, C. R., & Welker, K. M. (2011). Default mode network disruption secondary to a lesion in the anterior thalamus. *Archives of Neurology, 68,* 242–247.

Katzner, S., Nauhaus, I., Benucci, A., Bonin, V., Ringach, D. L., & Carandini, M. (2009). Local origin of field potentials in visual cortex. *Neuron, 61,* 35–41.

Kirkland, K. L. (2002). High-tech brains: a history of technology-based analogies and models of nerve and brain function. *Perspectives in Biology and Medicine, 45,* 212–223.

Klee, M., & Rall, W. (1977). Computed potentials of cortically arranged populations of neurons. *Journal of Neurophysiology, 40,* 647–666.

Krnjevic, K., Dalkara, T., & Yim, C. (1986). Synchronization of pyramidal cell firing by ephaptic currents in hippocampus in situ. *Advances in Experimental Medicine and Biology, 203,* 413–423.

Lopes da Silva, F., & Van Rotterdam, A. (Eds.). (2005). *Biophysical Aspects of EEG and Magnetoencephalogram Generation.* Philadelphia: Lippincott Williams & Wilkins.

Lubenov, E. V. & Siapas, A. G. (2009). Hippocampal theta oscillations are traveling waves. *Nature, 459,* 534–539.

Mahon, S., Vautrelle, N., Pezard, L., Slaght, S. J., Deniau, J. M., Chouvet, G., et al. (2006). Distinct patterns of striatal medium spiny neuron activity during the natural sleep-wake cycle. *Journal of Neuroscience, 26,* 12587–12595.

Makeig, S., Bell, A. J., Jung, T.-P., & Sejnowski, T. J. (1996) Independent component analysis of electroencephalographic data. In D. Touretzky, M. Mozer, & M. Hasselmo (Eds). *Advances in Neural Information Processing Systems 8* (pp. 145–151). Cambridge, MA: MIT Press.

Makeig, S., Westerfield, M., Jung, T.-P., Enghoff, S., Townsend, J., Courchesne, E., et al. (2002). Dynamic brain sources of visual evoked responses. *Science, 295,* 690–694.

Makeig, S., Delorme, A., Westerfield, M., Jung, T.-P., Townsend, J., Courchesne, E., et al. (2004). Electroencephalographic brain dynamics following manually responded visual targets. *PLOS Biolog, 2,* 747–762.

Massimini, M., Huber, R., Ferrarelli, F., Hill, S., & Tononi, G. (2004). The sleep slow oscillation as a traveling wave. *Journal of Neuroscience, 24,* 6862–6870.

Milton, J. G., Chkcencheli, S. A., & Towle, V. L. (2007). Brain connectivity and spread of epileptic seizures. In V. K. Jirsa & R. McIntosh (Eds.), *Handbook of Brain Connectivity. Understanding Complex Systems* (pp. 477–503). Berlin: Springer.

Niedermeyer, E., & Lopes da Silva, F. (2005). *Electroencephalography: Basic Principles, Clinical Applications and Related Fields.* Philadelphia: Lippincott Williams & Wilkins.

Nunez, P. L., & Srinivasan, R. (2005). *Electric Fields of the Brain.* Oxford, UK: Oxford University Press.

Oren, I., Hajos, N., & Paulsen, O. (2010). Identification of the current generator underlying cholinergically induced gamma frequency field potential oscillations in the hippocampal CA3 region. *Journal of Physiology*, *588*, 785–797.

Petersen, C. C., Hahn, T. T., Mehta, M., Grinvald, A., & Sakmann, B. (2003). Interaction of sensory responses with spontaneous depolarization in layer 2/3 barrel cortex. *Proceedings of the National Academy of Sciences of the United States of America*, *100*, 13638–13643.

Rogers, B. P., Morgan, V. L., Newton, A. T., & Gore, J. C. (2007). Assessing functional connectivity in the human brain by fMRI. *Magnetic Resonance Imaging*, *25*, 1347–1357.

Rubino, D., Robbins, K. A., & Hatsopoulos, N. K. (2006). Propagating waves mediate information transfer in the motor cortex. *Nature Neuroscience*, *9*, 1549–1557.

Rulkov, N. F., Timofeev, I., & Bazhenov, M. (2004). Oscillations in large-scale cortical networks: map-based model. *Journal of Computational Neuroscience*, *17*, 203–223.

Sanchez-Vives, M. V., & McCormick, D. A. (2000). Cellular and network mechanisms of rhythmic recurrent activity in neocortex. *Nature Neuroscience*, *3*, 1027–1034.

Seigneur, J., & Timofeev, I. (2011). Synaptic impairment induced by paroxysmal ionic conditions in neocortex. *Epilepsia*, *52*, 132–139.

Steriade, M., Nuñez, A., & Amzica, F. (1993a). Intracellular analysis of relations between the slow (<1 Hz) neocortical oscillations and other sleep rhythms of electroencephalogram. *Journal of Neuroscience*, *13*, 3266–3283.

Steriade, M., Nuñez, A., & Amzica, F. (1993b). A novel slow (<1 Hz) oscillation of neocortical neurons *in vivo*: depolarizing and hyperpolarizing components. *Journal of Neuroscience*, *13*, 3252–3265.

Steriade, M., Timofeev, I., & Grenier, F. (2001). Natural waking and sleep states: a view from inside neocortical neurons. *Journal of Neurophysiology*, *85*, 1969–1985.

Thimm, J., Mechler, A., Lin, H., Rhee, S., & Lal, R. (2005). Calcium-dependent open/closed conformations and interfacial energy maps of reconstituted hemichannels. *Journal of Biological Chemistry*, *280*, 10646–10654.

Timofeev, I., Grenier, F., & Steriade, M. (2001). Disfacilitation and active inhibition in the neocortex during the natural sleep-wake cycle: an intracellular study. *Proceedings of the National Academy of Sciences of the United States of America*, *98*, 1924–1929.

Timofeev, I., Bazhenov, M., Seigneur, J., & Sejnowski, T. (in press). Neuronal synchronization and thalamocortical rhythms in sleep, wake and epilepsy. In J. Noebels, M. Avoli, M. A. Rogawski, R. W. Olsen, & A. V. Delgado-Escueta (Eds.), *Jasper's Basic Mechanisms of the Epilepsies* (4th edition). New York: Oxford University Press.

Trevelyan, A. J. (2009). The direct relationship between inhibitory currents and local field potentials. *Journal of Neuroscience*, *29*, 15299–15307.

Volgushev, M., Chauvette, S., Mukovski, M., & Timofeev, I. (2006). Precise long-range synchronization of activity and silence in neocortical neurons during slow-wave sleep. *Journal of Neuroscience*, *26*, 5665–5672.

Whitmer, D., Worrell, G., Stead, M., Lee, I. K., & Makeig, S. (2009). Utility of independent component analysis for interpretation of intracranial EEG. *Frontiers in Human Neuroscience*, *4*, 184.

Wilson, C. J., & Kawaguchi, Y. (1996). The origins of two-state spontaneous membrane potential fluctuations of neostriatal spiny neurons. *Journal of Neuroscience*, *16*, 2397–2410.

9 Mapping the Multiscale Information Content of Complex Brain Signals

Vasily A. Vakorin and Anthony R. McIntosh

Summary

There is growing evidence that variability in brain signals is an expression of the critical dynamics of neural networks. Characterization of this variability in the framework of complex systems brings a valuable new perspective to empirical studies. A number of techniques have recently been developed under the integrative framework of information theory, nonlinear dynamics, and theory of complex systems to support the collection of empirical evidence to unravel the principles of brain dynamics. This chapter mainly focuses on the quantification of the complexity of the brain signals, such as electroencephalogram (EEG) or magnetoencephalogram (MEG) measurements. Specifically, we describe the definition, interpretation, and applications of sample entropy estimated at different timescales. Discussion of the relations between sample entropy and other statistics such as spectral power, autocorrelation, nonstationarity, and graph measures is also included.

9.1 Brain as a Complex System

Many theoretical aspects of brain function focus on describing the properties of the structure and dynamics of the large-scale neuronal networks supporting a specific cognitive or behavioral task. Under this account, two complementary principles have been articulated in the literature: functional segregation and integration. Evidence in support of functionally segregated organization at different levels of the neural hierarchy is extensive. In contrast to modular deployment of local specialization, neuronal groups are interconnected between each other at many levels to support the emergence of coherent cognitive and behavioral states (Churchland & Sejnowski, 1988). One possible paradigm to address the relations between specialization and integration is to consider the brain as a complex system (Jirsa & McIntosh, 2007). This approach focuses on complexity, a broadly defined property characterizing a highly variable system with many parts whose behaviors strongly depend on the behavior of other parts (Deisboeck & Kresh, 2006). A distinctive feature of a complex system is that a set of properties of this system cannot obviously be derived from the properties of the individual parts.

The progress in complex systems, in particular with applications in neuroscience, was based primarily on techniques for building and understanding mathematical models, with reference to particular types of brain signals, as well as on measuring complexity as it is. Several chapters in this book serve as examples of the modeling endeavors to explore brain integration. This chapter essentially deals with the methods facilitating the collection of empirical evidence in support of the principles characterizing brain dynamics. Specifically, we will mainly focus on time series analysis, inspired by information theory and nonlinear dynamics. More specifically, we will discuss the definition, interpretation, and applications of a statistic termed sample entropy able to quantify the signal complexity.

9.2 Information-Theoretic Tools

Information theory, which began as a branch of applied mathematics and communication engineering involving the quantification of information, offers in some sense unique tools for design and estimation of complexity measures. The concepts developed within the framework of information theory represent fundamental measures for describing the variability of signals and uncertainty in observed variables, as well as the interdependence of different variables. Information-theoretic tools have proved to be important and sensitive enough for studying complex systems and are crucial for understanding complexity measures (Baddeley, Hancock, & Fldik, 2000).

Entropy $H(x)$ is a measure of uncertainty associated with a single random variable μ_x (Shannon, 1949). This term typically refers to the Shannon entropy, which quantifies the expected amount of the information in a signal. A mathematical definition of entropy begins from a set of axioms defining the general properties of information. First, the information is a function of the probability distribution of μ_x only, that is, $H(X) = H(p_1,..., p_n)$, where p_i is the probability to be in the state i. Second, the information reaches its maximum for the uniform distribution (highest unpredictability). Third, expending the probability space with events of zero probability should not change the information. Finally, joint entropy of two independent variables is equal to the sum of the individual entropies. If all these axioms are satisfied, the entropy will be in the form of

$$H_\alpha(x) = \frac{1}{1-\alpha} \log \sum_{\substack{i \\ \text{(states)}}} p_i^\alpha \tag{9.1}$$

with any non-negative real number α. This is called the Rényi entropy and is defined up to a multiplicative constant. In its turn, the choice of this constant is equivalent to the choice of the base of the logarithm used. When $\alpha \to 1$, the Rényi entropy converges to

$$H_1(x) = - \sum_{\substack{i \\ \text{(states)}}} p_i \log[p_i], \tag{9.2}$$

which is the Shannon entropy.

For a given time series $x(t)$, $t = 1,..., N$, Shannon entropy can be used to quantify the average information received with measurements of $x(t)$, presumably associated with a random variable. This can be implemented with a box counting approach, based on partitioning of data space into the bins of size δ. The probability distribution is then estimated as relative frequencies of the occurrence of data samples in particular finite-size bins. In this case, the Shannon entropy is given by

$$H_1(x,\delta) = - \sum_{\substack{i \\ \text{(bins)}}} p_i(x,\delta) \log[p_i(x,\delta)], \tag{9.3}$$

with $p_i(x,\delta)$ being the probability of finding a data sample in the ith bin.

For two time series $x_1(t)$ and $x_2(t)$, $t = 1,..., N$, their joint entropy can be defined as

$$H_1(x_1,x_2,\delta) = - \sum_{\substack{i \\ \text{(bins)}}} p_i(x_1,x_2,\delta) \log[p_i(x_1,x_2,\delta)], \tag{9.4}$$

where $p_i(x_1,x_2,\delta)$ is the probability of a data sample falling into a bin of size δ, specified in the two-dimensional space spanned by $x_1(t)$ and $x_2(t)$. In a similar way, one can define the joint entropy of m time series $x_1(t),...,$ $x_{m-1}(t)$ and $x_m(t)$. Specifically, the joint entropy is

$$H_1(x_1,...,x_m,\delta) = - \sum_{\substack{i \\ \text{(bins)}}} p_i(x_1,...,x_m,\delta) \log[p_i(x_1,...,x_m,\delta)]. \tag{9.5}$$

In addition, the conditional entropy $H_1(x_1|x_2, \delta)$ of $x_1(t)$ given $x_2(t)$ can be defined as the amount of information contained in $x_1(t)$ provided that the knowledge about $x_2(t)$ is excluded. Specifically,

$$H_1(x_1 \mid x_2, \delta) = H_1(x_1, x_2, \delta) - H_1(x_2, \delta). \tag{9.6}$$

In the case of a multivariate signal $[x_1(t), \ldots, x_m(t)]$, we have

$$H_1(x_m \mid x_1, \ldots, x_{m-1}, \delta) = H_1(x_1, x_2, \ldots, x_m, \delta) - H_1(x_1, \ldots, x_{m-1}, \delta), \tag{9.7}$$

which is the conditional entropy of $x_m(t)$ given $[x_1(t), \ldots, x_{m-1}(t)]$.

9.3   Information and Nonlinear Dynamics

According to a recent theory, cognitive operations are the result of generation and transformation of cooperative modes of neural activity (Bressler, 1995, 2002; McIntosh, 1999). Specifically, the principles emphasize the integrative capacity of the brain in terms of ensembles of coupled neural systems interacting in a nonlinear way (Nunez, 1995; Jirsa & McIntosh, 2007). Typically, in a nonlinear analysis of electroencephalogram (EEG) or magnetoencephalogram (MEG), one assumes that an individual time series represents the manifestation of an underlying multidimensional nonlinear dynamic model (Stam, 2005). In other words, we need to reconstruct, from a time series of observations, the dynamics in the multidimensional state space of the underlying model. It can be done with time delay embedding

$$\mathbf{x}_m(t) = [x_1(t), x_2(t), \ldots, x_m(t)] \equiv \{x(t), x(t+\tau), \ldots, x[t+(m-1)\tau]\}, \tag{9.8}$$

wherein a time series $x(t)$ is converted to a sequence of vectors in an m-dimensional space. We note that the ultimate goal is not to reconstruct an orbit in the state space that is closest to the true one. However, Takens' embedding theorem states that if the embedding dimension m is sufficiently high, the macrocharacteristics of a dynamic system such as the entropy can be reconstructed (Takens, 1981).

Given time delay embedding (9.8), the Kolmogorov entropy (Kolmogorov, 1959; Sinai, 1959), which is a measure of the mean rate of information generated by a dynamic system, is defined as

$$\begin{aligned}
K_1 &= \lim_{\substack{m\to\infty \\ \delta\to 0}} \frac{1}{\tau}[H_1(x_m \mid x_1, \ldots, x_{m-1}, \delta)] \\
&= \lim_{\substack{m\to\infty \\ \delta\to 0}} \frac{1}{\tau}[H_1(x_1, x_2, \ldots, x_m, \delta) - H_1(x_1, x_2, \ldots, x_{m-1}, \delta)] \\
&\equiv \lim_{\substack{m\to\infty \\ \delta\to 0}} \frac{1}{\tau}[H_1(\mathbf{x}_m, \delta) - H_1(\mathbf{x}_{m-1}, \delta)].
\end{aligned} \tag{9.9}$$

K_1 measures the unpredictability of a system. In particular, it represents the uncertainty that remains in the next event, provided that complete knowledge of its history is given.

Estimating the Kolmogorov entropy would require the knowledge about the values of the joint entropies, which can be computed as

$$H_1(\mathbf{x}_m,\delta) = -\sum_{\substack{i \\ (\text{bins})}} p_i(\mathbf{x}_m,\delta)\log[p_i(\mathbf{x}_m,\delta)] = -\sum_{\substack{t \\ (\text{data points})}} \log[p_{i(t)}(\mathbf{x}_m,\delta)],$$

(9.10)

where $p_{i(t)}(\mathbf{x}_m,\delta)$ is the probability of finding a state vector $\mathbf{x}_m(t)$ in the ith bin represented by a box of diameter δ. In its turn, $p_{i(t)}(\mathbf{x}_m,\delta)$ can be approximated by the probability $P_t(\mathbf{x}_m,r)$ of being in the m-dimensional state space within a radius r (or diameter $\delta = 2r$), centered around the state vector $\mathbf{x}_m(t)$ observed at time t (Grassberger & Procaccia, 1983; Prichard & Theiler, 1995). Thus, we have

$$H_1(\mathbf{x}_m,\delta) \approx -\sum_{\substack{t \\ (\text{datapoints})}} \log[P_t(\mathbf{x}_m,r)] = -\log[C_1(\mathbf{x}_m,r)],$$

(9.11)

where $C_1(\mathbf{x}_m,r)$ is a so-called correlation integral estimated as

$$C_1(\mathbf{x}_m,r) = \frac{1}{n(n-1)} \times \sum_{i=1}^{n}\left\{\sum_{j\neq i}^{n}\Theta[r-\|\mathbf{x}_m(i)-\mathbf{x}_m(j)\|]\right\}.$$

(9.12)

Here, n is the number of state vectors, Θ is the Heaviside function, and $\|\cdot\|$ stands for the maximum norm distance between two state vectors $\mathbf{x}_m(i)$ and $\mathbf{x}_m(j)$, observed at the times i and j. The correlation integral $C_1(\mathbf{x}_m,r)$ is interpreted as the likelihood that the distance between two randomly chosen points, $\mathbf{x}_m(i)$ and $\mathbf{x}_m(j)$ in the m-dimensional space spanned by $\mathbf{x}_m(t)$, is smaller than r. The function $\sum_{i\neq j}\Theta[r-\|\mathbf{x}_m(i)-\mathbf{x}_m(j)\|]$ for a given point i represents the number of points j such that the distance between the state vectors $\mathbf{x}_m(i)$ and $\mathbf{x}_m(j)$ is less than r.

Thus, the Kolmogorov entropy can be estimated as

$$K_1 \approx \lim_{\substack{m\to\infty \\ r\to 0}} \frac{1}{\tau}\{\log[C_1(\mathbf{x}_{m-1},r)] - \log[C_1(\mathbf{x}_m,r)]\}.$$

(9.13)

Estimation of K_1 at finer and finer partitions of the state space ($r \to 0$) would require more and more data points ($n \to \infty$). Grassberger and Procaccia (1983) suggested to use the K_2 entropy defined as

$$K_2 = \lim_{r\to 0}\lim_{m\to\infty}\lim_{n\to\infty}\frac{1}{\tau}\{\log[C_1(\mathbf{x}_{m-1},r)]-\log[C_1(\mathbf{x}_m,r)]\}, \tag{9.14}$$

which is a lower bound for K_1.

The Kolmogorov entropy K_1, as well as K_2, thus represent an important step for characterizing dynamic systems. However, they cannot be used for measuring the complexity of natural (neural) systems, as the amount of data needed to compute the limits in (9.14) is beyond that which is available in practice.

9.4 Approximate and Sample Entropy

A statistic called approximate entropy (ApEn) was proposed to quantify the complexity of short and noisy time series (Pincus, 1991, 1995). Specifically, K_2 was approximated by ApEn using fixed parameters m and r as well as $\tau = 1$, measured in data points. The condition $\tau = 1$ implies that the observed time series of the length N can be associated with a time delay embedding $\mathbf{x}_m(t) = \{x(t), x(t-1), \dots, x(t-m+1)\}$, where $t = 1, \dots, N-m+1$. We can define the function $C_i^m(r)$ as

$$C_i^m(r) = \frac{1}{N-m+1}\sum_{j=1}^{N-m+1}\Theta[r-\|\mathbf{x}_m(i)-\mathbf{x}_m(j)\|], \tag{9.15}$$

which represents the probability that a randomly chosen state vector $\mathbf{x}_m(j)$ will be found within the sphere of radius r, centered at $\mathbf{x}_m(i)$, where i is fixed. Averaging the natural logarithm of the functions $C_i^m(r)$ across all the state vectors, we have a function

$$\Phi^m(r) = \frac{1}{N-m+1}\sum_{i=1}^{N-m+1}\ln[C_i^m(r)]. \tag{9.16}$$

Approximate entropy was defined as

$$\text{ApEn}(m,r) = \lim_{N\to\infty}[\Phi^m(r)-\Phi^{m+1}(r)], \tag{9.17}$$

which can be estimated as

$$\text{ApEn}(m,r,N) = \Phi^m(r)-\Phi^{m+1}(r). \tag{9.18}$$

ApEn is approximately equal to the negative average natural logarithm of conditional probability that two delay vectors, which are close in an m-dimensional state space (meaning that the distance between them is less than the scale length r), will remain close in an $(m + 1)$-dimensional state space.

The algorithm for computing ApEn counts each state vector as matching (compared with) itself. A direct consequence of such a practice is that the approximate entropy becomes a biased statistic. Specifically, the expected values of ApEn(m,r,N) is less than ApEn(m,r), especially for relatively small N.

A statistic called sample entropy was proposed to correct this bias (Richman & Moorman, 2000). Specifically, two alterations were made. First, self-matches were excluded when computing the function $C_i^m(r)$. Second, only the first $(N - m)$ m-dimensional state vectors $\mathbf{x}_m(i)$ were considered, which ensured that for all $1 \leq i \leq N-m$, the m-dimensional state vectors $\mathbf{x}_{m+1}(i)$ can be defined. Specifically, similar to $C_i^m(r)$, the function $B_i^m(r)$ is defined as $1/(N - m - 1)$ multiplied by the number of state vectors $\mathbf{x}_m(j)$ located within r of $\mathbf{x}_m(j)$:

$$B_i^m(r) = \frac{1}{N-m-1} \sum_{\substack{j\,\text{such that}\\ j \neq i}}^{N-m} \Theta\big[r - \| \mathbf{x}_m(i) - \mathbf{x}_m(j) \|\big], \qquad (9.19)$$

where j goes from 1 to $N - m$, and $j \neq i$ to exclude self-matches. Then, similar to (9.16), averaging across $(N - m)$ vectors, we have

$$B^m(r) = \frac{1}{N-m} \sum_{i=1}^{N-m} B_i^m(r). \qquad (9.20)$$

Similarly, the equivalent of $B_i^m(r)$ in an $(m + 1)$-dimensional representation of the original time series $x(t)$, the function $A_i^m(r)$, is given by $1/(N - m - 1)$ times the number of state vectors $\mathbf{x}_{m+1}(j)$ located within r of $\mathbf{x}_{m+1}(j)$:

$$A_i^m(r) = \frac{1}{N-m-1} \sum_{\substack{j\,\text{such that}\\ j \neq i}}^{N-m} \Theta\big[r - \|\mathbf{x}_{m+1}(i) - \mathbf{x}_{m+1}(j)\|\big], \qquad (9.21)$$

which can be averaged across $(N - m)$ points as

$$A^m(r) = \frac{1}{N-m} \sum_{i=1}^{N-m} A_i^m(r). \qquad (9.22)$$

Sample entropy is defined then as follows:

$$\text{SampEn}(m,r) = \lim_{N \to \infty} \big\{ \ln\big[B^m(r)\big] - \ln\big[A^m(r)\big] \big\}, \qquad (9.23)$$

which is estimated as

$$\text{SampEn}(m,r,N) = \ln\left[B^m(r)\right] - \ln\left[A^m(r)\right] = -\ln\left[\frac{A^m(r)}{B^m(r)}\right]. \tag{9.24}$$

It should be noted that the ratio $A^m(r)/B^m(r)$ is precisely the conditional probability that two events will remain within the distance r of each other in an $(m + 1)$-dimensional space, provided that they were close (less than r) in an m-dimensional space. The statistic $\text{SampEn}(m,r,N)$ is computed as the negative natural logarithm of such a probability. A greater likelihood of remaining close (less than r) results in smaller values for the SampEn statistic, indicating less irregularities. Conversely, higher values are associated with the signals having more complexity and less regular patterns in their representations.

9.5   Estimation of Sample Entropy

Estimation of the sample entropy is based on the reconstruction of multivariate dynamics underlying the observed time series. In general, time delay embedding is a crucial and nontrivial step. There are many competing approaches proposed in the literature, and all of them are heuristic and somewhat mutually exclusive. Estimating the autocorrelation function provides one approach for choosing the embedding delay τ. A number of studies proposed different information-theoretic criteria for selecting the embedding parameters optimally. Lai and Lerner (1998) numerically argued that the correct selection of τ is optimal, whereas selecting m is not. Kim, Eykholt, & Slas (1998) concluded that it is the embedding window $m \times \tau$ that is crucial in the issue of estimating correlation dimension, a measure based on computing correlation integrals. Small and Tse (2004) proposed a robust criterion for reconstructing the underlying dynamics from a finite time series in the presence of noise. They concluded that only the embedding window is significant, whereas the lag τ is model dependent.

Another point to bear in mind is that signaling in the brain is not instantaneous, and propagation of neural activity takes time (Desmedt & Cheron, 1980). Thus, coupled nonlinear systems with time delay in coupling play an important role for modeling neural dynamics (Niebur, Schuster, & Kammen, 1991; Ghosh, Rho, McIntosh, Ktter, & Jirsa, 2008; Deco, Jirsa, McIntosh, Sporns, & Ktter, 2009). A particular class of systems, which can create patterns of arbitrary dimension, are time delay feedback systems. The dimension of the state space of such systems is infinite. This would be in parallel to the definition of SampEn, which is closely related to the Kolmogorov entropy defined for $m \to \inf$. In the literature on estimating the complexity of the brain signals, a typical choice for the parameter m is $m = 2$. However, estimating the complexity of the neuromagnetic somatosensory steady-state response, Vakorin et al. (2010) used relatively large values of m, when SampEn became stable ($m = 5$). In this case, a completely data-driven pipeline, wherein the source activity was estimated on a relatively fine grid encompassing the whole brain, revealed the activation pattern similar to those based on modeling the MEG data with a set of dipoles. This effect was not clear when $m = 2$.

With regard to the embedding delay τ, the original definition of the sample entropy implies $\tau = 1$. A natural extension would be to include the estimation of SampEn as a function of the parameter τ (Kaffashi, Foglyano, Wilson, & Loparo, 2008). The point is that sample entropy is, by construction, a measure of predictability. Predictability based on linear stochastic fluctuations can be compared across different signals estimating the autocorrelation function. In some cases, the autocorrelation of time series does not decay quickly. In turn, the influence of long-range linear correlations on computing nonlinear invariants is not minimized. Consequently, the correct quantification of the complexity of the underlying system is compromised, thus providing spurious results for comparative analysis of time series with short- and long-range autocorrelations. Kaffashi et al. (2008) computed the sample entropy both for the original time series and the surrogate data, which had approximately the same linear characteristics (such as the autocorrelation function and the distribution of the signal amplitudes) as the original data, but with the destroyed nonlinear properties. Their simulations based on the Lorenz and Rössler systems showed that when τ is close to 1, the difference in SampEn between the original and surrogate data was insignificant. These results suggest that for small τ, the sample entropy reflects mostly the linear properties of the signal.

9.6 Multiscale Entropy

An alternative approach that implicitly controls for the embedding delay τ is based on down-sampling the original time series by factors 2, 4, 8, ... Down-sampling would alleviate the effects of linear correlations between consecutive samples. A similar idea was previously implemented by Zhang (1991), who introduced a complexity measure based on the

Shannon entropy of various scales. Specifically, the coarse-grained signal $y(t)$ at the scale θ was defined as

$$y^{(\theta)}(t) = \int_{t-\theta/2}^{t+\theta/2} dt' x(t'), \tag{9.25}$$

wherein the fluctuations at scales smaller than θ are eliminated. Costa, Goldberger, and Peng, (2002) proposed to unify the sample entropy with an idea of coarse-grained signals in case of finite time series. Specifically, the original time series $x(i)$, where $i = 1,...,N$, are first divided into non-overlapping windows of length θ, where $\theta = 1, 2, 3,...$. Then, the data points are averaged inside each window. Thus, the amplitude of the coarse-grained time series $y^{(\theta)}(t)$ at timescale θ is calculated according to

$$y^{(\theta)}(t) = \frac{1}{\theta} \sum_{i=(t-1)\theta+1}^{i=t\theta} x(i), \ 1 \le t \le N / \theta. \tag{9.26}$$

The trivial case of $\theta = 1$ represents the original time series. The length of $y^{(\theta)}(t)$ decreases with θ and is equal to N/θ. Finally, the sample entropy can be computed as a function of the scale factor θ. This is known as the multiscale entropy (MSE). Estimation of the MSE curves have become a popular choice to characterize the complexity of the brain signals.

A few things are worth noting here. First, higher values of θ, which is somewhat equivalent to higher τ, should alleviate linear stochastic effects in the time series. At the same time, it implies that the sample entropy, which is related to the mean rate of the information produced by a dynamical system, is averaged over larger intervals, defined by τ in (9.9). Finally, down-sampling the data by averaging the data points within a time window of length θ is equivalent to the low-pass filter with θ determining the filter cutoff. Such an approach has its own advantages and flaws. On the one hand, various patterns of synchronized and coordinated oscillations in the brain could operate at different frequency regimes. Thus, having a mechanism able to discriminate different frequency components, as captured by the MSE curves, would be beneficial for a comparative analysis of the brain signals. On the other hand, such nonlinear relations between the scale factor θ and the corresponding frequency band make the interpretations of the MSE curves less trivial. Later we will discuss the observed relations between the MSE and spectral power of the brain signals.

9.7   Applications of Multiscale Entropy

A number of studies used the approximate and sample entropy statistics to quantify the variability of the brain signals both for the electrode measurements (Abasolo et al., 2005; Abasolo, Hornero, Espino, Alvarez, & Poza, 2006) and source dynamics (Misic, Mills, Taylor, & McIntosh, 2010; Vakorin et al. 2010). In particular, MSE has been successfully applied to map increasing complexity with development in children (McIntosh, Kovacevic, & Itier, 2008; Lippé, Kovacevic, & McIntosh, 2009). It has also been applied to discriminate different modes of visual perception (Misic et al., 2010). Other applications of the MSE approach can be found in studies on normal brain activity in resting and cognitive states, in particular as a function of age, in an analysis of degenerative brain diseases (Alzheimer's disease), and in epilepsy (Protzner, Valiante, Kovacevic, McCormick, & McAndrews, 2010).

Misic et al. (2010) showed that the variability of neuromagnetic activity, which was sensitive to the task content, was also highly region specific. Specifically, children (6–16 years old) and adults (20–41 years old) performed a one-back face recognition task with inverted and upright faces. The temporal variability of neural activity represented by approximately 600 sources covering the whole brain was estimated computing the sample entropy statistic at scales 1–14 (original sampling rate 625 Hz). During development, neuromagnetic activity became more complex across the whole brain, with most robust increases in medial parietal regions. The complexity of source dynamics was higher for younger children and adults performing the upright face recognition task than with inverted faces. Figure 9.1A shows a data-driven statistical contrast, capturing the difference between upright and inverted conditions. This effect was significant only in the right fusiform gyrus, as can be seen figure 9.1B. Such results are consistent with the idea that a greater propensity is acquired for configural and holistic processing as the brain develops. Thus, transient changes in functional integration modulated by task demand can be extracted from the variability of regional brain activity.

McIntosh et al. (2008) analyzed the relations between maturation and variability of the brain signals in children (8–15 years) and young adults (20–33 years). EEG sampled at 500 Hz was recorded when the participants performed a rapid face recognition task. Specifically, during each trial, a novel or familiar face was presented, and the participants responded by pressing one of two buttons depending on whether they recognized the face or not. The MSE curves were computed as a measure

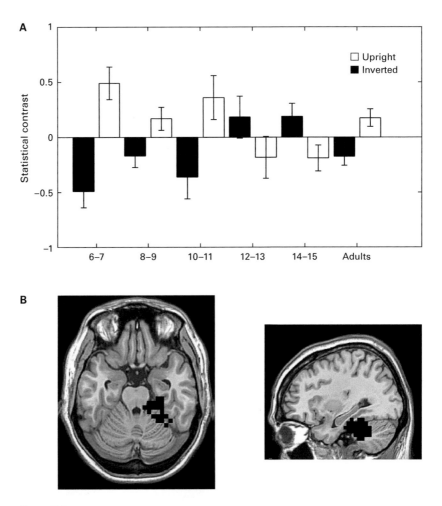

Figure 9.1
Inversion effect captured by the multiscale entropy. (A) A multivariate statistical data-driven contrast that accounts for most of the variance of MSE estimates. (B) Statistical maps showing brain regions that robustly support differences in the MSE curves between upright and inverted faces across all age groups (6–7, 8–9, 10–11, 12–13, 14–16 years old and adults).

of the signal complexity, in addition to the pre- and post-stimulus dimensionality estimation of trial-to-trial variability, determined as a minimum number of principal components capturing 90% of the variance across trials. For both MSE and principal component analysis (PCA), a robust gradual increase in the brain variability measures was observed across age groups (see figure 9.2, plate 24). The maturation-related increase in entropy was essentially expressed for all the electrodes and at all scales (1–14). Given similar age-related differences at all timescales, the area under the MSE curve was computed as a cumulative index of maturational changes in the variability of the brain signals. It was found that brain signal variability, which increased with age, negatively correlated with response time variability and positively correlated with accuracy. In other words, increased brain variability that characterizes brain maturation was associated with more stable and accurate behavior.

Similar results were obtained in characterizing EEG signal complexity during early development (Lippé et al., 2009). Typically, developing infants and children from 1 to 60 months old participated in the study. The subjects were separated into four age groups. In addition, adults between 20 and 30 years participated in the study. The visual and auditory evoked potentials were measured in response to a black-and-white

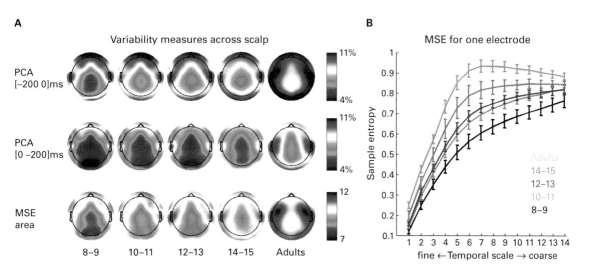

Figure 9.2 (plate 24)
Within-subject brain variability across age groups. (A) Group mean results across the scalp for the pre- and post-stimulus PCA dimensionality estimate and sample entropy averaged across all the scales. (B) Group mean MSE curves for channel O2 (error bars represent standard errors). Similar MSE curves were obtained for all channels and showed age-related increase in sample entropy at all scales.

reversing checkerboard presented binocularly for 500 ms and a 50 ms broadband noise presented in free-field binaurally in a soundproof room. A typical methodological issue faced by such studies is the need to compare the developmental trajectories of visual and auditory systems. They cannot be compared directly in terms of the event-related potentials because of morphological and spatial differences of their waveforms. Complexity measures, such as MSE, do not depend on these specific features and thus provide a tool directly to compare the sensory systems of different modality. The age-related differences in MSE were estimated at the timescales 1–4 (sampling frequency 250 Hz). For both conditions, age-related differences in MSE were significant and stably expressed across all temporal scales. At the same time, differences in the signal complexity for the auditory and visual responses were found only for the infants and children, but not for the adults. Notably, from 1 to 60 months, complexity was greater for the response to visual stimuli than for that to auditory stimuli.

A number of studies applied the MSE approach to explore the differences in the EEG signals between normal subjects and patients with Alzheimer's disease (AD). Park, Kim, Kim, Cichocki, & Kim (2007) used the resting-state EEG and reported the MSE curves (scales 1–16, original sampling frequency 200 Hz) averaged over channels and individuals for three groups: normal population, AD patients, and subjects with mild cognitive impairment (MCI). The MSE curves for the three groups have common features. Specifically, the sample entropy reached its maximum at scales 5–7 and then gradually decreased. Severe AD patients had a significantly lower level of the sample entropy values than that of the normal group at scale 2–16. The maximal difference in the complexity was observed at scales 6–8. At the same time, the main difference in the MSE curve between MCI and normal subjects was the shift of the peak in SampEn toward coarse timescales for the MCI subjects. Thus, a crossover in the MSE curves was observed, with higher complexity at fine timescales for the normal subjects.

Escudero, Abásolo, Hornero, Espino, & López (2006) performed the MSE analysis of the spontaneous EEG recordings from the AD patients and control subjects, measured in an awake state with eyes closed. The sample entropy was computed at scales 1–12 (sampling rate 256 Hz). The EEG background activity for most of the electrodes and scale factors was less complex in AD patients than that in control subjects. The results denoted the existence of a crossover in the MSE curves between normal and AD groups approximately at scales 10–12. Mizuno et al. (2010) used longer time series in a study where EEG was recorded for AD patients and age- and sex-matched healthy subjects with the eyes closed. The sampling rate was 200 Hz, and the sample entropy was computed at scales 1–20. Similar to Park et al. (2007), the sample entropy for both groups increased first, then decreased as scale factor increased. However, the peak in the MSE curve was reached around scale 4 and 7 for the control and AD subjects, respectively. Thus, a crossover in MSE was clearly observed for all the electrodes, and the sample entropy for the control subjects was higher at fine timescales (2–6) and smaller at coarse timescales (9–20).

Many studies explored the nonlinear nature of epileptic seizures and demonstrated the pathologic loss of complexity of the epileptogenic signal (Lehnertz & Elger, 1997). Strong evidence was collected that epileptic seizures represent highly nonlinear effects of brain dynamics (Lehnertz & Elger, 1997). Among other statistics to characterize the nonlinear features of the epileptogenic EEG, multiscale entropy was used by Protzner et al. (2010), who studied patients shown to have right mesial temporal seizure onsets. Specifically, the MSE was computed based on EEG dynamics measured in epileptogenic (right) and healthy (left) hippocampi (sampling rate 500 Hz, scales 1–8). EEG was recorded during performance of memory tasks; namely, scene recording and recognition, known to be sensitive to mesial temporal integrity. Reduced signal complexity was found in epileptogenic hippocampus compared with the healthy one at all the scales. The difference in sample entropy was robust only for the scene encoding task, but not for recognition.

9.8   Complexity and Spectral Power

As we described earlier, sample entropy characterizes time series complexity in terms of their regularity. This statistic is also a good candidate for defining a criterion for the detection of nonlinear deterministic phenomena. However, sample entropy can represent not only the uncertainty associated with information presumably generated by a nonlinear system underlying the observed signal but also the variability related to the instrumental or physiologic noise described as stochastic processes. It is worth noting that filtered noise can mimic low-dimensional dynamics and chaos (Rapp, Albano, Schmah, & Farwell, 1993).

The primary candidate for the "linear'" confounding effects is the spectral power. A number of studies reported the existence of reliable correlations between sample entropy and power. For example, Bruce,

Bruce, & Vennelaganti (2009) compared the regularity and spectral power of the EEG signals between middle-aged and elderly healthy female subjects in wake, nonrapid, and rapid eye movement sleep. The regularity was quantified as sample entropy of the original signal ($\theta = 1$). The sample entropy was negatively correlated with delta power and positively correlated with beta power. A better predictor of sample entropy was found to be related to the power ratio of higher to lower frequencies: (alpha + beta)/(delta + theta). As discussed by Kaffashi, Foglyano, Wilson, & Loparo (2008), the linear properties of a signal may significantly contribute to the sample entropy at fine timescales (small θ).

Similar observations have been made in the studies on aging. As previously discussed, McIntosh et al. (2008) showed that sample entropy increased at scales 1–14 with brain maturation. At the same time, they reported age-related decreases in spectral power in lower frequencies (<10 Hz), combined with increase in higher frequencies (>15 Hz). The brain signals having stronger lower-frequency components may show relatively less variability, and therefore lower relative complexity. Increasing the relative magnitude of the Fourier coefficients for low frequencies in the adult EEG led to MSE estimates that were close to those for children. Results similar to those of McIntosh et al. (2008) were found by Lippé et al. (2009), wherein changes in complexity of the EEG signals seemed to parallel differences in relative spectral power. Specifically, for both visual and auditory conditions, development-related higher values of the sample entropy at all the scales were accompanied by significant and robustly expressed decreases in power across lower frequencies (<5 Hz) and increases across higher frequencies (>7 Hz). Essentially, changes in power for both conditions replicated a previously reported shift toward higher frequencies during brain development. In particular, an interaction between increased involvement of alpha rhythms in development and overall redistribution of power toward higher frequencies can be mentioned as a reason for loss of stability and observing a crossover in spectral power across different age groups.

The neuropathology of AD was characterized by the relations between MSE and spectral power, similar to normal aging. Specifically, Mizuno et al. (2010) showed significant increases in theta and decreases in beta band in AD patients compared with those of the healthy control subjects. To investigate the relations between MSE and power, scale factors were binned into four groups. Sample entropy at fine and coarse timescales was significantly correlated with relative spectral power for beta and theta frequency rhythms.

Another study, which reported differences in MSE and power between AD and healthy populations, investigated how spectral features are expressed in MSE (Park et al., 2007). Specifically, the authors estimated the MSE curves based on synthetic signals, consisting of a pure sine wave of various frequencies (5–20 Hz), superimposed on $1/f$ noise. We used similar signals and, in addition to MSE (scales 1–50, sampling rate 250 Hz), computed the autocorrelation of coarse-grained time series at lag of one data point, which is consistent with the embedding delay of $\tau = 1$, as used in the definition of SampEn. Figure 9.3A summarizes the main results. At small scales, a decrease in autocorrelation values is accompanied by a corresponding increase in sample entropy,

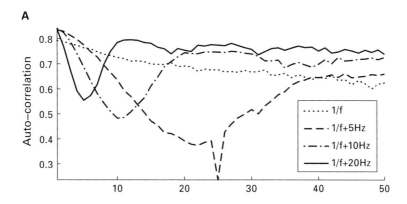

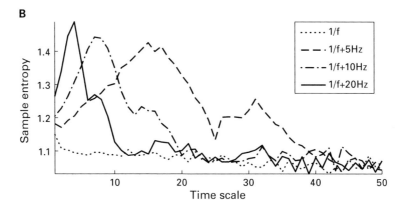

Figure 9.3
Autocorrelation at lag 1 (A) and sample entropy (B) of synthetic signals considered at different timescales. The synthetic signals are constructed as a pure sine wave of various frequencies, corrupted by $1/f$ noise.

inducing a local peak in MSE. This local maximum is shifting from fine toward coarse timescales as the frequency of a sinusoidal rhythm decreases. Thus, considering two signals, say 5-Hz and 20-Hz rhythms corrupted with $1/f$ noise, we observe a crossover in the corresponding MSE curves, similar to that based on brain signals. At coarse scales, the sinusoidal component is filtered out through the coarse-graining procedure (9.26). As can be seen, the sample entropy tends asymptotically to reach its baseline value associated with the complexity of $1/f$ noise. As noticed in Park et al. (2007), a range of timescales spanning approximately one period of a sine wave is sufficient for the sample entropy values to become stable.

One of the questions remaining is whether differences in the MSE curves based on the signals from different brain states can be completely explained by differences in spectral power. Vakorin and McIntosh (2011) explored this issue using resting-state EEG collected in the eyes-closed condition with age as a perturbation factor. Specifically, typically developing adolescents participated in the study when they were 10, 11.5, and 13 years old. Sample entropy at scales 1–50 (sample rate 500 Hz) was estimated for the original signals and for artificial data that had the same power distribution as the original data. Specifically, the artificial (surrogate) signals were constructed by applying the Fourier transform to the original EEG signals, randomizing the phase of the Fourier components, and then applying the inverse Fourier transform. Critically, the spectral power was kept the same, but the nonlinear components, if any, would be destroyed.

Two primary conclusions were made. First, the null hypothesis that there is no difference in MSE between the original and surrogate data was rejected at a 99.9% confidence interval. Specifically, the difference between sample entropy values was robust and increased toward coarse scales. This effect was robustly expressed across most of the electrodes. As expected, the sample entropy values for the surrogate signals, $SampEn_{surr}$, were higher than those for the original data, $SampEn_{orig}$, as the phase randomization makes the time series less regular and more unpredictable. Second, the complexity of both the original and surrogate data increased as a function of age. Specifically, Vakorin and McIntosh (2011) tested age-related changes of differences in sample entropy between the surrogate and original data (normalized with respect to the sample entropy values for the surrogate signals) in relation to brain development. It was found that the relative difference ($SampEn_{surr} - SampEn_{orig}$)/$SampEn_{surr}$ decreased with age (see figure 9.4). These results

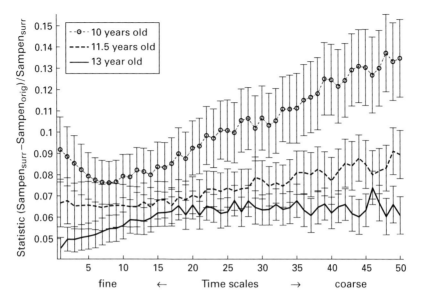

Figure 9.4
Age-relative changes of the relative difference in sample entropy between the original data and the same data with randomized phase (surrogate time series) as a function of timescales. The curves shown for one electrode are averaged across a group of subjects. Error bars: standard errors.

would support the idea that the brain signals become more "noisy" in development.

9.9   Complexity and Nonstationarity

At the large-scale level, the brain noise, which is in general understood as the variability of the brain signals, can be characterized from two perspectives: complexity and metastability (Fingelkurts & Fingelkurts, 2004). These two frameworks are essentially complementary, as they are believed to reflect the variability of the dynamic repertoire of neural systems. Metastability is the principle describing the brain's ability to deviate off the equilibrium state and stay in another state for an extended period of time. Typically, it is a result of the integration of many functional modules, producing coordinated neural oscillations. Statistically, metastability can be described by exploring the nonstationary phenomena in the EEG or MEG signals (Kaplan, Fingelkurts, Fingelkurts, Borisov, & Darkhovsky, 2005).

A number of studies previously characterized the changes in non-stationarity of brain signals during brain maturation (Koenig et al., 2002). Vakorin et al. (2011) analyzed the changes in nonstationarity as well as complexity of brain signals during early adolescence using resting-state EEG collected in two conditions: eyes open and eyes closed. The nonstationarity analysis was performed on an electrode-by-electrode basis, separately for each subject and condition. Specifically, the time series representing the electrode potentials were initially divided into relatively small segments. Each segment was fitted to a basic polynomial model, and the segment similarity was computed in the space of model parameters. Then, a clustering algorithm was applied to unify the segments of similar behaviors into clusters, representing quasi-stationary mental states. Thus, nonstationarity of the EEG signals was estimated in terms of the mean segment length and the number of mental states. At the same time, complexity of the same time series was quantified as sample entropy estimated at different timescales using the MSE approach.

It was found that in general, nonstationarity increases with age. In particular, the mean segment length was decreased with brain maturation, which is in accordance with previous findings (Koenig et al., 2002). This effect was widespread across the electrodes. However, in contrast to the studies, wherein the number of states was explicitly kept constant across different age groups (Koenig et al., 2002), Vakorin et al. (2011) showed that the number of states also increased with age. This effect was localized in the parieto-occipital area. Furthermore, the mean segment length negatively correlated with the complexity, with the values of correlations being stronger at coarse timescales (see figure 9.5A, plate 25). At the same time, positive correlations were found between the number of mental states and spectral power, reaching a distinctive peak in the alpha frequency band for the electrodes localized in the parieto-occipital area (see figure 9.5B, plate 25). Thus, a significant difference in signal complexity between two brain states can be observed not only due to nonlinearity and spectral properties but also due to nonstationarity of the brain signals or a combination of all the factors.

9.10   Complexity and Network Structure

There was an attempt to relate the functional embedding of a brain region to the complexity of neural activity from that region. Specifically, Misic, Vakorin, Paus, & McIntosh (2011) used resting-state EEG mea-

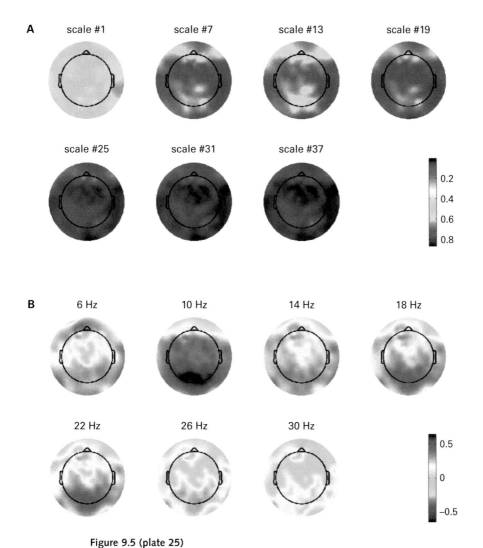

Figure 9.5 (plate 25)
Distribution of the correlations: (A) between complexity of the brain signals, quantified as sample entropy and the mean stationary segment length, controlling for the number of states; (B) between the number of stationary states and spectral power, with the effect of the mean stationary segment length removed.

sured in the eyes-closed and eyes-open conditions to link sample entropy to the characteristics describing the neural networks from a position of graph theory. More specifically, the undirected graphs of functional networks were constructed by computing the correlations between all pairs of electrodes, preserving a portion of the strongest edges and setting all others to zero. Two statistics were computed to characterize the structural properties of the newly constructed networks: the degree and efficiency of each node (electrode). The degree of a node was determined by counting the number of nonzero connections to other electrodes. Efficiency, a measure of topological proximity to other nodes, was computed as the inverse of the harmonic mean of the minimum path length between a given node and all other nodes. At the same time, the complexity of neural activity of each node was computed by integrating sample entropy values across all scales (1–20, original sampling rate 500 Hz).

For different threshold correlation values, Misic et al. (2011) found that the complexity of neural activity positively correlated with the degree of the network and the efficiency (see figure 9.6). In other words, the more connections a node of the functional network has, the higher the complexity of this node. In addition, higher complexity of specific nodes was associated with shorter minimum path lengths between these nodes and the rest of the networks. These results would indicate that the variability observed in neural dynamics not only represents the information processed locally but also reflects some properties of the functional organization of the brain.

9.11   Conclusion

Sample entropy can be viewed as a statistic used to detect the existence of nonlinear dynamics associated with observed time series. Typically, one can assume that one observes nonlinear systems in different states, and the goal is to describe these differences. Although different, two initial conditions would not be differentiated at certain experimental precision. However, they may evolve into distinguishable states after some finite time. Thus, one could say that a system that is sensitive to initial conditions produces information. Sample entropy can detect these effects, as it is ultimately related to the Kolmogorov entropy, which is interpreted as the mean rate of information generated by a dynamic system.

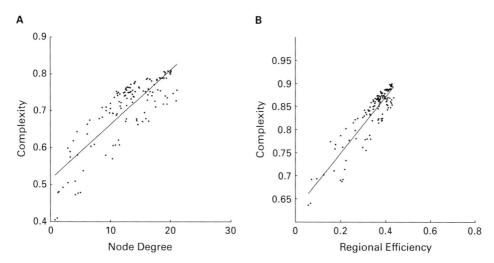

Figure 9.6
Values of sample entropy are integrated across scales and correlated with functional network parameters: node degree (A) and local efficiency (B). Each point is associated with one electrode. Statistics are averaged across a group of subjects. Graphs were obtained by proportional thresholding, leaving 10% of the strongest connections.

In practice, however, sample entropy is sensitive not only to nonlinear deterministic effects but also to linear stochastic effects. As we discussed earlier, the brain's rhythmic activity contributes differentially to sample entropy values at different timescales, depending on the frequency of oscillations. In addition, we have seen that changes in sample entropy are in parallel with changes in linear characteristics of a signal such as autocorrelation. Also, nonstationarity could be a factor contributing to what is observed as the presence of nonlinear effects. Specifically, different amplitude values for the alternating segments of varying length is an example of nonlinear static transformations compared with the nonlinear dynamics of the systems underlying EEG or MEG signals.

However, we believe that it would be unreasonable simply to reduce sample entropy to autocorrelation, spectral power, nonstationarity, or any of their combinations. The general idea is that the brain signals found in EEG or MEG are primarily due to combined contributions from many sources with high coherence. The situation is complicated by the fact that all these sources are intrinsically coupled. In addition, the network consistently undergoes reorganization, either as a result of experience or in response to damage to one or more nodes of the network. As stated by Nunez and Shrinivasan (2005), "when the number of connections between members of the neural group becomes sufficiently large, new characteristic frequencies may emerge."

Estimation of spectral power answers the question of how many components a given signal contains at specific frequencies. However, sample entropy is designed to be dependent not only on how many of the oscillatory components are present but also on how they interact between each other. Autocorrelation alone is not an answer to the question of what is measured by sample entropy. Indeed, these two statistics may correlate with each other. In some sense, it is an expected result as both of them reflect the regularity of the signals. But regularity that is based on the notion of information content of the signals reflecting the coupled coherent neural ensembles is different from that based on the cross-correlation of a signal with itself. The situation is somewhat similar in cases of nonstationarity. In general, from the statistical point of view, nonstationarity has an influence on estimation of the sample entropy statistic as a measure of complexity. However, from the physiologic point of view, nonstationarity itself, as observed in the brain signals, is a direct consequence of complex behavior of the interacting neural ensembles. Nonstationarity measures and statistics designed to quantify signal complexity seem to represent different facets of the same brain dynamics.

References

Abasolo, D., Hornero, R., Espino, P., Alvarez, D. & Poza, J. (2006). Entropy analysis of the EEG background activity in Alzheimer's disease patients. Physiological Measurement, 27, 241–253.

Abasolo, D., Hornero, R., Espino, P., Poza, J., Sanchez, C. I., & de la Rosa, R. (2005). Analysis of regularity in the EEG background activity of Alzheimer's disease patients with Approximate Entropy. Clinical Neurophysiology, 1160(8), 1826–1834.

Baddeley, R., Hancock, P., & Fldik, P. (Eds.). (2000). Information Theory and the Brain. Cambridge, UK: Cambridge University Press.

Bressler, S. L. (1995). Large-scale cortical networks and cognition. Brain Research. Brain Research Reviews, 200(3), 288–304.

Bressler, S. L. (2002). Understanding cognition through large-scale cortical networks. Current Directions in Psychological Science, 110(2), 58–61.

Bruce, E. N., Bruce, M. C., & Vennelaganti, S. (2009). Sample entropy tracks changes in electroencephalogram power spectrum with sleep state and aging. Journal of Clinical Neurophysiology, 260(4), 257–266.

Churchland, P. S., & Sejnowski, T. J. (1988). Perspectives on cognitive neuroscience. Science, 2420(4879), 741–745.

Costa, M., Goldberger, A. L., & Peng, C. K. (2002). Multiscale entropy analysis of physiologic time series. Physical Review Letters, 89, 062102.

Deco, G., Jirsa, V., McIntosh, A. R., Sporns, O., & Ktter, R. (2009). Key role of coupling, delay, and noise in resting brain fluctuations. Proceedings of the National Academy of Sciences of the United States of America, 1060(25), 10302–10307.

Deisboeck, T. S., & Kresh, J. Y. (Eds.). (2006). *Complex Systems in Science in Biomedicine*. Berlin: Springer.

Desmedt, J. E., & Cheron, G. (1980). Central somatosensory conduction in man: neural generators and interpeak latencies of the far-field components recorded from neck and right or left scalp and earlobes. *Electroencephalography and Clinical Neurophysiology*, *500*(5–6), 382–403.

Elger, C. E., & Lehnertz, K. (1998). Seizure prediction by non-linear time series analysis of brain electrical activity. *European Journal of Neuroscience*, *10*, 786–789.

Escudero, J., Abásolo, D., Hornero, R., Espino, P., & Lápez, M. (2006). Analysis of electro-encephalograms in Alzheimer's disease patients with multiscale entropy. *Physiological Measurement*, *27*, 1091–1106.

Fingelkurts, A. A., & Fingelkurts, A. A. (2004). Making complexity simpler: multivariability and metastability in the brain. International Journal of Neuroscience, *1140*(7), 843–862.

Ghosh, A., Rho, Y., McIntosh, A. R., Ktter, R., & Jirsa, V. (2008). Cortical network dynamics with time delays reveals functional connectivity in the resting brain. *Cognitive Neurodynamics*, *20*(2), 115–120.

Grassberger, P., & Procaccia, I. (1983). Estimation of the Kolmogorov entropy from a chaotic signal. *Physical Review A.*, *28*, 2591–2593.

Jirsa, V. K., & McIntosh, A. R. (2007). *Handbook of Brain Connectivity*. Berlin: Springer-Verlag.

Kaffashi, F., Foglyano, R., Wilson, C. G., & Loparo, K. A. (2008). The effect of time delay on approximate and sample entropy calculations. *Physica D. Nonlinear Phenomena*, *2370*(23), 3069–3074.

Kaplan, A.Ya., Fingelkurts, Al. A., Fingelkurts, An. A., Borisov, S. V., & Darkhovsky, B. S. (2005). Nonstationary nature of the brain activity as revealed by EEG/MEG: methodological, practical and conceptual challenges. *Signal Processing*, *85*, 2190–2212.

Kim, H. S., Eykholt, R., & Slas, J. D. (1998). Delay time window and plateau onset of the correlation dimention for small data sets. *Physical Review E: Statistical Physics, Plasmas, Fluids, and Related Interdisciplinary Topics*, *58*, 5676–5682.

Koenig, T., Prichep, L., Lehmann, D., Valdes Sosa, P., Braeker, E., Kleinlogel, H., et al. (2002). Millisecond by millisecond, year by year: normative EEG microstates and developmental stages. *NeuroImage*, *160*(1), 41–48.

Kolmogorov, A. N. (1959). Entropy per unit time as a metric invariant of automorphism. *Doklady of Russian Academy of Sciences*, *124*, 754–755.

Lai, Y. C., & Lerner, D. (1998). Effective scaling regime for computing the correlation dimention from chaotic time series. *Physica D. Nonlinear Phenomena*, *115*, 1–18.

Lehnertz, K., & Elger, C. E. (1997). Neuronal complexity loss in temporal lobe epilepsy: effects of carbamazepine on the dynamics of the epileptogenic focus. *Electroencephalography and Clinical Neurophysiology*, *1030*(3), 376–380.

Lippé, S., Kovacevic, N., & McIntosh, A. R. (2009). Differential maturation of brain signal complexity in the human auditory and visual system. *Frontiers in Human Neuroscience*, *3*, 48.

McIntosh, A. R. (1999). Mapping cognition to the brain through neural interactions. *Memory (Hove, England)*, *70*(5–6), 523–548.

McIntosh, A. R., Kovacevic, N., & Itier, R. J. (2008). Increased brain signal variability accompanies lower behavioral variability in development. *PLoS Computational Biology*, *40*(7), e1000106.

Misic, B., Mills, T., Taylor, M. J., & McIntosh, A. R. (2010). Brain noise is task-dependent and region-specific. *Journal of Neurophysiology*, *104*, 2667–2676.

Misic, B., Vakorin, V. A., Paus, T., & McIntosh A. R. (2011). Functional embedding predicts the variability of neural activity. *Frontiers in Systems Neurosceince*, *5*, 90.

Mizuno, T., Takahashi, T., Raymond, Y. C., Kikuchi, K., Murata, T., Takahashi, K., et al. (2010). Assessment of EEG dynamical complexity in Alzheimer's disease using multiscale entropy. *Clinical Neurophysiology*, *1210*(9), 1438–1446.

Niebur, E., Schuster, H. G., & Kammen, D. M. (1991). Collective frequencies and metastability in networks of limit-cycle oscillators with time delay. *Physical Review Letters*, *67*, 2753–2756.

Nunez, P. L. (1995). *Neocortical Dynamics and Human Brain Rhythms*. Oxford, UK: Oxford University Press.

Nunez, P. L., & Shrinivasan, R. (2005). *Electric Fields in the Brain: The Neurophysics of EEG*. Oxford, UK: Oxford University Press.

Park, J. H., Kim, S., Kim, C. H., Cichocki, A., & Kim, K. (2007). Multiscale entropy analysis of EEG from patients under different pathological conditions. *Fractals 15*(4), 399–404.

Pincus, S. M. (1991). Approximate entropy as a measure of system complexity. *Proceedings of the National Academy of Sciences of the United States of America*, *88*, 2297–2301.

Pincus, S. M. (1995). Approximate entropy (ApEn) as a complexity measure. *Chaos (Woodbury, N.Y.)*, *50*(1), 110–117.

Prichard, D., & Theiler, J. (1995). Generalized redundancies for time series analysis. *Physica D. Nonlinear Phenomena*, *84*, 476–493.

Protzner, A. B., Valiante, T. A., Kovacevic, N., McCormick, C., & McAndrews, M. P. (2010). Hippocampal signal complexity in mesial temporal lobe epilepsy: a noisy brain is a healthy brain. *Archives Italiennes de Biologie*, *1480*(3), 289–297.

Rapp, P. E., Albano, A. M., Schmah, T. I., & Farwell, L. A. (1993). Filtered noise can mimic low-dimensional chaotic attractors. *Physical Review E: Statistical Physics, Plasmas, Fluids, and Related Interdisciplinary Topics*, *470*(4), 2289–2297.

Richman, J. S., & Moorman, J. R. (2000). Physiological time-series analysis using approximate entropy and sample entropy. *American Journal of Physiology. Heart and Circulatory Physiology*, *2780*(6), H2039–H2049.

Shannon, C. E. (1949). *The Mathematical Theory of Communication*. Urbana, IL: University of Illinois Press.

Sinai, Ya. G. (1959). On the notion of entropy of a dynamical system. *Doklady of Russian Academy of Sciences*, *124*, 768–771.

Small, M., & Tse, C. K. (2004). Optimal embedding parameters: a modeling paradigm. *Physica D. Nonlinear Phenomena*, *194*, 283–296.

Stam, C. J. (2005). Nonlinear dynamical analysis of EEG and MEG: review of an emerging field. *Clinical Neurophysiology*, *1160*(10), 2266–2301.

Takens, F. (1981). Detecting strange attractors in turbulence. In D. A. Rand & L.-S. Young (Eds.), *Dynamical Systems and Turbulence*, Lecture Notes in Mathematics, Vol. 898. New York: Springer-Verlag.

Vakorin, V. A., & McIntosh, A. R. (2011) On spectral power and complexity of resting-state EEG signals in development. Submitted.

Vakorin, V. A., McIntosh, A. R., Misic, B., Krakovska, O., & Paus, T. (2011). Exploring age-related changes in dynamical nonstationarity in electroencephalographic signals during early adolescence. Submitted.

Vakorin, V. A., Ross, B., Krakovska, O. A., Bardouille, T., Cheyne, D., & McIntosh, A. R. (2010). Complexity analysis of the neuromagnetic somatosensory steady-state response. *NeuroImage*, *510*(1), 83–90.

Zhang, Y.-C. (1991). Complexity and 1/f noise. A phase space approach. *Journal de Physique I France*, *I*, 971–977.

10 Connectivity and Dynamics of Neural Information Processing

Viktor Jirsa, Raoul Huys, Ajay Pillai, Dionysios Perdikis, and Marmaduke Woodman

Summary

Brain function arises from the complex interactions of brain networks, in which neural activity needs to be tightly coordinated. How this coordination is achieved is largely unknown, although various proposals thereof have been made. Here, we review some of the approaches to neural information processing in brain networks and propose a novel concept termed *structured flows on manifolds* (SFMs) describing function as a low-dimensional dynamic process emerging from coupled neurons. Initially, we develop this concept and demonstrate its validity in networks of coupled populations. In a second step, we provide proof of concept for this formalism in networks of spiking neurons. Then, we show how sets of SFMs can capture the dynamic repertoire of complex behaviors and develop novel forms of functional architectures based on hierarchies of timescales. We illustrate these concepts using the example of handwriting.

10.1 Introduction

Functionally meaningful processes like perception–action and cognition arise from the complex interactions of brain networks that are in contact with the environment. Proper brain function requires the coordination of regional activity across the (large-scale) brain network, which may occur in the form of synchronization of oscillatory activity and is amendable to changes via recruitment or disengagement of regional activity. These mechanisms are fundamental in establishing the precise temporal relationships between neural responses that are in turn relevant for memory, perception, and consciousness. For example, synchronization of cortical areas is thought to be involved in the so-called binding of object features to a common percept (Gray, Konig, Engel, & Singer, 1989). Input from multiple sensory modalities such as vision, hearing, and touch is combined to give rise to a coherent percept (King & Calvert, 2001;

Calvert, Spence, & Stein, 2004; Thesen, Vibell, Calvert, & Osterbauer, 2004) through the activation of multisensory integration areas. In the case of movement, the brain controls large groups of muscles and combines sensory information from the environment and musculature to execute purposeful motor behavior (Kelso, 1982). Although these processes are undoubtedly complex, they are nevertheless significantly lower-dimensional than the network activity generating it. Furthermore, such functional behaviors are reproducible, hence have a deterministic component, and are not limited to transitions between functional states. The latter implies that whatever the coordinated network activity is, it has to account for the emergence of functions related to transient, metastable, multistable, and multifunctional patterns.

The current literature suggests that large-scale brain networks engage and disengage in a dynamic fashion to form functionally connected networks (Friston, 1994; Tononi, Sporns, & Edelman, 1994; Horwitz, Tagamets, & McIntosh, 1999; Büchel & Friston, 2000; Bressler & Kelso, 2001; Friston, 2002). Besides the theory of heteroclinic channels (see chapter 7 in this volume) and related approaches (Ashwin et al. 2003, 2007), no other approaches even get close to address the transient nature of functional dynamics. Heteroclinic channels are low-dimensional mathematical objects that are defined by a sequence of successive metastable states. Under certain conditions, all the trajectories in the neighborhood of these states remain in the channel, ensuring robustness and reproducibility in a wide range of parameters. A certain degree of asymmetry in the connectivity of the network giving rise to a heteroclinic channel is necessary to guarantee the existence of such a channel. Though heteroclinic channels are powerful tools to describe transient dynamics of perception and cognition, it remains unknown how other functional but nontransient processes shall be captured by a network dynamics. We hypothesize that functional processes extend far beyond computation of states, which is a concept well known as attractor dynamics in the network community. Upon a stimulus signal, an attractor network changes its activity such that it settles into an activity pattern, typically a fixed-point attractor. The reaching of the attractor is then identified with the emergence of a percept or the recognition of a visual or auditory object. Under this view, only the final state matters for the (perceptual) process, not the trajectory toward the attractor. We propose, in contrast, that the actual trajectories are relevant for the function and represent the process involved in a particular function or behavior. The ensemble of trajectories captures a system's behavior, and the ensemble of behaviors identifies a system's dynamic repertoire, which in conjunction with a selection and competition process offers a new entry point toward the understanding of functional architectures. In the following, we systematically develop this line of thought explicitly by traversing scales of abstraction from the very abstract, the definition of function, toward the concrete, that is, the application of handwriting.

10.2 Structured Flows as Functional Units of Processes

The proposition that function is reflected in structured flows echoes the idea that complex processes (or behaviors) are decomposable into so-called (functional) primitives, a notion that is widely adhered to in the biological and life sciences. For instance, the vocalization of singing birds contains functional elements occurring over distinct timescales (Kiebel, Daunizeau, & Friston, 2008), such as notes and groups of notes (syllables). These elements appear to be represented in the bird's forebrain in a hierarchical fashion (Yu & Margoliash, 1996) that, when appropriately put together, may entice another bird nearby to sing along (or otherwise). Human communication is arguably decomposable in a similar vein; in speech perception, phonemes constitute the meaningful categories relevant for communication (see Tuller, Nguyen, Lancia, & Vallabha, 2011, and references therein). In artificial intelligence, perception–action architectures may use primitives to acquire complex skills via sequential learning cycles (Shevchenko, Windridge, & Kittler, 2009). In the investigation of human movement, the idea that (functional) primitives are used as building blocks to construct complex perceptual–motor behavior is widely adhered to also, even though their identification has been (and still is) debated at length (cf. Huys, Jirsa, Studenka, Rheaume, & Zelaznik, 2008; Sternad, 2008; and references in both). Nevertheless, the human movement sciences may have shown the largest advances in this respect due to the comparative ease of recording movement time series. For this reason, we shall elaborate on this in more detail later. First, however, we will briefly outline a few notions from dynamical systems theory that are required for the remainder of this chapter.

A phase flow constitutes the direction and strength of the evolution of a point in the phase (or state) space; that is, the space spanned by the (state) variables required to predict the system's future given the present state. For instance, the state space of a movement along a single (physical) dimension is the space spanned by the system's position x and its time derivative, the velocity $\dot{x}$. According to dynamical systems theory, every deterministic, time-continuous and autonomous system can be unambiguously described through its flow in phase space. In that regard, autonomous systems have no explicit time dependency; the system's evolution depends solely on its state variables. In contrast, the behavior of non-autonomous systems is additionally shaped by a time-dependent impact. The flow in phase space (also referred to as the vector field) uniquely describes the direction of the system's evolution as a function of its current state, $(x, \dot{x})$, for the example above. Whereas the phase flow prescribes a system's dynamics, a trajectory is an actualization of the system's evolution in phase space governed by its flow. Phase flows are structured: Each position in the phase space has a unique flow direction associated with it, and the flow's topology defines the system's qualitative behavior. In one-dimensional systems—the flow is defined on a line—only fixed points can occur, that is, points where the system's rate of change is zero ($\dot{x} = 0$); if stable [unstable], all trajectories eventually converge toward it [diverge away from it]. Fixed points in two-dimensional systems come in a larger variety as the flow is no longer necessarily directed straight toward (or away) from the fixed point but may also approach (or recede from) it spiraling (in which case they are called spirals) or approach along one direction and recede along another direction (in which case they are called saddles; cf. figure 4.1B in chapter 4 of this volume). In addition, two-dimensional spaces allow for so-called limit cycles, which are closed orbits that may be stable or unstable, as well as separatrices, which are structures dividing the phase space in regions with locally distinct phase flows. In three (and higher)-dimensional systems, the dynamical repertoire expands and may include strange attractors allowing for chaotic behavior. In figure 10.1 (plate 26), three two-dimensional phase flows are illustrated with different phase flow topologies. We note here once again that the phase space is typically much higher-dimensional in neural systems. To display low-dimensional dynamics in this high-dimensional space, the trajectory needs to be attracted to a lower-dimensional subspace, the so-called manifold, and then execute its dynamics within this subspace. Such imposes constraints upon the general dynamics and thus the neural system generating it. In the remainder of this chapter, we will discuss these constraints and refer to dynamics restricted to a particular attractive subspace with a characteristic flow as a *structured flow on manifold* (SFM).

We here refrain from elaborately motivating why it would be appropriate to cast cognitive function in terms of mathematical objects (but see, for instance, Meijer & Roth, 1988; Haken, 1995; Kelso, 1995; Port & van

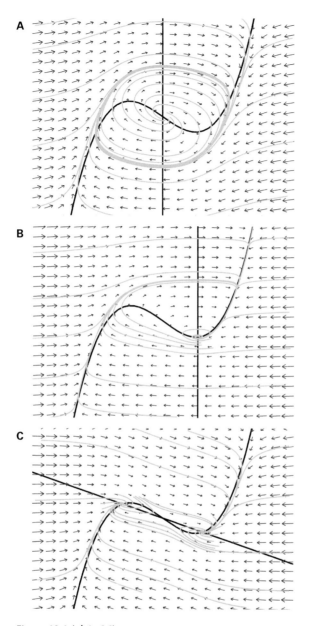

Figure 10.1 (plate 26)

Phase flows of the excitator system. The flows are depicted via the black arrows; the nullclines are subsets of phase space points, in which the flow is zero in either the vertical or horizontal direction, and are represented by the magenta and red lines (for the horizontal and vertical component of the flow, respectively); trajectories are represented by the blue lines. Fixed points are located at the crossing of both nullclines, where the flow in both directions is zero by definition. (A) Stable limit cycle containing an unstable spiral (fixed point). (B) Monostable system containing a stable fixed point and a separatrix. The latter is located just below left to the fixed point, where the two trajectories strongly converge. (C) Bistable system: An unstable fixed point with two stable fixed points with a separatrix in between. Systems with separatrices can be viewed as having threshold properties: A trajectory will be executed only if the system crosses it. Note that for all cases, quantitative changes in the flow may be induced by variation of the nullclines that do not affect the flow's topology.

Gelder, 1998; van Gelder, 1998; Beer, 2000; and references therein). Rather, we will briefly present empirical evidence from human movement sciences in support of the idea that structured phase flows underwrite functional processes. The investigation of rhythmic movements and rhythmic sensorimotor coordination in terms of (coupled) limit cycles has a rich history in the movement sciences (Kugler, Kelso, & Turvey, 1980; Kelso, Holt, Rubin, & Kugler, 1981; Haken, Kelso, & Bunz, 1985; Kay, Kelso, Saltzman, & Schöner, 1987; Beek & Beek, 1988; Kelso, Delcolle, & Schöner, 1990; Kay, Saltzman, & Kelso, 1991; Kelso, 1995; Beek, Rikkert, and van Wieringen, 1996; Mottet & Bootsma, 1999; Daffertshofer, Huys, & Beek, 2004; Huys, Daffertshofer, & Beek, 2004; Post, de Groot, Daffertshofer, & Beek, 2007). Until recently, the identification of the limit cycle ingredients (i.e., attractor identification) was achieved via perturbation and/or approximation methods. Of late, however, methods were developed allowing for the reconstruction of phase flows from experimentally recorded time series (Friedrich & Peinke, 1997; Daffertshofer, 2010). We used these techniques to investigate the structural layout (i.e., topology) of phase spaces underlying movement trajectories in different task contexts (Huys, Studenka, Rheaume, Zelaznik, & Jirsa, 2008; Huys, Fernandez, Bootsma, & Jirsa, 2010; Huys, Studenka, Zelaznik, & Jirsa, 2010). As an entry point, we searched for the existence of fixed points versus limit cycles in repetitive finger "tapping" (without surface contact; Huys, Studenka, et al. 2008. Corresponding model simulations showed that monostable (i.e., fixed point and separatrix) systems (Jirsa & Kelso, 2005) (see also figure 10.1, plate 26) could not produce repetitive movements at high frequencies. In the experiment, participants executed auditory-paced flexion–extension finger movements at frequencies from 0.5 Hz to 3.5 Hz under various instructions. The reconstructed phase flows clearly distinguished conditions in which a fixed point flow structured the phase space (*discrete system*) versus those in which a limit cycle flow did so (*rhythmic system*) (identified at movement frequencies roughly below versus above ~1.5 Hz; see figure 10.2, plate 27). By implication—owing to theorems from dynamical systems theory (Strogatz, 2001)—discrete and rhythmic movements belong to distinct classes that cannot be reduced to each other (for details, see Huys, Jirsa, et al., 2008; Huys, Studenka et al., 2008). These results were corroborated in subsequent studies investigating Fitts's task (i.e., involving accuracy constraints; Huys, Fernandez, et al., 2010) and circle drawing (which constitutes a four-dimensional phase space; Huys, Studenka, et al., 2010). Furthermore, an indication for the existence of a separatrix, as posed in

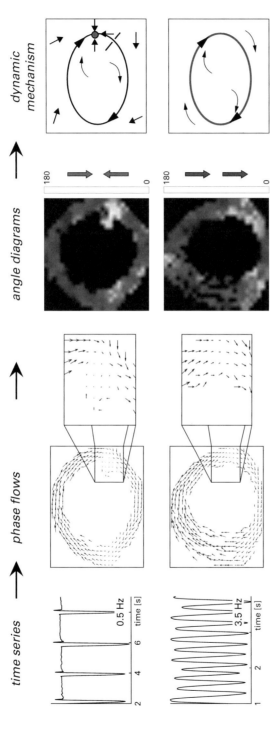

Figure 10.2 (plate 27)
Phase flows from experimental data. The upper and lower panels depict results from finger movements and 0.5 Hz and 3.5 Hz, respectively. Time series of position data are shown in the leftmost panels. To their right, corresponding reconstructed phase flows are shown (with position and velocity on the horizontal and vertical axes, respectively), represented by the arrows. The flow is bounded in both conditions. In the enlarged subpanel, it can be seen that the flow locally converges to a point in the 0.5-Hz condition but not in the 3.5-Hz condition. The angle diagrams depict the maximal angles between neighboring vectors (arrows) for each state, which more clearly visualizes the local convergence of the flow (in red) in the upper panel (only). The rightmost panels provide a scheme of the dynamic mechanisms involved in each case: Whereas movements emerge autonomously in the "rhythmic" system, an additional input is required to "kick" the system across the separatrix (black line perpendicular to the trajectory, in the top-right figure) to execute individual movements in the "discrete" system.

the monostable system (see figure 10.1, plate 26), was recently reported by Fink and colleagues (Fink, Kelso, & Jirsa, 2009), who examined false starts (i.e., the inappropriate timed beginning of a behavioral act) in a movement-perturbation experiment.

These results indicate that phase flows, structured through qualitatively distinct topologies, are used in a manner that depends on the specific task constraints at hand (next to quantitative "contextual" flow adjustments under a given topology as, e.g., in the context of Fitts's task; Mottet & Bootsma, 1999; Huys, Fernandez, et al., 2010). Trivially, the set comprising the discrete and rhythmic processes is but a limited subset of all behavioral processes possible. The structured flow on a manifold (SFM) approach, which in principle allows for numerous structured flows, overcomes this limitation. In that regard (and see later), the phase flows discussed earlier form a subset (i.e., specific realizations) of SFMs. In particular, we propose that the (embedded) nervous system instantiates SFMs rather than trajectories (i.e., specific "task" realizations), which renders processes flexible yet stable and minimizes the system's need to have detailed "knowledge" about initial conditions.

10.3   Structured Flows on Manifolds

SFMs have essentially three conceptual components: (1) a part of the dynamics that gives rise to the manifold or constrains the dynamics to a particular subspace; (2) a subsequent slow dynamics that governs the flow on this manifold; and (3) a fast dynamics that collapses onto the manifold. Mathematically, we can construct a general system of this nature as follows:

$$\dot{\xi}_j = -f(\xi_j, \xi_i)\xi_j + \mu g(\xi_j, \xi_i)$$
$$\dot{\xi}_i = -\xi_i + N(\xi_j, \xi_i),$$

(10.1)

where $f(.) = 0$ defines the manifold, and g(.) describes the subsequent flow; the set of ξ_i represents the fast variable dynamics toward the manifold, and the flow on the manifold is governed by the set of ξ_j representing the slow variable dynamics. The smallness parameter μ ($0 < \mu \ll 1$) establishes a timescale hierarchy and ensures that the dynamics of g(.) will always be slow in comparison to the timescale of ξ_i and $f(.)$. By choice of an appropriate function $f(.)$, we can constrain the manifold to be attractive, and its flow is described by g(.) on the manifold. Systems of this form contain an *inertial manifold* used in the reduction of infinite-dimensional dynamical systems to finite-dimensional spaces. The inertial manifold itself can be considered a global analogue of the center manifold. Whereas the center manifold theorem forms the mathematical basis of the adiabatic elimination leading to the enslaving principle of synergetics (Haken, 1983, 1995), there is not yet such a general theoretical basis for inertial manifolds. As such, systems exhibiting inertial manifolds have to be dealt with on a case-by-case basis.

Figure 10.3 (plate 28) shows some examples of SFMs in higher-dimensional phase spaces (only three dimensions though are visualized). The manifolds and its flow are generated by equation (10.1), where the SFMs are two-dimensional in all cases. In the top-left corner of the figure, every point on the manifold (in blue) is a fixed point, hence all trajectories are attracted to the manifold, but then remain there, as the flow is zero on the manifold. The network scheme under the corresponding SFM indicates that all weights are identical in this case (all links have the same thickness), which is equivalent to $\mu = 0$. If this symmetry of connectivity is broken, $\mu \neq 0$, in the network, then this leads to a nonzero flow as indicated in the right-top of the figure and its corresponding network scheme. In this particular example, the structured flow is composed of a coexisting limit cycle and fixed point separated by a separatrix on the manifold. Trajectories (in blue) allow visualization of this topology. Another example of the same flow topology but a nonplanar manifold is shown on the bottom of figure 10.3 (plate 28). Generally, different network realizations (through connectivity) can give rise to the same functional dynamics. The actual difference across realizations will manifest itself in the transient dynamics toward the manifold. This property allows for an enormous redundancy and flexibility, which allows for rapid network reorganizations through plastic changes to preserve function if needed.

Equation (10.1) provides guidelines for deriving constraints imposed upon networks of coupled neural populations or ensembles of spiking neurons. These constraints identify the parameter regimes for the emergence of certain SFMs. In the following, we consider the constraints imposed upon ensembles of spiking neurons.

10.4   Emergence of SFMs from Spiking Neuron Networks

We model (individual) neurons using the FitzHugh–Nagumo neuron model; in the absence of input, it may oscillate or rest at a stable fixed

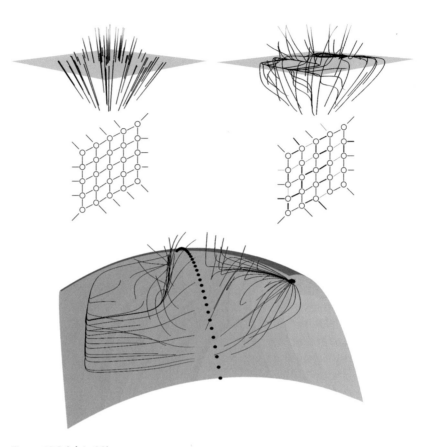

Figure 10.3 (plate 28)
Examples of manifolds with different types of flow dynamics. A graphical illustration of
the key concept behind SFMs. In a high-dimensional space, the dynamics collapses onto a
manifold and primarily remains on the manifold during function. The blue lines indicate
trajectories with different initial conditions that evolve fast toward the manifold. Top row,
left: SFM with a planar manifold and flow zero. This is accomplished when all connections
are of equal strength in the network (see the network scheme underneath). Top row, right:
same situation as on the left, but now with symmetry breaking (as illustrated in the network
scheme underneath) establishing a flow with coexisting limit cycle and fixed point. Bottom
row: SFM with a nonplanar manifold and a flow composed of a limit cycle and a fixed point
separated by a separatrix (dots).

point (quiescent) if the intrinsic excitability is not above its threshold. Adding afferent synaptic input I_{syn}, the neural and synaptic dynamics yields

$$\dot{x}_i = \left(x_i - \frac{x_i^3}{3} + y_i \right) \tau_f$$

$$\dot{y}_i = -\left[x_i + a_i + (x_i - x_0)I_{\text{syn}}^i - I_{\text{stim}} \right]/\tau_f \qquad (10.2)$$

$$\dot{q}_i = \left[(1 - q_i)H(x_i - x_{\text{thr}}) - \kappa q_i \right]/\tau_s,$$

where x_i and y_i are the fast and slow variables of the ith neuron, respectively; $I_{\text{syn}}^i = \sum_j g_{ij}q_j$ is the total postsynaptic current received by the ith neuron with connectivity weight matrix $G = (g_{ij})$; q_i represents the synaptic action (i.e., the proportion of active postsynaptic channels); a_i is the intrinsic excitability; I_{stim} is the input to this neuron [which is constant at the timescale of the (x,y) dynamics]; x_0 determines whether the synaptic input is excitatory ($x_0 = 0$) or inhibitory ($x_0 = -2$); τ_f, τ_s are timescale constants; $H(.)$ is the Heaviside function; x_{thr} sets the spiking threshold; and κ determines the synaptic action's rate of decay.

To focus on a network's dynamics firing rate, we follow a line of reasoning similar to Nowotny and Rabinovich (2007), who performed a mean field approximation to eliminate the neural dynamics from a network of three neurons with synaptic couplings. Note that for the moment, we ignore the indices of the variables but reintroduce them later on. To express the network dynamics in terms of firing rate [i.e., eliminate the (x,y) component to enhance focus on the firing rate], we wish to find a function $F(.)$ that approximates the effect of the (x,y) subsystem on q. Naturally, we will lose all information about the spike timings and replace the effect on q by a mean field. One way to do so is to express the firing rate through the parameters present in the neural model. Thereto, we set $\dot{y} = 0$ to derive

$$\hat{x} = (x_0 I_{\text{syn}} + I_{\text{stim}} - a)/(1 + I_{\text{syn}}), \qquad (10.3)$$

which is an expression that (in the absence of noise) determines whether the neuron is oscillating or not. As $\hat{x}$ crosses -1, the dynamics of (x,y) exhibits a bifurcation from a fixed-point dynamics to a limit cycle [i.e., the real part of the eigenvalues of the Jacobian evaluated at the fixed point (x_0,y_0) become positive]. Because the nullclines of q and x do not depend on I_{syn}, $\hat{x}$ parameterizes the qualitative behavior of the (x,y) subsystem (see figure 10.4).

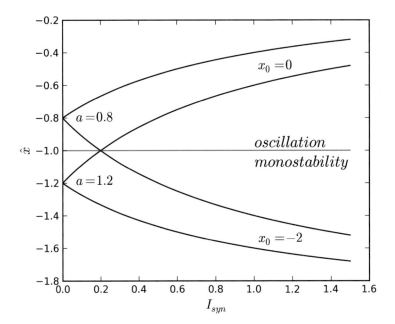

Figure 10.4
The value of $\hat{x}$ parameterizes the response of individual neurons to synaptic input.

In moving toward the approximation $F(\hat{x}) \approx H(x - x_{\mathrm{thr}})$, so as to obtain a mean field firing rate model, we first consider a population of neurons with a normal distribution of excitabilities $\alpha \to \alpha_i$ (with mean μ_a), giving us a new mean estimate

$$\mu_{\hat{x}} = (x_0 I_{\mathrm{syn}} + I_{\mathrm{stim}} - \mu_a)/(1 + I_{\mathrm{syn}}), \tag{10.4}$$

as a function of the current I_{syn}. This expression allows us to parameterize the firing rate $F(.)$ (i.e., the proportion of firing neurons in the population) by integrating over the probability distribution PDF above the critical $\hat{x}_c = -1$,

$$F(\mu_{\hat{x}}, \sigma_{\hat{x}}) = \int_{\hat{x}_c}^{\infty} \mathrm{PDF}(\hat{x}, \mu_{\hat{x}}, \sigma_{\hat{x}}) d\hat{x}, \tag{10.5}$$

which produces a sigmoidal response function whose slope is inversely related to the distribution's variance. As $\mu_{\hat{x}}$ depends on I_{syn}, we can write

$$\dot{q}_i = \left[(1 - q_i) f_i(I_{\mathrm{syn}}, \sigma_{\hat{x}}) - \kappa q_i \right] / \tau_s. \tag{10.6}$$

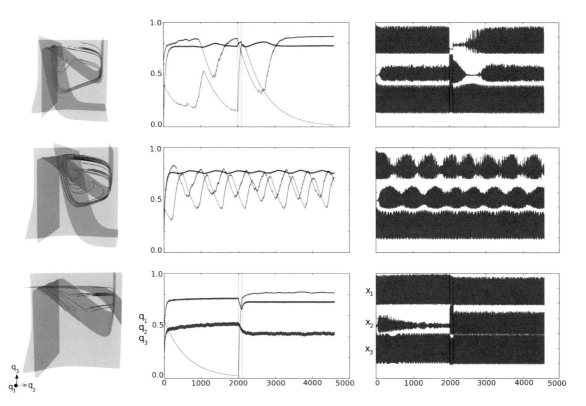

Figure 10.5 (plate 29)
Phase flows in a spiking network. The three rows, from top to bottom, demonstrate the emergence of the same flows as in figure 10.1 (plate 26), that is, a monostable flow, a limit cycle, and a bistable flow, arising in a three-neuron network. Left column: The phase space structure is shown via surfaces of the q_1, q_2, and q_3 nullclines (light blue); the trajectories reveal the essential flow. Middle column: The time course of synaptic action (q_{1-3}) in the network, with the vertical red lines delimiting perturbations delivered via I_{stim}. Right column: The time courses of each neuron's membrane potential (x_{1-3}) indicating spiking activity.

We introduce a symmetry breaking (through the parameters of the functions F_i), which determines the phase space structure of the network dynamics.

We numerically illustrate our approach by imposing the dynamics of an excitator system (Jirsa & Kelso, 2005) on a network of three neurons with the dynamics defined by equation (10.2). Figure 10.5 (plate 29) shows the membrane potentials of a network of three spiking neurons as well as their corresponding synaptic actions (right and middle column, respectively). It can be clearly seen that the network is able to generate three distinct phase flows (left column) that are generated through the symmetry breaking in the functions F_i. In other words, SFM may arise in biologically plausible neural networks.

10.5   Functional Architectures: SFM and Timescale Hierarchies

Above, we outlined a perspective on the emergence of low-dimensional structured phase flows from neural networks (SFM) and provided evidence for their utilization in relatively simple (motor) behavioral tasks. As said (briefly), such SFM may well serve as the building blocks suggested to underlie more complex behaviors and processes and may be truly identified as "primitives" using theorems from dynamical systems theory. Consistent with the notion of modes in synergetics (Haken, 1995, 2006), we refer to such primitives as functional modes. Importantly, by identifying functional modes through their topology, they combine invariant features with variation across different realizations (see figure 10.1, plate 26). In the following, we outline a framework for functional architectures underlying complex human function that has a set of functional modes (i.e., a dynamic repertoire) at its disposition. The modes are in competition with each other; the competition dynamics defines another temporal scale of organization.

10.5.1   Functional Architectures

In its most general formulation, we can describe a functional architecture through its flow in phase space $F(.)$ under additional operation (generally but not necessarily; for a detailed treatment, see Perdikis, Huys, & Jirsa, 2011a):

$$\dot{\mathbf{u}} = F[\mathbf{u}, \sigma(t)], \tag{10.7}$$

where $\mathbf{u}$ is the vector of the system's state variables, and $\sigma(t)$ represents a time-dependent influence—termed operational signal—that, if constant in time, $\dot{\sigma}(t) = 0$, renders the process autonomous. In the latter case, $F(.)$ is identical to the SFM of a particular functional mode. Let τ_u and τ_σ denote the timescales corresponding to a particular functional mode and operational signal $\sigma(t)$, respectively. $\sigma(t)$ may operate on various timescales relative to τ_f and may (in principle) span a continuum of scales. Four different (prototypical) instantiations of timescale separations can be envisioned: (1) $\sigma(t)$ may act much faster than the functional mode (i.e., $\tau_\sigma \ll \tau_u$), in which case we identify it with the Dirac function $\delta(t)$ (it acts as a "kick"); (2) $\sigma(t)$ may act on a timescale similar to that of the functional mode (i.e., $\tau_\sigma \ll \tau_u$), in which case $\sigma(t)$ may be said to operate the functional mode [we then rename it as $\eta(t)$]; (3) $\sigma(t)$ may act much slower than the functional mode ($\tau_\sigma \ll \tau_u$), in which case we rename it with $\xi(t)$; (4) $\sigma(t)$ may be constant, that is, $\dot\sigma(t) = 0$; thus effectively not act at all. A systematic treatment of the timescale separation and its use in functional architectures is found in Haken (1995).

In the implementation presented here, functional modes and operational signals $\xi(t)$ and $\delta(t)$ constitute a functional architecture where at each moment in time the "expressed" flow is given as a linear combination of all modes available in an agent's dynamical repertoire,

$$\dot{\mathbf{u}} = F(\mathbf{u},t) = \sum_i |\xi_i(t)| g_i(\mathbf{u}) + \delta(t), \tag{10.8}$$

where $\mathbf{u}$ is the state vector, and $g_i(.)$ is the vector field of the ith mode. ξ_i is constrained to positive values and acts as a weighting coefficient for the ith mode (operating slower than the modes except for fast transitions between them). Effectively, they "select" a particular component flow g_j (when $\xi_j = 1$ and all other $\xi_i = 0$, for $i \neq j$) via a pattern competition process.

Apart from this slow competition dynamics, the architecture provides for the optional involvement of the instantaneous $\delta(t)$ kicks (for instance, to cross a separatrix; cf. figure 10.1, plate 26). The functional architecture, thus, combines invariant features (the SFM) with those that are variable across repeated instances of a functional mode's appearance in an agent's behavior.

10.5.2 Functional Mode Competition

To avoid overlap of modes, we implement a winner-take-all (WTA) competition for the ξ_i dynamics,

$$\dot{\xi}_i = \frac{1}{\tau_c}\left(L_i - C_i \sum_k^N \xi_k^2 \right)\xi_i$$
$$L_i \in [0,1], \ \ C_i \in [1,+\infty), \tag{10.9}$$

where the time constant τ_c ensures fast competition, L_i controls the availability of a functional mode to partake in the competition, and C_i (jointly with L_i) determines its outcome. The mode decomposition based on a competition scheme follows previous work on the *synergetic computer* (Haken, 2004) and is well established in the literature of biological inspired computation (Grossberg, 1980). The architecture, however, does not critically depend on this competition; an alternative instantiation could be a winnerless competition based on transient heteroclinic sequences (see chapter 4 in this volume; Rabinovich & Huerta, 2008), as used in Woodman et al. (2010).

10.5.3 Serial Dynamics

To model serial behavior, additional "circuitry" is required to sequentially activate the functional modes taking part in the sequence. This is achieved by designing suitable dynamics for the L_i parameters that determine which functional modes may compete in the competition at each stage of the sequence and their activation duration (for details, see Perdikis, Huys, & Jirsa, 2011b). In addition, the C_i parameters determine which mode wins the competition at each stage and thus the specific order of the sequence. This *serial order* dynamics provides a "bottom-up" coupling from the functional space **u** to the slow operational signal $\dot{\xi}_i = f_\xi[L_i(\mathbf{u}), C_i(\mathbf{u})] = f_\xi^i(\mathbf{u})$. Thus, parallel representation of the sequence (encoded in arrays of L_i and C_i parameters) are combined with serial WTA processes at each competition stage similar in spirit to the well-established competitive queuing models of serial behavior (Bullock & Rhodes, 2003).

10.5.4 Implementation of Cursive Handwriting

As proof of concept, we illustrate the functional architecture in the context of serial motor behavior following the lines of thought developed by Perdikis, Huys, and Jirsa (2011b); in particular, cursive handwriting. $\mathbf{u} = [x \; y \; z]$ defines the state vector; functional modes correspond to characters modeled as three-dimensional SFMs. The manifold, a cylindrical spiral with an ellipsoid basis that unfolds along the x axis, is (without loss of generality) chosen to be common for all characters (for implementation reasons). The form of the functional dynamics as an instantiation of equation (10.8) reads

$$\tau_u \dot{x} = F_x(\mathbf{u}, t) = \mu \sum_i^N \left\{ |\xi_i| f_{x_i}[y, F_y(\mathbf{u}, t)] \right\}$$

$$\tau_u \dot{y} = F_y(\mathbf{u}, t) = \left[r^2 - (y-c)^2 - 4z^2 \right] \frac{(y-c)}{r^2} + \mu \sum_i^N |\xi_i| \left[z - \frac{(y-c)}{r^2}(y-c-r)(y-c+r) \right]$$

$$+ \delta_y \left(y, z, F_y, F_z, \sum_i^N |\xi_i| \right)$$

$$\tau_u \dot{z} = F_z(\mathbf{u}, t) = \left[r^2 - (y-c)^2 - 4z^2 \right] \frac{z}{r^2} + \mu \sum_i^N [|\xi_i| f_{z_i}(y, z)]$$

$$+ \delta_z \left(y, z, F_y, F_z, \sum_i^N |\xi_i| \right), \tag{10.10}$$

where r is the radius of the manifold, and y and z obey excitator-like dynamics (see earlier and Jirsa & Kelso, 2005), where for $f_z^{lc}(y,z) = -\mu_e^{lc}(y-c)$, $f_z^{mn}(y,z) = -\mu_e^{mn}(y-c\pm r)$, or $f_z^{bi}(y,z) = -\mu_e^{bi}(z)$, the system exhibits a limit cycle, the monostable system, or the bistable system, respectively. The smallness parameter μ introduces the timescale separation responsible for the fast contraction on the manifold, and $\mu_e^{lc/mn/bi}$ guarantees the timescale separation required for the threshold properties (see figure 10.1, plate 26). Further, the form of $f_{xi}(.)$ yields the desired letter shapes. Although this particular implementation is not unique (other choices may accomplish the same behavior equally well), it justly serves our purpose to demonstrate the functional architecture.

Notice that the dynamics of $\delta_{y,z}$ is a function of $\mathbf{u}$ and $\dot{\mathbf{u}}$ (as well as ξ_i) and together with $f_{\xi}(\mathbf{u})$ render the functional architecture autonomous. The architecture is characterized by a multiscale dynamics via the slow ξ_is, as a mode becomes temporarily stable during its activation and subsequently destabilizes to give way to the next one in the sequence. Finally, the functional dynamics drives the dynamics in the handwriting workspace (the xy plane).

Figure 10.6 (plate 30) demonstrates a simulation of the "handwritten" word *flow* generated by the functional architecture. The system produces the word to which it converges after a first transitive effort (due to random initial conditions). The dynamical repertoire consists of $N = 37$ functional modes. Monostable flows are used to generate the f [with a point attractor at $(y^*,z^*) = (4, 0)$], the l and o [point attractors at $(y^*,z^*) = (0, 0)$] (where $\delta_{y,z}$ triggers one cycle per stimulus), and a limit cycle flow for the w. Auxiliary linear point attractor phase flows are used at the beginning and ending of the flow properly to set the initial and final conditions.

10.6   Discussion

We elaborated our perspective on the emergence of functionally meaningful processes that we conceptualized in terms of trajectories shaped by low-dimensional phase flows. We showed how such functional dynamics may arise from (in principle high-dimensional) neural (spiking) networks as SFM and provided evidence for their implication in the control of (motor) behavior. Finally, we laid out a framework for functional architectures based on SFM in conjunction with additional dynamics at various timescales for the generation of complex processes. The implications of the outlined perspective are multiple and relevant for—but not

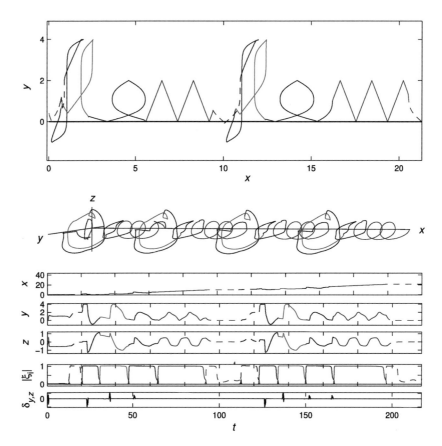

Figure 10.6 (plate 30)
The word *flow* is generated by the functional architecture. From top to bottom: The output trajectory on the handwriting workspace (*xy* plane); the trajectory in the three-dimensional (functional) *xyz* phase space; time series of the *x*, *y*, and *z* output dynamics; time series of the slow sequential dynamics $|\xi_i|$; and time series of the "instantaneous" $\delta_{y,z}$ kicks. The different colors distinguish the four main functional modes (blue for *f*, green for *l*, magenta for *o*, and cyan for *w*), while the initial and final auxiliary flows are depicted in dashed blue and dashed cyan, respectively. The short segments of black at the beginning of the time series depict the part of the trajectory where none of the flows participating in the sequence dominate, and all ξ_is of the nonparticipating (inhibited) modes are depicted with a red line.

limited to—the neurosciences and behavioral sciences alike. In the following, we will discuss some of these implications.

We have shown that networks of spiking neurons may give rise to SFM, which is a major leap forward in granting biological realism to the SFM approach. In addition, it substantiates the hypothesis that neural networks may code for flows, which has (at least) two important implications. First, it contrasts the (common) idea that nervous system functioning is geared toward instantiating specific "solutions" (trajectories, in the language here used) but rather suggests that it "sets up" an appropriate "functional organization" (the SFM) that renders accomplishing a desired goal likely under perturbations of any kind (i.e., "internal" as well as "external" to the agent). Second, if confirmed, it unambiguously settles the discussion whether dynamics are merely descriptors of functional processes or represent causal ingredients underlying their control.

Indeed, functional architectures as expressed through SFMs are robust against small parameter variations. When noise drives the network dynamics in absence of external stimuli, then for a given structured flow on the manifold, the network activations express themselves as they would in contexts of specific cognitive tasks. One may speculate that such occurs during rest or daydreaming. During resting-state activity of large-scale brain dynamics, surprisingly coherent spatiotemporal patterns have been observed intermittently that resemble task-related brain activations (see chapter 1 in this volume). Studies of resting-state networks propose that noise explores the dynamic repertoire of the brain, of which SFMs would be a prime candidate for its manifestation (Deco, Jirsa, & McIntosh, 2011).

Finally, similar to our approach, the two traditional approaches to cognitive modeling (symbolic dynamics and connectionism) define functional units and a set of operations on them (commonly referred to as "computation"). In symbolic dynamics, information is represented explicitly as organized symbols, and computation takes the form of syntactic rules combining them (Newel, 1990). In connectionist models, patterns of activation, distributed across the nodes of large networks, allow for parallel computations (Kremer, 2001). So-called hybrid cognitive architectures combine symbolic knowledge representation with connectionist learning algorithms (Sun & Alexandre, 1997). In all but a few cases (Rabinovich & Huerta, 2008; Kozma & Freeman, 2009; Rabinovich & Muezzinoglu, 2009), however, the functional units are considered as static patterns or "states." Even in cases in which processes are modeled dynamically and dealt with in real time, they are eventually broken into a succession of "discrete" states and treated as such (cf. the recurrent neural networks literature: Kolen & Kremer, 2001; Maass, Natschlager, & Markram, 2002; Carpenter & Grossberg, 2003). In contrast, we explicitly aim to refurnish a process with its defining feature, namely temporal evolution. Indeed, the emphasis on (cognitive) *processes* rather than states is compatible with (temporal) change across (time-invariant) "content" and may resolve the (apparent) conflict of continuously evolving experiences (Damasio, 2000) versus discrete (conscious) units (James, 1890) and place cognition on an ontological footing consistent with physics and everyday experience alike.

Acknowledgments

The research leading to these results received funding in part from the European Union Seventh Framework Program (FP7/2007- 2013) under grant agreement no. 269921 (BrainScaleS) and from the Brain NRG Phase II, James S McDonnell Foundation.

References

Ashwin, P., Field, M., Rucklidge, A. M., & Sturman, R. (2003). Phase resetting effects for robust cycles between chaotic sets. *Chaos, 13*, 973–81. Available at http://www.ncbi.nlm.nih.gov/pubmed/12946190.

Ashwin, P., Orosz, G., Wordsworth, J., & Townley, S. (2007). Dynamics on networks of cluster states for globally coupled phase oscillators. *SIAM Journal of Applied Dynamic Systems 6*, 728–758.

Beek, P. J., & Beek, W. J. (1988). Tools for constructing dynamical models of rhythmic movement. *Human Movement Science, 7*, 301–342.

Beek, P. J., Rikkert, W. E. I., & van Wieringen, P. C. W. (1996). Limit cycle properties of rhythmic forearm movements. *Journal of Experimental Psychology: Human Perception & Performance, 22*, 1077–1093.

Beer, R. (2000). Dynamical approaches to cognitive science. Trends in Cognitive Sciences, *4*, 91–99.

Bressler, S. L., & Kelso, J. A. S. (2001). Cortical coordination dynamics and cognition. Trends in Cognitive Sciences, *5*, 26–36.

Büchel, C., & Friston, K. J. (2000). Assessing interactions among neuronal systems using functional neuroimaging. Neural Networks, *13*, 871–882.

Bullock, D., & Rhodes, B. J. (2003). Competitive queuing for planning and serial performance. In M. A. Arbib (Ed.), *The Handbook of Brain Theory and Neural Networks* (pp. 241–244). Cambridge, MA: MIT Press.

Calvert, G. A., Spence, C., & Stein, B. E. (2004). *The Handbook of Multisensory Processes.* Cambridge, MA: MIT Press.

Carpenter, G. A., & Grossberg, S. S. (2003). Adaptive resonance theory. In M. A. Arbib (Ed.), *The Handbook of Brain Theory and Neural Networks* (pp. 87–90) Cambridge, MA: MIT Press.

Daffertshofer, A. (2010). Benefits and pitfalls in analyzing noise in dynamical systems—on stochastic differential equations and system identification. In R. Huys & V. K. Jirsa (Eds.). *Nonlinear Dynamics in Human Behavior* (pp. 35–68). Berlin: Springer-Verlag.

Daffertshofer, A., Huys, R., & Beek, P. J. (2004). Dynamical coupling between locomotion and respiration. Biological Cybernetics, *90*, 157–164.

Damasio, A. (2000). *The Feeling of What Happens: Body and Emotion in the Making of Consciousness*. San Diego: Harcourt.

Deco, G., Jirsa, V. K., & McIntosh, A. R. (2011). Emerging concepts for the dynamical organization of resting-state activity in the brain. Nature Reviews. Neuroscience, *12*, 43–56.

Fink, P. W., Kelso, J. A. S., & Jirsa, V. K. (2009). Perturbation-induced false starts as a test of the Jirsa-Kelso Excitator model. Journal of Motor Behavior, *41*, 147–157.

Friedrich, R., & Peinke, J. (1997). Statistical properties of a turbulent cascade. Physica D. Nonlinear Phenomena, *102*, 147–155.

Friston, K. J. (1994). Functional and effective connectivity in neuroimaging: a synthesis. Human Brain Mapping, *2*, 56–78.

Friston, K. J. (2002). Beyond phrenology: what can neuroimaging tell us about distributed circuitry? Annual Review of Neuroscience, *25*, 221–250.

Gray, C. M., Konig, P., Engel, A., & Singer, W. (1989). Oscillatory responses in cat visual cortex exhibit inter-columnar synchronization which reflects global stimulus properties. Nature, *338*, 334–337.

Grossberg, S. (1980). Biological competition: decision rules, pattern formation and oscillations. Proceedings of the National Academy of Sciences of the United States of America, *77*, 2338–2342.

Haken, H. (1983). *Synergetics: An Introduction. Nonequilibrium Phase Transitions and Self Organization in Physics, Chemistry and Biology*. Berlin: Springer.

Haken, H. (1995). *Principles of Brain Functioning: A Synergetic Approach to Brain Activity, Behavior and Cognition* (Springer Series in Synergetics). Berlin: Springer.

Haken, H. (2004). *Synergetic Computers and Cognition: A Top-Down Approach to Neural Nets*. Berlin: Springer Verlag.

Haken, H. (2006). *Information and Self-Organization: A Macroscopic Approach to Complex Systems* (Springer Series in Synergetics). Berlin: Springer.

Haken, H., Kelso, J. A. S., & Bunz, H. (1985). A theoretical model of phase transitions in human hand movements. Biological Cybernetics, *51*, 347–356.

Horwitz, B., Tagamets, M. A., & McIntosh, A. R. (1999). Neural modeling, functional brain imaging, and cognition. Trends in Cognitive Sciences, *3*, 91–98.

Huys, R., Daffertshofer, A., & Beek, P. J. (2004). The evolution of coordination during skill acquisition: the dynamical systems approach. In A. M. Williams & N. J. Hodges (Eds.), *Skill Acquisition in Sport: Research, Theory and Practice* (pp. 351–373). London: Routledge.

Huys, R., Fernandez, L., Bootsma, R. J., & Jirsa, V. K. (2010). Fitts' law is not continuous in reciprocal aiming. Proceedings. Biological Sciences, *277*, 1179.

Huys, R., Jirsa, V. K., Studenka, B. E., Rheaume, N., & Zelaznik, H. N. (2008). Human trajectory formation: taxonomy of movement based on phase flow topology. In A. Fuchs & V. K. Jirsa (Eds.), *Coordination: Neural, Behavioral and Social Dynamics* (pp. 77–92). Berlin: Springer-Verlag.

Huys, R., Studenka, B. E., Rheaume, N. L., Zelaznik, H. N., & Jirsa, V. K. (2008). Distinct timing mechanisms produce discrete and continuous movements. *PLoS Computational Biology, 4*, e1000061.

Huys, R., Studenka, B. E., Zelaznik, H. N., & Jirsa, V. K. (2010). Distinct timing mechanisms are implicated in distinct circle drawing tasks. *Neuroscience Letters, 472*, 24–28.

James, W. (1890). *The Principles of Psychology* (Vol. 1). Dover, NY: Dover Publications.

Jirsa, V. K., & Kelso, J. A. S. (2005). The excitator as a minimal model for the coordination dynamics of discrete and rhythmic movement generation. Journal of Motor Behavior, *37*, 35–51.

Kay, B. A., Kelso, J. A. S., Saltzman, E. L., & Schöner, G. (1987). Space-time behavior of single and bimanual rhythmical movements: data and limit cycle model. Journal of Experimental Psychology. Human Perception and Performance, *13*, 178–192.

Kay, B. A., Saltzman, E. L., & Kelso, J. A. S. (1991). Steady-state and perturbed rhythmical movements: A dynamical analysis. Journal of Experimental Psychology. Human Perception and Performance, *17*, 183–197.

Kelso, J. A. S. (Ed.). (1982). *Human Motor Behavior: An Introduction.* Hillsdale, NJ: Lawrence Erlbaum Associates.

Kelso, J. A. S. (1995). *Dynamic Patterns: The Self-Organization of Brain and Behavior.* Cambridge, MA: MIT Press.

Kelso, J. A. S., Delcolle, J. D., & Schöner, G. (1990). Action-perception as a pattern formation process. In M. Jeannerod (Ed.), *Attention and Performance XIII* (pp. 139–169). Hillsdale, NJ: Erlbaum.

Kelso, J. A. S., Holt, K. G., Rubin, P., & Kugler, P. N. (1981). Patterns of human interlimb coordination emerge from the properties of non-linear, limit cycle oscillatory processes: theory and data. Journal of Motor Behavior, *13*, 226–261.

Kiebel, S. J., Daunizeau, J., Friston, K. J. (2008). A hierarchy of time-scales and the brain. *PLoS Computational Biology*, *4*, e1000209.

King, A. J., & Calvert, G. A. (2001). Multisensory integration: perceptual grouping by eye and ear. Current Biology, *11*, R322–R325.

Kolen, J. F., & Kremer, S. C. (Eds.). (2001). *A Field Guide to Dynamical Recurrent Networks.* New York: Wiley-IEEE Press.

Kozma, R., & Freeman, W. J. (2009). The KIV model of intentional dynamics and decision making. Neural Networks, *22*, 277–285.

Kremer, S. C. (2001). Spatiotemporal connectionist networks: a taxonomy and review. Neural Computation, *13*, 249–306.

Kugler, P. N., Kelso, J. A. S., & Turvey, M. T. (1980). On the concept of coordinative structures as dissipative structures: I. Theoretical lines of convergence. In G. Stelmach & J. Requin (Eds.), *Tutorials in Motor Behavior* (pp. 3–47). Amsterdam: North-Holland.

Maass, W., Natschlager, T., & Markram, H. (2002). Real-time computing without stable states: a new framework for neural computation based on perturbations. Neural Computation, *14*, 2531–2560.

Meijer, O. G., & Roth, K. (1988). *Complex Movement Behaviour: The Motor-Action Controversy.* Amsterdam: North Holland.

Mottet, D., & Bootsma, R. J. (1999). The dynamics of goal-directed rhythmical aiming. Biological Cybernetics, *80*, 235–245.

Newel, A. (1990). *Unified Theories of Cognition.* Cambridge, MA: Harvard University Press.

Nowotny, T., & Rabinovich, M. I. (2007). Dynamical origin of independent spiking and bursting activity in neural microcircuits. Physical Review Letters, *98*, 128106.

Perdikis, D., Huys, R., & Jirsa, V. (2011a). Complex processes from dynamical architectures with time-scale hierarchy. PLoS ONE, *6*, e16589.

Perdikis, D., Huys, R., & Jirsa, V. K. (2011b) Time scale hierarchies in the functional organization of complex behaviors. *PLoS Computational Biology, 7*, e1002198.

Port, R. F., & van Gelder, T. (Eds.). (1998). *Mind as Motion: Explorations in the Dynamics of Cognition.* Cambridge, MA: MIT Press.

Post, A. A., de Groot, G., Daffertshofer, A., & Beek, P. J. (2007). Pumping a playground swing. Motor Control, *11*, 136–150.

Rabinovich, M. I., Huerta, R., Varona, P., & Afraimovich, V.S. (2008). Transient cognitive dynamics, metastability, and decision making. PLoS Computational Biology, *4*(5), e1000072.

Rabinovich, M. I., Muezzinoglu, M. K., Strigo, I., & Bystritsky, A. (2010). Dynamical principles of emotion-cognition interaction: mathematical images of mental disorders. *PLoS One, 5*, e12547.

Shevchenko, M., Windridge, D., & Kittler, J. (2009). A linear-complexity reparameterisation strategy for the hierarchical bootstrapping of capabilities within perception-action architectures. Image and Vision Computing, *27*, 1702–1714.

Sternad, D. (2008). Towards a unified theory of rhythmic and discrete movements—behavioral, modeling and imaging results. In A. Fuchs & V. K. Jirsa (Eds.), *Coordination: Neural, Behavioral and Social Dynamics* (pp. 105–133). Berlin: Springer-Verlag.

Strogatz, S. H. (2001). *Nonlinear Dynamics and Chaos: With Applications to Physics, Biology, Chemistry, and Engineering* (Studies in Nonlinearity). Boulder, CO: Westview Press.

Sun, R., & Alexandre, F. (Eds.). (1997). *Connectionist-Symbolic Integration: From Unified to Hybrid Approaches*. Hillsdale, NJ: Erlbaum.

Thesen, T., Vibell, J. F., Calvert, G. A., & Osterbauer, R. A. (2004). Neuroimaging of multisensory processing in vision, audition, touch, and olfaction. Cognitive Processing, *5*, 84–93.

Tononi, G., Sporns, O., & Edelman, G. M. (1994). A measure for brain complexity: relating functional segregation and integration in the nervous system. Proceedings of the National Academy of Sciences of the United States of America, *91*, 5033–5037.

Tuller, B., Nguyen, N., Lancia, L., & Vallabha, G. (2011). Nonlinear dynamics in speech perception. In R. Huys & V. K. Jirsa (Eds.), *Nonlinear Dynamics in Human Behavior* (pp. 135–150). Berlin: Springer.

van Gelder, T. (1998). The dynamical hypothesis in cognitive science. Behavioral and Brain Sciences, *21*, 615–628.

Woodman, M., Perdikis, D., Pillai, A. S., Dodel, S., Huys, R., Bressler, S. et al. (2010). Building neurocognitive networks with distributed functional architectures. In C. Hernandez et al. (Eds.), *From Brains to Systems* (pp. 101–109). Berlin: Springer.

Yu, A. C., & Margoliash, D. (1996). Temporal hierarchical control of singing in birds. *Science 273*, 1871–1875.

11 Transient Motor Behavior and Synchronization in the Cortex

Andreas Daffertshofer and Bernadette C. M. van Wijk

Summary

Bimanual coordination requires the functional integration of various cortical, subcortical, spinal, and peripheral neural structures. How is this integration accomplished? The answer to this question will not only add to our understanding of motor control but also help to unravel more general mechanisms underlying the information transfer across the cortex and beyond. To do so, however, experimental protocols and accompanying mathematical descriptions need to tackle transient behavior in addition to the conventionally addressed steady-state performance. The focus on transient switches allows for reducing mathematical descriptions to that of low-dimensional systems by means of a separation of timescales (center manifold approach) irrespective of the complexity of the dynamics under study. This applies to behavioral models, to models of macroscopic cortical activity, and to more local neural mass models. We outline seminal empirical findings regarding movement coordination, isolated switches between steady states, and a permanent loss of stability. To study neural information transfer explicitly, we further summarize some more recent findings of encephalographic recordings during such cascades of behavioral states. For the latter, we consider the dynamics of phases of oscillatory neural populations and link it to beta band oscillations whose envelope characteristics resemble the loss of stability of coordinated rhythmic movements.

11.1 Motor Behavior and Loss of Stability

Disentangling the information transfer across the human nervous system constitutes one of the greatest challenges in neuroscience. The study of motor behavior forms an expedient approach to this challenge, as it addresses intra- and inter-hemispheric interactions between bilateral motor areas while tuning outcome measures (i.e., motor performance) in a reproducible manner. The benefits of looking at motor activity (in general) and transient or unstable behavior (in particular) can be illustrated by a plethora of experimental paradigms from which we here only highlight some "simple" hand and finger movements. We particularly consider inter-hemispheric interactions whose underlying fiber systems connecting the motor cortices through the corpus callosum is well documented (Boyd, Pandya, & Bignall, 1971; Pandya, Karol, & Heilbronn, 1971; Carson, 2005). Looking merely at this anatomic structure, the function of the inter-hemispheric interaction remains elusive (Ghacibeh et al., 2007). The same holds for looking at steady motor performance, probably because the fiber systems comprise both inhibitory and excitatory connections (Ferbert et al., 1992; Innocenti, 2009) that, as will be argued later, may or may not balance one another.

During unimanual movements, the contralateral motor cortex is more active than its ipsilateral counterpart and is considered the main controller of hand and finger movements (Brinkman & Kuypers, 1972; Gazzaniga, 1966). However, unimanual performance entails activities in both contralateral and ipsilateral motor cortices (Babiloni et al., 1999; Baraldi et al., 1999; Gribova, Donchin, Bergman, Vaadia, & Cardoso De Oliveira, 2002; Carson, 2005), which are clearly event-related, and their spatiotemporal patterns match (differences in strength aside) those observed during symmetric bimanual performances. This bilateral cortical activity may be induced through the aforementioned transcallosal pathways, which implies the presence of an instantaneous inter-hemispheric cross-talk. The motor control system has thus to account for this information transfer between hemispheres. Especially when moving unimanually, the resulting ipsilateral activation needs to be reduced because, if the ipsilateral activity maps onto its contralateral cortico-spinal pathway, it may induce unintended mirror movements (Daffertshofer, van den Berg, & Beek, 1999; Gerloff & Andres, 2002; Serrien & Brown, 2002). In other words, during unimanual movements, one of the two end-effectors needs to be actively suppressed by inhibiting its contralateral motor area. Efficiency of performance demands a proper adjustment of inhibition with respect to its strength and timing. Given rhythmic motor and/or oscillatory neural activity, the latter implies phase locking between the participating units.

A proper balance between excitation and inhibition suppresses activity on one side of the body, whereas too weak/strong inhibition yields a symmetric/antisymmetric co-activation or synchronous versus alternating activity in the case of rhythmic motor performance (Dafertshofer, Peper, & Beek, 2005). Most probably, the central nervous system uses several ways to accomplish output suppression, which may involve thalamo-cortical loops, intra-hemispheric inhibition (e.g., between primary motor, premotor, and supplementary motor areas) (Donchin, Gribova, Steinberg, Bergman, & Vaadia, 1998; Carpenter, Georgopoulos, & Pellizzer, 1999; Gribova et al., 2002), or even more distant inhibitory circuits involving prefrontal areas. The precise structure of these under-pinnings can be identified by dis-balancing excitatory and inhibitory activity, which eventually yields transient behavior on the level of both neural populations and motor performance. In the following, this will be illustrated briefly by summarizing some seminal empirical findings before addressing selected dynamical models.

11.1.1 Behavioral Studies

Behavioral instabilities can be induced by having a subject tap his or her index finger in between the tones of an external acoustic stimulus train (i.e., syncopation) with a gradually decreasing inter-tone interval. At a particular inter-tone interval, an abrupt transition will occur to synchro-nization; that is, a mode of coordination in which the taps coincide with the tones. In this case, syncopation has become unstable, whereas syn-chronization becomes or remains stable. Simultaneous encephalographic recordings revealed that a phase transition occurred in the corresponding brain activity (Kelso et al., 1992; Daffertshofer, Peper, & Beek, 2000; Mayville et al., 2001). The term *phase transition* is adopted from thermo-dynamics and implies a qualitative change in the macroscopic order of the system under study. Capitalizing on the center manifold theorem, systems undergoing phase transitions can be analyzed in terms of low-dimensional dynamical systems, the so-called order parameter equations (Haken, 1983). Over the years, the concept of phase transitions provided a new basis for the construction of formal models of motor behavior and accompanying brain functioning (Haken, 1996) and corresponding experiments. Meyer-Lindenberg, Ziemann, Hajak, Cohen, & Berman (2002) established a link between the neural activity in premotor and supplementary motor areas and the degree of behavioral instability by transiently disturbing them using transcranial magnetic stimulations, which caused sustained transitions from less stable syncopated to more stable synchronized unimanual movements.

For bimanual coordination, Kelso, Holt, Rubin, & Kugler (1981) reported a by-now paradigmatic experiment on finger movements: When subjects start out moving their index fingers (or hands) rhythmically in anti-phase (simultaneous activation of non-homologous muscle groups),

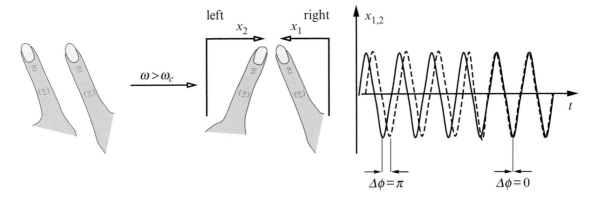

Figure 11.1
Phase transition from anti-phase to in-phase coordination in finger movements. When subjects start moving their index fingers in anti-phase, an increase of the movement frequency ω yields a switch to an in-phase pattern at a critical frequency ω_c; that is, the relative phase $\Delta\phi$ between the limbs switches from $\pm\pi$ to 0.

a gradual increase of the movement frequency yields a spontaneous, involuntary switch to an in-phase pattern (simultaneous activation of homologous muscle groups) at a certain critical frequency. Beyond this critical value, only the in-phase pattern can be stably performed. These coordinative states have been modeled by means of a single order parameter that heuristically coincides with the relative phase between the fingers (Haken, Kelso, & Bunz, 1985); see figure 11.1 and section 11.2.

During polyrhythmic performances, that is, during the production of rhythmic bimanual movements whose frequencies are related in a $P{:}Q$ ratio (P and/or $Q > 1$), interactions between limbs become even more apparent than in the iso-frequency (1:1) case because different frequency ratios vary considerably in their difficulty of performance (Summers, Rosenbaum, Burns, & Ford, 1993) even though the unimanual subtasks are equally simple. Interactions between the limbs result in a preference for frequency ratios that typically consist of small integers such as 1:2 or 1:3 (Peper, Beek, & van Wieringen, 1995). Peper and Beek (1998a, 1998b) studied interlimb interactions in subjects that tapped a 2:3 polyrhythm and found that amplitude of movement—and by this the coupling strength—is related reciprocally to movement tempo. Given that coupling depends on movement tempo, one can also consistently induce phase transitions, which allows for studying transient behavior and may lead to the reduction of dimensionality (i.e., the emergence of the aforementioned order parameters).

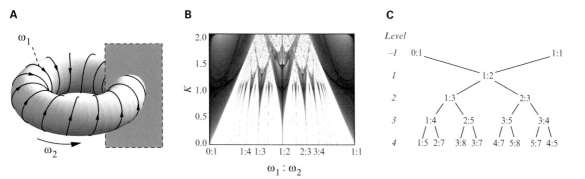

Figure 11.2
(A) Movement along the unit torus. Rational frequency ratios $\omega_1/\omega_2 = P/Q$ yield mode coupling corresponding to stable areas in the sine-circle map

$$\varphi_{n+1} = \left[\varphi_n + \frac{\omega_1}{\omega_2} - \frac{K}{2\pi} \sin\left(2\pi\varphi_n\right) \right] \mod 1,$$

provided the coupling strength K is chosen properly. Here, φ represents the phase of a forced oscillator and φ_n its value when passing the Poincaré section shown in the left panel. (B) Arnold tongues of the sine-circle map where the coupling strength K and the frequency ratio ω_1/ω_2 serve as bifurcation parameters; dark regions represent stable solutions. (C) Transitions between stable regimes occur according to the Farey principle that is here summarized in a tree-like scheme (Farey tree). In a Farey sequence of order n, all rational ratios with a denominator smaller than $n + 1$ are ordered within unity. According to Farey's theorem, the lowest-order rational ratio (i.e., the reduced fraction with the smallest denominator) situated between any two rational ratios h/k and h'/k' adjacent in the sequence is given by the mediant of the two parent ratios, $h''/k'' = (h + h')/(k + k')$. For a Farey sequence of a given order, every pair of adjacent ratios h''/k'' and h/k are unimodularly related; that is, $|\, h''k - hk'' \,| = 1$.

The stability and transitions in polyrhythmic performance have been interpreted in terms of the sine circle map. The circle map is a one-dimensional difference equation, which describes the influence of a periodic force on the phase of an oscillator (figure 11.2A). It displays regions of stable mode locking, so-called Arnold tongues (figure 11.2B), which represent resonance regimes whose widths are determined by both the initial frequency ratio and the strength of interaction (Jensen, Bak, & Bohr, 1983). In general, lower-order Arnold tongues are wider than higher-order ones and are, thus, more stable. If the coupling in this map is reduced, transitions between frequency locks occur from higher-order ratios $P':Q'$ to lower-order ones $P:Q$, with routes given by the Farey principle (figure 11.2C). Several experimentally observed transitions in rhythmic hand movements revealed indeed routes along branches in the so-called Farey tree e.g., (5:8 → 3:5 → 2:3 → 1:2 → 1:1), but others did not (for an overview, see Haken, Peper, Beek, & Daffertshofer, 1996). To account for the entire spectrum of dynamical features, another model has been developed as an alternative to the sine circle map as will be outlined in section 11.2.

Identifying models underlying (rhythmic) coordinated movements and their instabilities may crucially benefit from the study of the accompanying neural activity. Recall that phase transitions during rhythmic performance may coincide with an insufficient and thus poorly timed inhibition of certain neural populations. For rhythmic behavior, inhibition can be interpreted as anti-phase excitatory coupling between two units (e.g., primary vis-à-vis premotor or supplementary motor areas). Inhibition results in vanishing lump-sum activity at the movement frequency in the corresponding motor areas because two superimposed anti-phase–locked oscillations cancel. Deviations from such anti-phase locking yield a finite amount of overall activity, as cancellation is no longer guaranteed. In the following, we summarize some experimental findings that indeed indicate that during changes in movement coordination, the ipsilateral motor areas are less (or not) phase-locked.

11.1.2 Encephalographic Studies

Neurons synchronize their firing patterns in accordance with different behavioral states. On a larger scale, synchronous activities are considered to stem from mesoscale neural populations that oscillate at certain frequencies with certain amplitudes. Oscillatory activity may yield synchronization characteristics within a neural population or between populations (Salenius & Hari, 2003). The amplitude of a single oscillatory neural population reflects the degree of synchronization of its neurons; that is, it measures local synchrony. By looking at magneto- and/or electroencephalographic recordings (M/EEG), bimanual tapping has been found to be accompanied by frequency- and phase-locked activations of motor cortices in left and right hemispheres (Lang, Obrig, Lindinger, Cheyne, & Deecke, 1990; Daffertshofer, Peper, & Beek, 2000; Gerloff & Andres, 2002). For polyrhythmic movements, activity in various cortical areas at one of the two basic movement frequencies appeared to be linearly correlated with the motor output suggesting that bimanual patterns could be expressed as superposition of unimanual ones (Daffertshofer, Peper, Frank, & Beek, 2000). Activation patterns, however, changed profoundly when behavior became unstable. Starting with a frequency ratio of, for example, 3:8 or 5:8, an increase in overall tempo induced cascades of transitions to ratios consisting of small integers (e.g., 3:8 → 1:3 → 1:2 → 1:1).

In these experiments, spectral power in bilateral motor areas at both movement frequencies indicated the expected inter-hemispheric cross-talk in bimanual performance. A loss of coordination was primarily visible as transient increased power at the emerging, posttransition movement frequency of the finger that underwent the motor instability. At this frequency, the increase in power led to a pronounced activity in the hemisphere ipsilateral to the finger that underwent the movement instability. Before and after a phase transition, the spectral power at the frequency had equivalent (mirrored) spatial distributions, again indicating a dominance of neural activity at contralateral motor areas. In contrast, in the immediate vicinity of switches in coordination, that frequency component changed significantly by means of a drastic increase of spectral power in the ipsilateral motor areas. The spatial distributions of the spectral power respecting the stably performing limb remained roughly unaltered irrespective of an increasing tempo and reflected a permanent dominance of the contralateral hemisphere.

Further decomposition of encephalographic signals into spatial and temporal components and cross-spectral analyses revealed different spatial correlations within different frequency regimes (Houweling, Beek, & Daffertshofer, 2010). In correspondence to the movement cycles, a pattern of desynchronization and synchronization of beta activity (15–30 Hz) in motor cortex during the movement cycle changes while the movement tempo is increased (figure 11.3, plate 31).

This beta modulation decreases when the temporal distance between the episodes of event-related synchronization and desynchronization

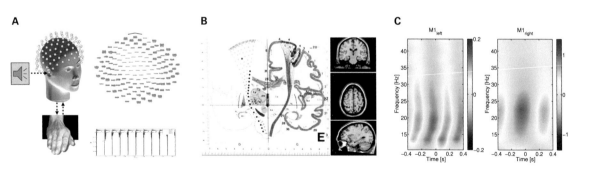

Figure 11.3 (plate 31)
(A) Scheme of magnetoencephalographic recordings (tapping to an acoustic metronome).
(B) Results of beamformer-based source localization of beta activity accompanying bimanual tapping; only the source in the left hemisphere is shown. (C) Time–frequency spectra of neural activity at primary motor areas ($M1_{left}$ and $M1_{right}$) during polyrhythmic tapping. Adapted from Houweling et al. (2010).

(ERS and ERD, respectively) diminish. This implies that coordination is limited by certain properties of the underlying neurophysiologic mechanism: The time required to build up local changes in synchronization within a neuronal ensemble may limit the central control of the muscles involved. In this case, the timescale of beta synchrony appears to form a key parameter for achieving timed phase synchrony in the motor cortex and along the neural axis. Once ERS/ERD cycles cannot be built-up properly, the movement phase starts slipping, and bilateral coordination collapses. In consequence, the timescale of beta synchrony forms an important constraint for the interactions between the cerebral hemispheres in that the time needed for the upregulation and downregulation of beta synchrony in rhythmic tapping forms a neurophysiologic bound for motor performance (Houweling et al., 2010). For the modeling in sections 11.3 and 11.4, this implies that during bimanual performance, inhibitory populations influence the beta amplitude modulation, which subserves the cortico-spinal information transfer. If cycles are too brief, inhibition is improper so that performance reduces in quality and becomes unstable.

As said, the power increase at the ipsilateral movement frequency can be interpreted as an improper intra-hemispheric phase-locking, which yields an effective loss of inter-hemispheric inhibition. A movement instability is accompanied by an increased cross-talk, indexed as the ratio between the amounts of spectral power at left and right movement frequencies within and between motor cortices (Daffertshofer, Peper, Frank, & Beek, 2000; Daffertshofer et al., 2005). That cross-talk is present at the movement frequency, suggesting that the bilateral phase locking over movement cycles is indeed mediated by beta oscillations and constrained by its phase dynamics.

The motor system is bilaterally activated during both bimanual and unimanual movements (Swinnen, 2002), and we seem to be innately equipped with the system calibrated for bilateral movement and have to learn to move unilaterally by suppression of activity through callosal pathways across the midline (Mayston, Harrison, & Stephens, 1999). Capitalizing on the interpretation of movement instabilities as phase transitions that may be captured mathematically in (simple) bifurcation schemes, Daffertshofer and coworkers (2005) proposed a mathematical model for the neural dynamics involved in rhythmic motor performance. This model will be discussed in section 11.3. To anticipate, this model describes how effective inhibition of inter-hemispheric interaction may result from excitatory transcallosal fibers projecting to primary and premotor areas and premotor areas inhibiting primary motor areas via intra-hemispheric cortico-cortical connections. According to the model, intra-hemispheric inhibition fails whenever phase coupling between motor areas becomes less strict. This yields a substantial amount of inter-hemispheric cross-talk and a destabilization of motor performance (Kelso et al., 1992). Before adding more details, however, we first summarize some mathematical models of behavioral instabilities, as the neural models outlined in sections 11.3 and 11.4 have to be able to address these dynamical structures, at least in their "macroscopic limit."

11.2 Behavioral Models

Rhythmic coordination tasks involving two (or more) moving limbs have been studied in terms of the dynamics of systems of coupled oscillators. Individual limb movements have been modeled as so-called limit-cycle oscillators typically involving low-order nonlinearities like Rayleigh and/or Van der Pol damping terms (Haken et al., 1985; Kay, Saltzman, Kelso, & Schöner, 1987). In addition, interactions between the limb movements have been modeled in terms of weak but nonlinear coupling functions that cause stable performance of in-phase and anti-phase coordination at low movement frequencies and stable performance of only in-phase coordination at high movement frequencies (Haken et al., 1985).

11.2.1 Steady States and Transitions

As mentioned earlier, in the immediate vicinity of a phase transition, the dynamics of coordinative patterns can be cast in the form of order parameter equations; that is, in the low-dimensional dynamics of one or a few collective variables that prescribe the entire dynamics of the system under study. In the case of interlimb coordination, the order parameter turns out to be the relative phase $\Delta\phi = \varphi_1 - \varphi_2$ between rhythmically moving limbs. Its stability properties are often captured by the dynamics

$$\Delta\dot{\phi} = -A\sin\Delta\phi - B\sin 2\Delta\phi, \tag{11.1}$$

where the dot notation refers to the derivative with respect to time. In this equation, B/A is the so-called control parameter that is meant to be controllable in an experimental setting. Here, B/A also acts as a bifurcation parameter. In line with the experimental findings, the movement frequency can be assumed to be reciprocally related to B/A: with increas-

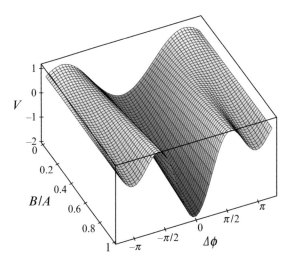

Figure 11.4
The evolution (11.1) of the relative phase between rhythmically moving fingers can be written as gradient dynamics,

$$\Delta\dot{\phi} = -\frac{dV}{d\Delta\phi}$$

with $V(\Delta\phi) = -A\cos\Delta\phi - \frac{1}{2}B\cos 2\Delta\phi.$

The minima of the potential $V(\Delta\phi)$, $\Delta\phi = 0$ and $\Delta\phi = \pm\pi$, represent the attractor states of relative phase; that is, the in-phase and anti-phase modes of coordination. To account for the transition from anti-phase to in-phase, the experimental control parameter frequency has to be capable of inducing changes in the potential landscape.

ing frequency, B/A decreases, resulting in a differential decrease in stability of the two distinct phase relations. This leads to the observed transition at a critical value of $B/A = 0.5$, at which the stable solution for anti-phase coordination is annihilated (figure 11.4).

In view of the various experimental findings outlined above, we extend the dynamics (11.1) in terms of a mathematical model that has been successfully used to describe the phenomena of frequency locking during polyrhythmic performance (Haken et al., 1996). This model appears particularly useful to account for the differential stability of various empirically observed frequency ratios and their loss of stability by means of phase. In fact, that model covers a broad spectrum of dynamical features of the empirical observations. However, as will be shown, the model's rich capacity does not come for free: The model incorporates a large set of parameters, particularly in the coupling function—the core when it comes to information transfer between units. Apart from the frequency dynamics, however, the phase dynamics may provide additional information about the more general validity of the model and, subsequently, about proper choices of model parameters.

We here estimate the generalized phase dynamics based on a system of two nonlinearly coupled self-sustaining oscillators (for an in-depth discussion, see Daffertshofer, Peper, Frank, & Beek, 2000), which reads

$$\ddot{x}_k = n(x_k, \dot{x}_k) + \frac{d}{dt} \left(\sum_{p=0}^{P} \sum_{q=0}^{Q} b_{pq}^{(k)} x_k^p x_l^q \right). \tag{11.2}$$

x_k describes for instance the moving limb's position ($k = 1, 2$). The function $n(x_k, \dot{x}_k)$ contains some nonlinearity guaranteeing self-sustained oscillations in the absence of any coupling between oscillators k and l (one typically uses the aforementioned Rayleigh and Van der Pol damping terms). Moreover, two (or more) oscillators are coupled to one another via the polynomial forms $\frac{d}{dt} x_k^p x_l^q$ that are weighted by some coupling parameters $b_{pq}^{(k)}$ (the parameters P and Q define the maximum frequency ratio to be incorporated in the model). As common in handling oscillators, the system (11.2) is transformed into a rotating coordinate system, and the frequency of the overall rhythm is rescaled to one. Put differently, one uses the Van der Pol transform

$$t = \tau/\Omega \quad \text{and} \quad \left\{ \begin{array}{l} x_k = r_k \cos(\omega_k \tau + \varphi_k) \\ y_k = -\omega_k r_k \sin(\omega_k \tau + \varphi_k) \end{array} \right\}$$

to define amplitudes r_k and phases φ_k. ω_k is the movement frequency of the limb k and represents an integer multiple of the frequency of the overall rhythm Ω. This system of oscillators can be averaged over a rhythmic cycle $2\pi/\Omega$ when assuming that its amplitude and phase change slowly compared with the oscillator's frequency Ω (and ω_k). That is, time-dependent amplitude and phase are fixed, the system is integrated over one period to remove all harmonic oscillations, and, subsequently, amplitude and phase are again considered to be time dependent (Guckenheimer & Holmes, 1990). We note that this procedure is also referred to as a combination of rotating wave approximation and slowly varying amplitude approximation (Haken, 1983). In the specific case of $P = Q = 5$, $\omega_1 = 5$, $\omega_2 = 3$, the generalized relative phase $\phi_{53} = 3\varphi_1 - 5\varphi_2$ then follows the dynamics

$$\dot{\phi}_{53} = \frac{25b_{54}^{(2)}r_1^4 + 20b_{34}^{(2)}r_1^2 + 9b_{45}^{(1)}r_1^2r_2^2 + 12b_{25}^{(1)}r_2^2}{512} r_1 r_2^3 \sin\phi_{53},$$

with which one can expect only a single steady phase relation between the two oscillators to be stable. In contrast, the relative phase $\phi_{32} = 2\varphi_1 - 3\varphi_2$ evolves according to

$$\dot{\phi}_{32} = \tfrac{1}{512}\big(96b_{42}^{(2)}r_1^4 + 96b_{22}^{(2)}r_1^2 + 72b_{24}^{(2)}r_1^2r_2^2 + 25b_{55}^{(1)}r_1^4r_2^4 +$$
$$+ 20b_{53}^{(1)}r_1^4r_2^2 + 40b_{35}^{(1)}r_1^2r_2^4 + 80b_{15}^{(1)}r_2^4 + 64b_{13}^{(1)}r_2^2\big)r_2 \sin\phi_{32} + \tfrac{3}{512}b_{45}^{(2)}\sin 2\phi_{32},$$

which allows for a stabilization of the relative phase at $\phi_{32} = \pm\pi$ apart from the in-phase solution $\phi_{32} = 0$. Note that this form is equivalent to (11.1); that is, to the Haken et al. (1985) model for the in-phase and anti-phase stability during isochronous movement. More details on these dynamics can be found in Daffertshofer, Peper, Frank, & Beek (2000). There it is shown that the dynamics of motor performance but also that of cortical activity display phenomena of multifrequency and generalized phase locking. A decomposition into spatial and temporal components of cortical activity and the subsequent cross-spectral analyses suggest that different spatial correlations are discernible within different frequency regimes. Dynamical interaction phenomena in the form of non-trivial correlations between and within hemispheres may occur at different spectral components; that is, at subharmonics and/or superharmonics of the movement frequency. Before addressing this in more detail, however, we first sketch the analysis of the accompanying transient regime; that is, the case in which explicit phase transitions as well as the emergence of so-called running solutions is dealt with.

11.2.2   Transients

The more general model for polyrhythmic motor performance was developed by Haken and coworkers (1996) to account for further features of empirical data: frequency locking, loss of stability, transitions to one or more lower-order frequency ratios, individual tendencies in these transition routes, which, as said, do not always agree with the Farey principle (cf. figure 11.2, right panel), as well as the emergence of free-running solutions. Running solutions here equal permanently transient (or unstable) states.

Starting with the oscillator dynamics (11.2), the averaging results in a phase dynamics that does not only display stability characteristics of the

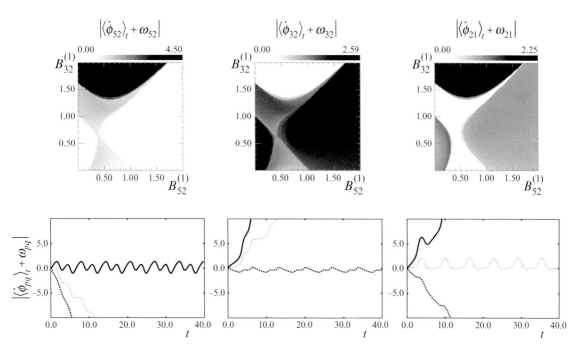

Figure 11.5
In general, the condition of frequency locking or "stability" can be expressed by $\phi_{pq} + \omega_{pq}t$ = const. + small oscillations; that is, $\langle \dot{\phi}_{pq} \rangle_t + \omega_{pq}t \to 0$, where $\langle \cdots \rangle_t$ denotes the average over time. The parameter range of "steady" states can be visualized by computing the time-averaged derivatives of ϕ_{pq} for different parameters. The resulting stability diagrams are coded such that instability corresponds to darker displays (upper panels); $B_{52}^{(2)} = 1$ and $B_{32}^{(2)} = 1$ as well as $B_{21}^{(1)} = B_{21}^{(2)} = 0.5$. Lower panels: Simulations of equation (11.3) with $p{:}q =$ (5:2, 3:2, 2:1), from left to right; we additionally set $B_{52}^{(1)} = 0.9$ and $B_{32}^{(1)} = 1$; solid lines ϕ_{52}; dashed lines ϕ_{32}; dotted lines ϕ_{21}.

phases but also indicates distinct regimes of frequency locking. In general, these equations obey the form for $j = 1, 2$,

$$\dot{\varphi}_j = \omega_j - \sum_{p=0}^{P} \sum_{q=0}^{Q} B_{pq}^{(j)} \sin \phi_{pq}, \tag{11.3}$$

with $\phi_{pq} = p{\cdot}(\omega_1 t + \varphi_1) - q{\cdot}(\omega_2 t - \varphi_2)$, and the integer values p and q are chosen according to the experimental observations sketched in, for example, Peper et al. (1995); see also figure 11.5.

In addition to steady states and isolated switches, the dynamics (11.3) also covers the fully transient regime including the aforementioned running solutions (lower panels in figure 11.5). As mentioned earlier, however, in order to appreciate this range, one has to identify a fairly large set of parameters $B_{pq}^{(j)}$, given the large set of possible polyrhythms that can be performed. Furthermore, as explained in Haken et al. (1996), these parameters also depend on the oscillators' amplitudes, which calls for a closer look at the phase-generating dynamics (11.2). If the oscillators describe limb movement, amplitude can be readily identified using the corresponding kinematics, which, however, does not imply that coupling is restricted to that level of description. On the contrary, the coupling between left and right sides of the body most likely involves neural dynamics all along the neural axis. In the following section, we hence discuss a model addressing the corresponding cortical underpinnings.

11.3   A Model for Cortical Areas

The differential stability in movement and cortical activity can be described by a model that builds on macroscopic descriptions of spatio-temporal patterning in the brain (e.g., neural mass models) (Wilson & Cowan, 1972; Freeman, 1975; Ermentrout & Cowan, 1979; Jirsa & Haken, 1996; Frank, Daffertshofer, Peper, Beek, & Haken, 2000; Wright et al., 2001; Haken, 2002). Emanating from large ensembles of mutually interacting neurons, averaging methods like mean-field approaches result in weakly nonlinear mapping from action potentials to dendritic currents. Because the latter can be considered as generators of extracellular fields, ensemble or field theoretical descriptions of the cortex yield the macroscopic dynamics of distinct cortical areas as recorded by M/EEG—see, for example, Jirsa, Jantzen, Fuchs, & Kelso (2002) for an in-depth discussion. To capture the main features of the empirical findings summarized in section 11.1, however, we first abstain from a more detailed ensemble theory by simply assuming that pulse rates and/or dendritic currents have oscillatory properties; see section 11.4 for more details on neural mass models.

We assume that the macroscopic activity in bilateral primary motor areas is the product of self-sustained but frequency- and phase-locked oscillations at the corresponding movement frequencies. Both cortices are linearly coupled with each other through transcallosal connections. In addition, two bilateral (premotor) areas are (bi-)linearly coupled to both contralateral and ipsilateral primary motor areas and respond (almost) instantaneously to their inputs. In turn, the activity of these additional units is mapped to the corresponding primary motor cortex (figure 11.6, middle panel; plate 32).

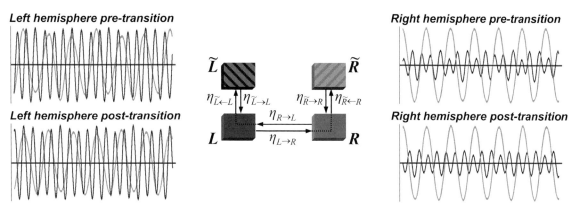

Left hemisphere pre-transition

Right hemisphere pre-transition

Left hemisphere post-transition

Right hemisphere post-transition

Figure 11.6 (plate 32)
Central panels: Cortical areas and scheme of connections between bilateral primary motor areas and premotor areas. Left and right panels: Simulations of neural activity in left/right hemispheres before and after a transition in bimanual coordination (upper and lower panels). Next to every unit, the time-dependent activities are depicted as being simulated using equations (11.4) and (11.5). Upper panels: 3:8 frequency locking ~ pretransition. Lower panels: 1:3 frequency locking ~ posttransition. The left panels show the evolution of the real parts of L (blue) and $\tilde{L}$ (green), and the right panels depict R (green) and $\tilde{R}$ (blue). The transition is realized by a reduction of the oscillators' amplitudes via a drop in $\gamma_{R,L}$. Upper panels, $\gamma_{R,L} = 0.5$; lower panels, $\gamma_{R,L} = 0.1$. Remaining parameters: $\omega_R = 1$, $\omega_L = 3/8$, $\kappa_R = \kappa_L = 0.5$, $\Delta\omega_{\tilde{R}} = \omega_R - \omega_L = -\Delta\omega_{\tilde{L}}$, $\eta_{L\to R} = \eta_{R\to L} = 0.01$, $\eta_{\tilde{R}\to R} = \eta_{\tilde{L}\to L} = 0.1$, $\eta_{\tilde{R}\leftarrow R} = \eta_{\tilde{L}\leftarrow L} = 0.25$. Adapted from Daffertshofer et al. (2005).

The time-dependent activity in right and left primary motor areas is summarized using the complex-valued quantities R and L, respectively. By choosing this complex-valued notion, we avoid the need for the Van der Pol transformation as in the more traditional oscillator approaches earlier. Then, the recorded activities are given by $|R|$ and $|L|$. The dynamics of these activities are (bi-)linearly coupled and, because we focus on rhythmic movements, R and L display self-sustained but frequency- and phase-locked oscillations at the distinct movement frequencies. Because of symmetry, calculations can be confined to one hemisphere, here the right one. For the sake of brevity, we cast the evolution of R into a Hopf normal form

$$\dot{R} - (\gamma_R - i\omega_R)R + |R|^2 R,$$

where ω_R represents the frequency and γ_R a factor of a linear "energy pump" of the unit R whose amplitude saturates due to the cubic damping of that unit. R receives input in two ways: First, it is directly driven by the activity in primary motor cortex of the opposite hemisphere, L, and second, an additional premotor or supplementary motor unit, denoted as $\tilde{R}$, inhibits the cross-talk by mediating the L-activity. The linear coupling reads $\propto \left(\tilde{R}_0 - \tilde{R}\right)^{*}(L - L_0)$, where $\tilde{R}_0$ and L_0 refer to coupling thresholds, which, for the sake of simplicity, will be ignored in the following. Thus, for the dynamics of R, we hence write

$$\dot{R} - (\gamma_R - i\omega_R)R + |R|^2 R = \eta_{L \to R}L - \eta_{\tilde{R} \to R}\tilde{R}^{*}L, \tag{11.4}$$

where $(\cdots)^{*}$ refers to conjugate complex values. The parameters $\eta_{L \to R}$ and $\eta_{\tilde{R} \to R}$ quantify the left/right coupling strengths and, as will be shown later, serve as bifurcation parameter tuning behavioral instabilities, similar to the parameter B/A in the dynamics (11.1). The unit $\tilde{R}$ receives input from both motor areas L and R. To stress the vital character of the (bi-)linear coupling, we further assume that the unit $\tilde{R}$ has simple intrinsic properties in that it behaves essentially like a linearly damped oscillatory system—we denote the coupling strength as $\eta_{\tilde{R} \leftarrow R}$ and ignore the direct coupling $\eta_{\tilde{R} \leftarrow L}$:

$$\dot{\tilde{R}} + \left(\kappa_{\tilde{R}} + i\Delta\omega_{\tilde{R}}\right)\tilde{R} = \eta_{\tilde{R} \leftarrow R}L^{*}R. \tag{11.5}$$

Next, we eliminate the oscillatory components by transforming $R = re^{-i\omega_R t}$ and $L = le^{-i\omega_L t}$ and further assume $\omega_R = P\Omega$ and $\omega_L = Q\Omega$ implying that R and L oscillate with a fixed frequency ratio $P{:}Q$ given a prescribed common frequency Ω; see also the discussion around equation (11.2). For stable performance of the polyrhythm $P{:}Q$, we additionally use $\Delta\omega_{\tilde{R}} = (P - Q)\Omega$, which allows for the transformation $\tilde{R} = \tilde{r}e^{-i\Delta\omega_{\tilde{R}}t} = \tilde{r}e^{i(q-p)\Omega t}$. The $\tilde{R}$-dynamics can thus be rewritten as $\dot{\tilde{r}} + \kappa_{\tilde{R}}\tilde{r} = \eta_{\tilde{R} \leftarrow R}l^{*}r$.

Recall that $\tilde{R}$ is driven by both L and R and inhibits the cross-talk $L{\to}R$. To enable this inhibition proper, we assume that the reaction time of the oscillations in that unit is sufficiently small; that is, $\tilde{R}$ is usually frequency- and phase-locked with L and R. Notice that if we do not presume such a frequency and phase locking, for instance, with respect to the left unit L, then $\tilde{R}$ will additionally oscillate with the frequency ω_L. In more general terms, $\tilde{R}$ follows instantaneously the dynamics of R and L because the timescale of $\tilde{r}$ is small compared with the timescales of R and L and that prescribed by the oscillations ω_R and ω_L. Importantly, in the case of such clearly separated timescales, $\tilde{r}$ basically acts as (amplitude-)filter and, accordingly, we can eliminate its dynamics adiabatically by means of $\dot{\tilde{r}} \approx 0$ (Haken, 1983). The adiabatic elimination yields

$$\dot{\tilde{r}} + \kappa_{\tilde{R}}\tilde{r} = \eta_{\tilde{R} \leftarrow R}l^{*}r \xrightarrow[\text{elimination}]{\text{adiabatic}} \tilde{r} \approx \frac{\eta_{\tilde{R} \leftarrow R}}{\kappa_{\tilde{R}}}l^{*}r.$$

When substituting this form into (11.5) and accounting for the aforementioned transformations, the amplitude dynamics in the right primary motor area reads

$$\dot{r} - \gamma_R r + |r|^2 r \approx \left(\eta_{L \to R} l - \frac{\eta^*_{\tilde{R} \leftarrow R} \eta_{\tilde{R} \to R}}{\kappa_{\tilde{R}}} l^2 r^* \right) e^{i(p-q)\Omega t}.$$

As R and L are still complex quantities, we recast them in terms of real-valued amplitudes and phases, $r = \rho e^{i\varphi_R}$ and $l = \lambda e^{i\varphi_L}$, which yields the following expression for the phase of the oscillation:

$$\dot{\varphi}_R = \eta_{L \to R} \frac{\lambda}{\rho} \sin\left[\varphi_L - \varphi_R + (p-q)\Omega t \right] \tag{11.6}$$
$$- \frac{\eta^*_{\tilde{R} \leftarrow R} \eta_{\tilde{R} \to R}}{} \lambda^2 \sin\left[2(\varphi_L - \varphi_R) + (p-q)\Omega t \right].$$

The dynamics (11.6) covers the phase evolution during stable polyrhythmic performance; that is, provided that the left and right motor areas are $P{:}Q$ frequency-locked. We note that if ω_R and ω_L are equal, or, equivalently, if $P = Q$, then by abbreviating

$$A = \frac{\eta_{L \to R} \lambda^2 - \eta_{R \to L} \rho^2}{\lambda \rho} \quad \text{and} \quad B = \frac{\eta^*_{\tilde{L} \leftarrow L} \eta_{\tilde{L} \to L}}{\kappa_{\tilde{L}}} \rho^2 - \frac{\eta^*_{\tilde{R} \leftarrow R} \eta_{\tilde{R} \to R}}{\kappa_{\tilde{R}}} \lambda^2,$$

the dynamics of the relative phase $\Delta\phi = \varphi_R - \varphi_L$ between R and L results in the Haken et al. (1985) model (11.1).

In contrast to purely behavioral studies, this model predicts that an increase in frequency affects the amplitudes of activity in the two primary motor areas, the strength of activity in premotor areas, and the degree of phase locking between the primary and premotor areas, and may therefore induce behavioral changes.

To summarize, cardinal differences in the intrinsic timescales of the synchronization dynamics in primary and premotor areas allow for a formal elimination of the evolution of the premotor activities. In consequence, two nonlinearly coupled oscillators can cover the combined dynamics if all four units (bilateral primary and premotor areas) are frequency- and phase-locked throughout stable performance. During phase transitions, however, strong residual activity appears in the ipsilateral hemisphere, locked to the finger that undergoes instability. The presence of this ipsilateral activity can be explained by decreasing differences in timescales between (the phase dynamics in) primary and premotor areas caused by an increasing movement frequency. If timescales do not separate, phase locking becomes improper yielding a loss of inhibition between ipsilateral primary and premotor areas. In the following, we outline how this (improper) phase locking may emerge in populations of neurons.

11.4 Neural Mass Models—From Coupled Oscillators to Network Activity

Modeling local populations of neurons in terms of averaged properties like their mean voltage and/or firing rates is very informative when studying neural synchronization dynamics. Mean field–like approaches have a long tradition and are typically referred to as neural mass modeling (Wilson & Cowan, 1972; Lopes da Silva, Hoeks, Smits, & Zetterberg, 1974; Freeman, 1975; Lopes da Silva, van Rotterdam, Barts, van Heusden, & Burr, 1976; Lopes da Silva, 1991; Jansen & Rit, 1995; Deco, Jirsa, Robinson, Breakspear, & Friston, 2008). Neural mass models have been used to study the origin of alpha rhythm, evoked potentials, pathologic brain rhythms, and the transition between normal and epileptic activity (Lopes da Silva et al., 1974; Jansen & Rit, 1995; Stam, Vliegen, & Nicolai, 1999; Stam, Pijn, Suffczynski, & Lopes da Silva, 1999; Valdes, Jimenez, Riera, Biscay, & Ozaki, 1999; David, Harrison, & Friston, 2005). Several studies considered small networks of two or three interconnected neural mass models (van Rotterdam, Lopes da Silva, van den Ende, Viergever, & Hermans, 1982; Schuster & Wagner, 1990a, 1990b; Wendling, Bartolomei, Bellanger, & Chauvel, 2001; David & Friston, 2003; Ursino, Zavaglia, Astolfi, & Babiloni, 2007) as well as larger networks of interconnected models (Sotero, Trujillo-Barreto, Iturria-Medina, Carbonell, & Jimenez, 2007; Ponten, Daffertshofer, Hillebrand, & Stam, 2010; Daffertshofer & van Wijk, 2011), an important step toward a proper description of interacting cortical areas as in models (11.4) and (11.5).

An interesting example of a neural mass model is the Wilson–Cowan model (Wilson and Cowan, 1972) because it can readily be derived from microscopic descriptions like integrate-and-fire neurons, but also from more general models like Haken's (2002) pulse-coupled neurons. The Wilson–Cowan model provides a comprehensive link toward an even more macroscopic description as its continuum limit resembles by now well-established neural field equations (Jirsa & Haken, 1996). That is, Wilson–Cowan units may be viewed as an intermediate but in some sense generic description of densely connected neural populations. For its oscillatory regime, one can generally deduce the corresponding phase dynamics (Schuster & Wagner, 1990a, 1990b; Aoyagi, 1995; Tass, 1999) in terms of a Kuramoto network of phase oscillators (Kuramoto, 1984; Strogatz, 2000; Acebron, Bonilla, Pérez Vicente, Ritort, & Spigler, 2005);

see also Daffertshofer and van Wijk (2011) for a recent study knotting these two seminal models together. In the following two sections, we will use the Kuramoto network to model transient phase synchronization behavior based on synaptic depression.

11.4.1 Steady States and Transitions

The collective behavior of a network of oscillators, whose states are captured by a single scalar phase φ_k, can, in a first approximation, be represented by the set of N coupled differential equations

$$\dot{\varphi}_k = \omega_k + \frac{\eta}{N} \sum_{l=1}^{N} D_{kl} \sin(\varphi_l - \varphi_k). \tag{11.7}$$

The dynamics (11.7) implies that the kth oscillator, with natural frequency ω_k, adjusts its phase according to input from other oscillators through a phase interaction function $\sin(\varphi_l - \varphi_k)$. The connectivity matrix D_{kl} is again scaled by an overall coupling strength, η. This coupling strength serves as a bifurcation parameter in that small values of η yield a network behavior that, in essence, agrees with the entirely uncoupled case (i.e., the phases are not synchronized), whereas η larger than a certain critical value η_c causes the phases to synchronize (Kuramoto, 1984; Strogatz, 2000; Acebron et al., 2005). The frequencies ω_k are distributed according to a specified probability density usually taken to be a symmetric, unimodal distribution (e.g., a Lorentz or a Gauss distribution) with mean ω_0. Although the sinusoidal interaction function is an approximation, it still permits a variety of highly nontrivial solutions. As such, the model (11.7) can be viewed as the canonical form for synchronization in extended, oscillatory media.

Strictly speaking, the system (11.7) does not represent the Kuramoto model in its original form as there the coupling between nodes k and l was considered isotropic and homogeneous (i.e., $D_{kl} = 1$ for all connections), by which the model reduces to

$$\dot{\varphi}_k = \omega_k + \frac{\eta}{N} \sum_{l=1}^{N} \sin(\varphi_l - \varphi_k). \tag{11.8}$$

As mentioned earlier, the effect of increasing η in the isotropic case is to increase the phase synchrony among the oscillators. Suppose the coupling is weak (i.e., smaller than the critical value, or $\eta \ll \eta_c$), then the oscillators' phases disperse, whereas for strong coupling ($\eta \gg \eta_c$), the oscillators become synchronous (i.e., the phases are locked at fixed differences). In the intermediate case ($\eta \approx \eta_c$), clusters of synchronous oscillators may emerge. However, many other oscillators, whose natural frequencies are at the tails of the distribution, are not locked into a cluster. In other words, as η increases, the interaction functions overcome the dispersion of natural frequencies ω_n resulting in a transition from incoherence to partial and then full synchronization (Acebron et al., 2005; Breakspear, Heitmann, & Daffertshofer, 2010).

11.4.2 Transients

More recently, the Kuramoto network (11.8) has been extended to the case in which the coupling parameter is no longer a constant value but depends on time. This dependence is either an externally prescribed trace (= external forcing) or, here more importantly, follows some dynamics that involves the current state of the coupled oscillators (= intrinsic forcing). We consider this more important because it may mimic the process of synaptic depression; that is, a form of short-term plasticity that is characterized by a decrease in synaptic strength due to a use-dependent desensitization of postsynaptic receptors (Zucker & Regehr, 2002). Synaptic depression can act as synaptic gain control mechanism (Abbott, Varela, Sen, & Nelson, 1997). Recently, Rothman, Cathala, Steuber, & Silver (2009) reported synaptic nonlinearities to be incorporated in neuronal gain modulation. They showed that when excitation is mediated by synapses with short-term depression, neuronal gain is controlled by an inhibitory conductance in a noise-independent manner, allowing for the driving and modulatory inputs to be multiplied together. The nonlinearity introduced by this depression transforms inhibition-mediated additive shifts in the input–output relationship into multiplicative gain changes. This is similar to the bilinear (hence multiplicative) input in the dynamics (11.5); see also the second equation in (11.9).

Synaptic depression has been included in computational studies of a neural model by Kilpatrick and Bressloff (Bressloff & Kilpatrick, 2010; Kilpatrick & Bressloff, 2010). In addition, Nadim, Manor, Kopell, & Marder (1999) showed that in a recurrent inhibitory network that includes an intrinsic oscillator, synaptic depression can give rise to two distinct modes of network operation. When the maximal conductance of the depressing synapse is small, the oscillation period is fully determined by the oscillator component. Increasing the maximal conductance beyond a threshold value activates a positive-feedback mechanism that greatly enhances the synaptic strength. There, the oscillation frequency is determined by the strength and dynamics of the depressing synapse. Because of the regenerative nature of the feedback, this circuit can be switched from one mode of operation to another by a very small change in the maximal conductance of the depressing synapse.

To model briefly these effects in the context of phase oscillators, we assume that the coupling in the Kuramoto model (11.8) depends on the overall state of synchrony[1] as quantified by the order parameter ρ (Kuramoto, 1984),

$$\dot{\varphi}_k = \omega_k + \chi \frac{\eta_0}{N} \sum_{l=1}^{N} \sin(\varphi_l - \varphi_k)$$

$$\dot{\chi} = -\frac{1}{\tau}\rho + \left(1 - [\tanh(\chi) - 1]^2\right)[\tanh(\chi) - 1] + \chi_0.$$

(11.9)

The order parameter ρ equals the phase divergence, phase-locking index, or the phase uniformity and is defined as $\rho = \left| \frac{1}{N} \sum_{k=1}^{N} e^{i\varphi_k} \right|$ (Mardia & Jupp, 2000). This dynamics results when starting off with a network of Wilson–Cowan oscillators that are coupled not only additively but also multiplicatively (Daffertshofer & van Wijk, submitted).

The model (11.9) leads to a drop in the overall coupling strength $\eta_0\chi$ as soon as the synchrony ρ is sufficiently large. In turn, when the coupling strength decreases, the synchronization vanishes, the phase oscillators diffuse, ρ becomes small again, and the coupling strength will again increase. This process induces oscillations of synchronization and desynchronization similar to the ERS/ERD cycles mentioned in section 11.1.2. Importantly, the relaxation time τ prescribes the onset of the oscillations, whereas the *mean coupling strength* η_0 defines the value of the frequency of the ERS/ERD cycles: The stronger the coupling, the longer it takes to desynchronize the phase oscillators, and the ERS/ERD cycle frequency is decreased; see figure 11.7 (plate 33) for numerical examples and recall the importance of (the separation of) timescales in models (11.4) and (11.5).

Controlling movement via changes in distributed spectral processing in the beta band may be beneficial for its high temporal resolution. The production of a beta cycle requires rapid changes in synchronization within a functional (cluster of) neuronal ensembles (Pfurtscheller & da Silva, 1999). In the experiment by Houweling and coworkers (2010), the upregulation and downregulation of beta synchrony was directly related to the movement frequency. Moreover, as frequency increased, both ERS/ERD shifted in time toward the motor event. This idea challenges

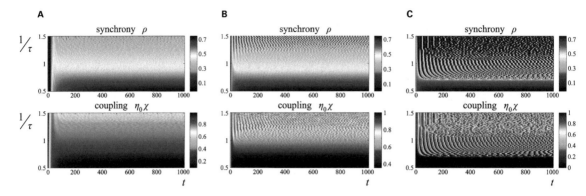

Figure 11.7 (plate 33)
Simulations of the model (11.9) for different parameters η_0. An increase in coupling leads to a spontaneous synchronization between phase oscillators, but by the same token an increase in synchrony yields a drop in coupling. Beyond a critical value of the damping $1/\tau$, oscillations between synchronization and desynchronization occur provided the overall coupling is sufficiently large (B and C). $N = 200$. (A) $\eta_0 = 0.1$; (B) $\eta_0 = 0.5$; (C) $\eta_0 = 1.0$.

the notion of ERS as a simple response to recalibrate the underlying network ("rebound"). As the target frequency increases, ERS and ERD start overlapping each other, which evidently limits performance. Put differently, the time required to establish interactions between neural populations serves as a very natural constraint on motor performance. On this account, beta modulations not only facilitate but also limit the ability to perform coordination tasks.

11.5   Conclusion

Combining steady states, transitions, and transient behavior is without doubt a prerequisite for unraveling the "full" dynamic range of motor performance and its neural underpinnings. We illustrated this by modeling rhythmic bimanual coordination tasks that show transitions from anti-phase to in-phase patterns and from complex to simpler polyrhythmic frequency ratios with increasing movement tempo. Computational models that explain the neural dynamics underlying these transitions in bimanual coordination prove to be valuable in understanding intra- and inter-hemispheric coupling between motor areas. Notably, these cortical interactions would not have been evident from looking at steady-state performance alone. It is only when transitions in behavior are induced that the intra-hemispheric canceling of inter-hemispheric cross-talk fails, and hints of its presence become apparent.

A closer look at the neural dynamics reveals that rhythmic movements are accompanied by periodic changes of synchronization and desynchronization of beta oscillations (i.e., ERS/ERD cycles). Whereas synchrony emerges spontaneously, which is well described by the dynamics of the Kuramoto network, desynchronization requires a drop in interneural coupling strength, an effect that we here identified as synaptic depression. Incorporating this as synchrony-dependent coupling yields the empirically observed ERS/ERD cycles during rhythmic movement.

Acknowledgments

We would like to thank Peter Beek, Tjeerd Boonstra, and Lieke Peper for the fruitful discussions about movement coordination and its neural underpinnings. Particular thanks go to Sanne Houweling for providing substantial material for this chapter. This work received financial support in part from the Netherlands Organisation for Scientific Research (NWO grant no. 021–002–047).

Note

1. The recent extension of the Kuramoto model as proposed by Aoki and Aoyagi (2009), however, does not address this characteristic because their dynamics,

$$\dot{\varphi}_k = \omega_k + \tfrac{\eta}{N} \sum_{l=1}^{N} C_{kl} \sin(\varphi_l - \varphi_k + \alpha)$$

$$\dot{C}_{kl} = \varepsilon \sin(\varphi_l - \varphi_k + \beta),$$

exhibits three kinds of asymptotic behavior: a two-cluster state, a coherent state with a fixed phase relation, and a chaotic state with frustration; the latter most likely because of the additional phase shift α and β.

References

Abbott, L. F., Varela, J. A., Sen, K., & Nelson, S. B. (1997). Synaptic depression and cortical gain control. *Science*, *275*(5297), 220–224.

Acebron, J., Bonilla, L., Pérez Vicente, C., Ritort, F., & Spigler, R. (2005). The Kuramoto model: a simple paradigm for synchronization phenomena. *Reviews of Modern Physics*, *77*, 137–185.

Aoki, T., & Aoyagi, T. (2009). Co-evolution of phases and connection strengths in a network of phase oscillators. *Physical Review Letters*, *102*(3), 034101.

Aoyagi, T. (1995). Network of neural oscillators for retrieving phase information. *Physical Review Letters*, *74*(20), 4075–4078.

Babiloni, C., Carducci, F., Pizzella, V., Indovina, I., Romani, G. L., Rossini, P. M., et al. (1999). Bilateral neuromagnetic activation of human primary sensorimotor cortex in preparation and execution of unilateral voluntary finger movements. *Brain Research*, *827*(1–2), 234–236.

Baraldi, P., Porro, C. A., Serafini, M., Pagnoni, G., Murari, C., Corazza, R., et al. (1999). Bilateral representation of sequential finger movements in human cortical areas. *Neuroscience Letters*, *269*(2), 95–98.

Boyd, E. H., Pandya, D. N., & Bignall, K. E. (1971). Homotopic and nonhomotopic interhemispheric cortical projections in the squirrel monkey. *Experimental Neurology*, *32*(2), 256–274.

Breakspear, M., Heitmann, S., & Daffertshofer, A. (2010). Generative models of cortical oscillations: neurobiological implications of the kuramoto model. *Frontiers Hum Neurosci*, *4*, 190.

Bressloff, P. C., & Kilpatrick, Z. P. (2010). Effects of synaptic depression and adaptation on spatiotemporal dynamics of an excitatory neuronal network. *Physica D. Nonlinear Phenomena*, *239*(9), 547–560.

Brinkman, J., & Kuypers, H. G. (1972). Splitbrain monkeys: cerebral control of ipsilateral and contralateral arm, hand, and finger movements. *Science*, *176*(34), 536–539.

Carpenter, A. F., Georgopoulos, A. P., & Pellizzer, G. (1999). Motor cortical encoding of serial order in a context-recall task. *Science*, *283*(5408), 1752–1757.

Carson, R. G. (2005). Neural pathways mediating bilateral interactions between the upper limbs. *Brain Research*, *49*(3), 641–662.

Daffertshofer, A., & van Wijk, B. C. M. (2011). On the influence of amplitude on the connectivity between phases. *Frontiers in Neuroinformatics*, *5*(6), 1–12.

Daffertshofer, A., & van Wijk, B. C. M. (Submitted). Multiplicative interactions between neural mass models—synchrony dependent coupling.

Daffertshofer, A., Peper, C. E., & Beek, P. J. (2000). Spectral analyses of event-related encephalographic signals. *Physics Letters. [Part A]*, *266*(4–6), 290–302.

Daffertshofer, A., Peper, C. E., & Beek, P. J. (2005). Stabilization of bimanual coordination due to active interhemispheric inhibition: a dynamical account. *Biological Cybernetics*, *92*(2), 101–109.

Daffertshofer, A., van den Berg, C., & Beek, P. J. (1999). A dynamical model for mirror movements. *Physica D. Nonlinear Phenomena*, *132*, 243–266.

Daffertshofer, A., Peper, C. E., Frank, T. D., & Beek, P. J. (2000). Spatio-temporal patterns of encephalographic signals during polyrhythmic tapping. *Human Movement Science*, *19*(4), 475–498.

David, O., & Friston, K. J. (2003). A neural mass model for MEG/EEG: coupling and neuronal dynamics. *NeuroImage*, *20*(3), 1743–1755.

David, O., Harrison, L., & Friston, K. J. (2005). Modelling event-related responses in the brain. *NeuroImage*, *25*(3), 756–770.

Deco, G., Jirsa, V. K., Robinson, P. A., Breakspear, M., & Friston, K. (2008). The dynamic brain: from spiking neurons to neural masses and cortical fields. *PLoS Computational Biology*, *4*(8), e1000092.

Donchin, O., Gribova, A., Steinberg, O., Bergman, H., & Vaadia, E. (1998). Primary motor cortex is involved in bimanual coordination. *Nature*, *395*(6699), 274–278.

Ermentrout, G. B., & Cowan, J. D. (1979). Temporal oscillations in neuronal nets. *Journal of Mathematical Biology*, *7*(3), 265–280.

Ferbert, A., Priori, A., Rothwell, J. C., Day, B. L., Colebatch, J. G., & Marsden, C. D. (1992). Interhemispheric inhibition of the human motor cortex. *Journal of Physiology*, *453*, 525–546.

Frank, T. D., Daffertshofer, A., Peper, C. E., Beek, P. J., & Haken, H. (2000). Towards a comprehensive theory of brain activity: coupled oscillator systems under external forces. *Physica D. Nonlinear Phenomena*, *144*(1–2), 62–86.

Freeman, W. J. (1975). *Mass Action in the Nervous System*. New York: Academic Press.

Gazzaniga, M. S. (1966). Visuomotor integration in split-brain monkeys with other cerebral lesions. *Experimental Neurology*, *16*(3), 289–298.

Gerloff, C., & Andres, F. G. (2002). Bimanual coordination and interhemispheric interaction. *Acta Psychologica*, *110*(2–3), 161–186.

Ghacibeh, G. A., Mirpuri, R., Drago, V., Jeong, Y., Heilman, K. M., & Triggs, W. J. (2007). Ipsilateral motor activation during unimanual and bimanual motor tasks. *Clinical Neurophysiology*, *118*(2), 325–332.

Gribova, A., Donchin, O., Bergman, H., Vaadia, E., & Cardoso De Oliveira, S. (2002). Timing of bimanual movements in human and non-human primates in relation to neuronal activity in primary motor cortex and supplementary motor area. *Experimental Brain Research*, *146*(3), 322–335.

Guckenheimer, J., & Holmes, P. (1990). *Nonlinear Oscillations, Dynamical Systems, and Bifurcations of Vector Fields*. New York: Springer.

Haken, H. (1983). *Synergetics. An Introduction*. Berlin: Springer.

Haken, H. (1996). *Principles of Brain Functioning*. Berlin: Springer.

Haken, H. (2002). *Brain Dynamics*. Berlin: Springer.

Haken, H., Kelso, J. A., & Bunz, H. (1985). A theoretical model of phase transitions in human hand movements. *Biological Cybernetics*, *51*(5), 347–356.

Haken, H., Peper, C. E., Beek, P. J., & Daffertshofer, A. (1996). A model for phase transitions in human hand movements during multifrequency tapping. *Physica D. Nonlinear Phenomena*, *90*(1–2), 179–196.

Houweling, S., Beek, P. J., & Daffertshofer, A. (2010). Spectral changes of interhemispheric crosstalk during movement instabilities. *Cerebral Cortex*, *20*(11), 2605–2613.

Innocenti, G. M. (2009). Dynamic interactions between the cerebral hemispheres. *Experimental Brain Research*, *192*(3), 417–423.

Jansen, B. H., & Rit, V. G. (1995). Electroencephalogram and visual evoked potential generation in a mathematical model of coupled cortical columns. *Biological Cybernetics*, *73*(4), 357–366.

Jensen, M. H., Bak, P., & Bohr, T. (1983). Complete devils staircase, fractal dimension, and universality of mode-locking structure in the circle map. *Physical Review Letters*, *50*(21), 1637–1639.

Jirsa, V. K., & Haken, H. (1996). Field theory of electromagnetic brain activity. *Physical Review Letters*, *77*(5), 960–963.

Jirsa, V. K., Jantzen, K. J., Fuchs, A., & Kelso, J. A. (2002). Spatiotemporal forward solution of the EEG and MEG using network modeling. *IEEE Transactions on Medical Imaging*, *21*(5), 493–504.

Kay, B. A., Saltzman, E. L., Kelso, J. A. S., & Schöner, G. (1987). Space-time behavior of single and bimanual rhythmical movements—data and limit-cycle model. *Journal of Experimental Psychology. Human Perception and Performance*, *13*(2), 178–192.

Kelso, J. A., Holt, K. G., Rubin, P., & Kugler, P. N. (1981). Patterns of human interlimb coordination emerge from the properties of non-linear, limit cycle oscillatory processes: theory and data. *Journal of Motor Behavior*, *13*(4), 226–261.

Kelso, J. A., Bressler, S. L., Buchanan, S., DeGuzman, G. C., Ding, M., Fuchs, A., et al. (1992). A phase transition in human brain and behavior. *Physics Letters. [Part A]*, *169*(3), 134–144.

Kilpatrick, Z. P., & Bressloff, P. C. (2010). Spatially structured oscillations in a two-dimensional excitatory neuronal network with synaptic depression. *Journal of Computational Neuroscience*, *28*(2), 193–209.

Kuramoto, Y. (1984). *Chemical Oscillations, Waves, and Turbulence*. New York: Springer.

Lang, W., Obrig, H., Lindinger, G., Cheyne, D., & Deecke, L. (1990). Supplementary motor area activation while tapping bimanually different rhythms in musicians. *Experimental Brain Research*, *79*(3), 504–514.

Lopes da Silva, F. (1991). Neural mechanisms underlying brain waves: from neural membranes to networks. *Electroencephalography Clinical Neurophysiology, 79*(2), 81–93.

Lopes da Silva, F. H., Hoeks, A., Smits, H., & Zetterberg, L. H. (1974). Model of brain rhythmic activity. The alpha-rhythm of the thalamus. *Kybernetik, 15*(1), 27–37.

Lopes da Silva, F. H., van Rotterdam, A., Barts, P., van Heusden, E., & Burr, W. (1976). Models of neuronal populations: the basic mechanisms of rhythmicity. *Progress in Brain Research, 45*, 281–308.

Mardia, K. V., & Jupp, P. E. (2000). *Directional Statistics*. Chichester, UK: John Wiley & Sons.

Mayston, M. J., Harrison, L. M., & Stephens, J. A. (1999). A neurophysiological study of mirror movements in adults and children. *Annals of Neurology, 45*(5), 583–594.

Mayville, J. M., Fuchs, A., Ding, M., Cheyne, D., Deecke, L., & Kelso, J. A. (2001). Event-related changes in neuromagnetic activity associated with syncopation and synchronization timing tasks. *Human Brain Mapping, 14*(2), 65–80.

Meyer-Lindenberg, A., Ziemann, U., Hajak, G., Cohen, L., & Berman, K. F. (2002). Transitions between dynamical states of differing stability in the human brain. *Proceedings of the National Academy of Sciences of the United States of America, 99*(17), 10948–10953.

Nadim, F., Manor, Y., Kopell, N., & Marder, E. (1999). Synaptic depression creates a switch that controls the frequency of an oscillatory circuit. *Proceedings of the National Academy of Sciences of the United States of America, 96*(14), 8206–8211.

Pandya, D. N., Karol, E. A., & Heilbronn, D. (1971). The topographical distribution of interhemispheric projections in the corpus callosum of the rhesus monkey. *Brain Research, 32*(1), 31–43.

Peper, C. E., & Beek, P. J. (1998a). Are frequency-induced transitions in rhythmic coordination mediated by a drop in amplitude? *Biological Cybernetics, 79*(4), 291–300.

Peper, C. E., & Beek, P. J. (1998b). Distinguishing between the effects of frequency and amplitude on interlimb coupling in tapping a 2:3 polyrhythm. *Experimental Brain Research, 118*(1), 78–92.

Peper, C. E., Beek, P. J., & van Wieringen, P. C. W. (1995). Multifrequency coordination in bimanual tapping: asymmetrical coupling and signs of supercriticality. *Journal of Experimental Psychology. Human Perception and Performance, 21*, 1117–1138.

Pfurtscheller, G., & da Silva, F. H. L. (1999). Event-related EEG/MEG synchronization and desynchronization: basic principles. *Clinical Neurophysiology, 110*(11), 1842–1857.

Ponten, S. C., Daffertshofer, A., Hillebrand, A., & Stam, C. J. (2010). The relationship between structural and functional connectivity: graph theoretical analysis of an EEG neural mass model. *NeuroImage, 52*(3), 985–994.

Rothman, J. S., Cathala, L., Steuber, V., & Silver, R. A. (2009). Synaptic depression enables neuronal gain control. *Nature, 457*(7232), 1015–1018.

Salenius, S., & Hari, R. (2003). Synchronous cortical oscillatory activity during motor action. *Current Opinion in Neurobiology, 13*(6), 678–684.

Schuster, H. G., & Wagner, P. (1990a). A model for neuronal oscillations in the visual cortex. 1. Mean-field theory and derivation of the phase equations. *Biological Cybernetics, 64*(1), 77–82.

Schuster, H. G., & Wagner, P. (1990b). A model for neuronal oscillations in the visual cortex. 2. Phase description of the feature dependent synchronization. *Biological Cybernetics, 64*(1), 83–85.

Serrien, D. J., & Brown, P. (2002). The functional role of interhemispheric synchronization in the control of bimanual timing tasks. *Experimental Brain Research, 147*(2), 268–272.

Sotero, R. C., Trujillo-Barreto, N. J., Iturria-Medina, Y., Carbonell, F., & Jimenez, J. C. (2007). Realistically coupled neural mass models can generate EEG rhythms. *Neural Computation, 19*(2), 478–512.

Stam, C. J., Vliegen, J. H., & Nicolai, J. (1999). Investigation of the dynamics underlying periodic complexes in the EEG. *Biological Cybernetics*, *80*(1), 57–69.

Stam, C. J., Pijn, J. P., Suffczynski, P., & Lopes da Silva, F. H. (1999). Dynamics of the human alpha rhythm: evidence for non-linearity? *Clinical Neurophysiology*, *110*(10), 1801–1813.

Strogatz, S. H. (2000). From Kuramoto to Crawford: exploring the onset of synchronization in populations of coupled oscillators. *Physica D. Nonlinear Phenomena*, *143*(1–4), 1–20.

Summers, J. J., Rosenbaum, D. A., Burns, B. D., & Ford, S. K. (1993). Production of polyrhythms. *Journal of Experimental Psychology. Human Perception and Performance*, *19*(2), 416–428.

Swinnen, S. P. (2002). Intermanual coordination: from behavioural principles to neural-network interactions. *Nature Reviews. Neuroscience*, *3*(5), 348–359.

Tass, P. A. (1999). *Phase Resetting in Medicine and Biology*. Berlin: Springer.

Ursino, M., Zavaglia, M., Astolfi, L., & Babiloni, F. (2007). Use of a neural mass model for the analysis of effective connectivity among cortical regions based on high resolution EEG recordings. *Biological Cybernetics*, *96*(3), 351–365.

Valdes, P. A., Jimenez, J. C., Riera, J., Biscay, R., & Ozaki, T. (1999). Nonlinear EEG analysis based on a neural mass model. *Biological Cybernetics*, *81*(5–6), 415–424.

van Rotterdam, A., Lopes da Silva, F. H., van den Ende, J., Viergever, M. A., & Hermans, A. J. (1982). A model of the spatial-temporal characteristics of the alpha rhythm. *Bulletin of Mathematical Biology*, *44*(2), 283–305.

Wendling, F., Bartolomei, F., Bellanger, J. J., & Chauvel, P. (2001). Interpretation of inter-dependencies in epileptic signals using a macroscopic physiological model of the EEG. *Clinical Neurophysiology*, *112*(7), 1201–1218.

Wilson, H. R., & Cowan, J. D. (1972). Excitatory and inhibitory interactions in localized populations of model neurons. *Biophysical Journal*, *12*(1), 1–24.

Wright, J. J., Robinson, P. A., Rennie, C. J., Gordon, E., Bourke, P. D., Chapmar, C. L., et al. (2001). Toward an integrated continuum model of cerebral dynamics: the cerebral rhythms, synchronous oscillation and cortical stability. *Biosys*, *63*(1–3), 71–88.

Zucker, R. S., & Regehr, W. G. (2002). Short-term synaptic plasticity. *Annual Review of Physiology*, *64*, 355–405.

12   Free Energy and Global Dynamics

Karl J. Friston

Summary

In this chapter, we will look at the role of neuronal dynamics from a purely functional perspective and ask: How can we understand self-organized neuronal activity in relation to what the brain is doing? We will take a fairly abstract approach and consider neuronal dynamics in terms of optimization, namely, considering dynamics in terms of an underlying function that is being minimized. By considering the imperatives for neuronal processing in terms of perceptual inference, this turns out to be relatively easy, because all inference can be cast as finding a model of (sensory) input with the greatest evidence. This introduces the notion that the brain entails a model of its sensorium, which is optimized to explain sensory data. Crucially, this model may contains prior beliefs about the itinerant and sequential nature of events in the world that may be encoded by central pattern generators, which show exactly the same winnerless competition discussed in earlier chapters. In what follows, we look at these issues from the point of view of variational free energy minimization and Bayesian inference, where prior expectations call on autonomous dynamics that underwrite the way we perceive the world and act upon it.

12.1   Introduction

This chapter provides a theoretical perspective on global brain dynamics from the point of view of the free-energy principle. This principle has been chosen as a global brain theory that is formulated explicitly in terms of dynamical systems. We will see that the free-energy principle emerges when we consider the ensemble dynamics of biological systems like ourselves. When we look closely what this principle implies for the behavior of systems like the brain, one finds a fairly simple explanation for action and behavior. More specifically, free energy provides a natural explanation for active inference and the Bayesian brain hypothesis.

Within the Bayesian brain framework, the ensuing dynamics can be separated, in a principled way, into those serving perceptual inference, learning, and attention. Dynamics here are central, both to understand the nature of self-organizing systems and to explain the adaptive nature of neuronal dynamics and plasticity in terms of optimization.

Within this context, we will attempt a teleological explanation of dynamics; namely, what do they do in the context of adaptive behavior and perception. The premise here is that the brain is trying to optimize something (specifically, free energy) and uses a generalized gradient descent to perform this optimization. In other words, one can understand neuronal dynamics as optimizing a quantity through the method of steepest ascent, which can be described with a (complicated) set of ordinary differential equations. It is these equations that give rise to the itinerant (wandering) dynamics that have been described in previous chapters. In what follows, we will see how the optimization of free energy leads naturally to optimal action and perception. Crucially, the nature of this optimization rests heavily on the brain's internal or generative model of the world that it navigates. This model includes prior beliefs about the causal structure and dynamics in this world, which constrain both perception and action. This adds a second level of dynamics that reflect our prior expectations about the trajectories of states and their attractors in our environment. This chapter considers itinerant dynamics and how we can understand them in terms of prior beliefs about sensorimotor trajectories. In particular, we will look at action–observation in the context of handwriting and how it rests on stable heteroclinic channels. This is one of many examples of how itinerant dynamics are embedded in generative models of the sensorium. It is particularly relevant in the context of this book, given we appeal to the same normal forms considered in previous chapters. Here, we disclose their fundamental role in shaping action and perceptual inference.

This chapter comprises two parts. In the first, we provide a didactic overview of the free-energy principle, motivating it from basic principles. We will consider the underlying imperative that applies to all biological agents, namely, to conserve themselves by minimizing surprise, and how this calls upon the minimization of free energy. We then unpack the free-energy principle in terms of its implication for action and perception. This leads to active inference and perceptual inference, of the sort considered by the Bayesian brain hypothesis. We illustrate the key aspects of this treatment with a few selected examples and conclude by thinking about the timescales over which the dynamics of free-energy minimization may be manifest. The second part of this chapter presents a particular example in greater detail. This example considers handwriting in terms of itinerant expectations about sequences of movements. Not only does it provide a plausible account of sensorimotor execution, but it also touches upon the cognitive neuroscience of action–observation and how we represent ourselves and others.

12.2   The Free-Energy Principle

In recent years, there has been growing interest in free-energy formulations of brain function (Dayan, Hinton, & Neal 1995; Friston, 2005), not just from the neuroscience community, where it has caused some puzzlement (Thornton, 2010), but also from fields as far apart as psychotherapy (Carhart-Harris & Friston, 2010) and social politics (Grist, 2010). The free-energy principle has been described as a unified brain theory (Huang, 2008) and may have broader implications for how we interact with our environment. This section describes the origin of the free-energy formulation, its underlying premises, and the implications for how we represent and interact with the world. Table 12.1 provides a glossary of the quantities that we will be dealing with.

The free-energy principle is a simple postulate that has complicated ramifications. It says that all agents or biological systems (like us) must minimize free energy. This postulate is as simple and fundamental as Hamilton's law of least action and the celebrated H-theorems in statistical physics (Lifshitz & Pitaevskii, 1981). The principle was originally formulated as a computational account of perception (Friston, 2005) that borrows heavily from statistical physics and machine learning (Feynman, 1972; Hinton & van Camp, 1993; MacKay, 1995). However, its explanatory scope includes action and behavior (Friston, Daunizeau, & Kiebel, 2009) and may be linked, at a fundamental level, to our very existence: In brief, the free-energy principle takes well-known statistical ideas and applies them to problems in population (ensemble) dynamics and self-organization (Ashby, 1947; Nicolis & Prigogine, 1977; Haken, 1983; Kauffman, 1993). In applying these ideas, many aspects of our brains, how we perceive and the way we act, become understandable as necessary and self-evident attributes of biological systems. To see this, consider the following problem.

How, in a changing and unpredictable world, do biological agents resist a natural tendency to disorder and thermodynamic equilibrium? All the physics that we know, such as the fluctuation theorem (which generalizes

Table 12.1
Generic variables and quantities in the free-energy formation of active inference under the Laplace assumption (i.e., generalized predictive coding)

Variable	Description
$m \in \mathcal{M}$	**Generative model or agent:** In the free-energy formulation, each agent or system is taken to be a model of the environment in which it is immersed. $m \in M$ corresponds to the form (e.g., degrees of freedom) of a model entailed by an agent, which is used to predict sensory signals.
$a \subset \vartheta$	**Action:** These variables are states of the world that correspond to the movement or configuration of an agent (i.e., its effectors).
$\tilde{s}(t) = s \oplus s' \oplus s'' \oplus \dots \in S$	**Sensory signals:** These generalized sensory signals or samples comprise the sensory states, their velocity, acceleration, and temporal derivatives to high order. In other words, they correspond to the trajectory of an agent's sensations.
$\mathcal{L}(\tilde{s}\,|\,m) = -\ln p(\tilde{s}\,|\,m)$	**Surprise:** This is a scalar function of sensory samples and reports the improbability of sampling some signals under a generative model of how those signals were caused. It is sometimes called (sensory) surprisal or self-information. In statistics, it is known as the negative log-evidence for the model.
$H(S\,|\,m) \propto \int dt \mathcal{L}(\tilde{s}(t)\,|\,m)$	**Entropy:** Sensory entropy is, under ergodic assumptions, proportional to the long-term time average of surprise.
$\mathcal{G}(\tilde{s},\vartheta) = -\ln p(\tilde{s},\vartheta\,|\,m)$	**Gibbs energy:** This is the negative log of the density specified by the generative model; namely, surprise about the joint occurrence of sensory samples and their causes.
$\mathcal{F}(\tilde{s},\tilde{\mu}) = \mathcal{G}(\tilde{s},\tilde{\mu}) + \frac{1}{2}\ln\|\mathcal{G}_{\tilde{\mu}\tilde{\mu}}\|$ $\geq \mathcal{L}(\tilde{s}\,|\,m)$	**Free energy:** This is a scalar function of sensory samples and a proposal density, which upper bounds surprise. It is called free energy because it is the expected Gibbs energy minus the entropy of the proposal density. Under a Gaussian (Laplace) assumption about the form of the proposal density, free energy reduces to the simple function of Gibbs energy shown.
$\mathcal{S}(\tilde{s},\tilde{\mu}) = \int dt \mathcal{F}(\tilde{s},\tilde{\mu})$ $\geq H(S\,|\,m)$	**Free action:** This is a scalar functional of sensory samples and a proposal density, which upper bounds the entropy of sensory signals. It is the time or path integral of free energy.
$q(\vartheta) = \mathcal{N}(\tilde{\mu},\mathcal{C})$ $\tilde{\mu} = \mu \oplus \mu' \oplus \mu'' \oplus \dots$ $\mathcal{C} = \mathcal{G}_{\tilde{\mu}\tilde{\mu}}^{-1}$	**Proposal density:** This is also known as a variational ensemble or recognition density and becomes (approximates) the conditional density over hidden causes of sensory samples when free-energy is minimized. Under the Laplace assumption, it is specified by its conditional expectation and covariance.

Table 12.1
(continued)

Variable	Description
$\boldsymbol{\vartheta} = \{\mathbf{u}, \boldsymbol{\varphi}, a\}$ $\vartheta = \{u, \varphi\}$ $u = \{x, v\}$ $\varphi = \{\theta, \gamma\}$	**True (bold) and hidden (italics) causes:** These quantities cause sensory signals. The true quantities exist in the environment, and the hidden homologues are those assumed by the generative model of that environment. Both are partitioned into time-dependent variables and time-invariant parameters.
$\theta \subset \varphi \subset \vartheta$	**Hidden parameters:** These are the parameters of the mappings (e.g., equations of motion) that constitute the deterministic part of a generative model.
$\gamma \subset \varphi \subset \vartheta$	**Log-precisions:** These parameters control the precision (inverse variance) of fluctuations that constitute the random part of a generative model.
$x(t) = x^{(1)} \oplus x^{(2)} \oplus x^{(3)} \dots$ $\subset u \subset \vartheta$	**Hidden states:** These hidden variables encode the hierarchical states in a generative model of dynamics in the world.
$v(t) = v^{(1)} \oplus v^{(2)} \oplus v^{(3)} \dots$ $\subset u \subset \vartheta$	**Hidden causes:** These hidden variables link different levels of a hierarchical generative model.
$g(x^{(i)}, v^{(i)}, \theta)$ $f(x^{(i)}, v^{(i)}, \theta)$	**Deterministic mappings:** These are equations at the ith level of a hierarchical generative model that map from states at one level to another and map hidden states to their motion within each level. They specify the deterministic part of a generative model.
$\omega^{(i,v)}$ $\omega^{(i,x)}$	**Random fluctuations:** These are random fluctuations on hidden causes and the motion of hidden states. Gaussian assumptions about these fluctuations furnish the probabilistic part of a generative model.
$\tilde{\Pi}^{(i,v)} = R^{(i,v)} \otimes \Pi(\gamma^{(i,v)})$ $\tilde{\Pi}^{(i,x)} = R^{(i,x)} \otimes \Pi(\gamma^{(i,x)})$	**Precision matrices:** These are the inverse covariances among (generalized) random fluctuations on the hidden cases and motion of hidden states.
$R^{(i,v)}$ $R^{(i,x)}$	**Roughness matrices:** These are the inverse of a matrix encoding serial correlations among (generalized) random fluctuations on the hidden cases and motion of hidden states.
$\tilde{\varepsilon}^{(i,v)} = \tilde{v}^{(i-1)} - \tilde{g}^{(i)}$ $\tilde{\varepsilon}^{(i,x)} = \mathcal{D}\tilde{x}^{(i)} - \tilde{f}^{(i)}$	**Prediction errors:** These are the prediction errors on the hidden causes and motion of hidden states evaluated at their current conditional expectation.
$\xi^{(i,v)} = \tilde{\Pi}^{(i,v)}\tilde{\varepsilon}^{(i,v)}$ $\xi^{(i,x)} = \tilde{\Pi}^{(i,x)}\tilde{\varepsilon}^{(i,x)}$	**Precision-weighted prediction errors:** These are the prediction errors weighted by their respective precisions.

the second law of thermodynamics; Evans, 2003), suggests that random fluctuations in our environment will ultimately change our physical states to the point we cease to exist (i.e., we should gently decompose or evaporate). And yet, biological systems seem to violate these laws, maintaining precise physiologic states for long periods of time (Bernard, 1974). In other words, they occupy a small number of states with a high probability and avoid a large number of other states. In short, they appear to resist thermodynamic imperatives. Mathematically, we can summarize this remarkable capacity by saying biological agents maintain a low entropy distribution on the states that they could occupy. Entropy is just the average surprise or negative log probability of an agent being in a particular state (see table 12.1). In short, the question we need to address is how biological systems minimize their average surprise. Surprise here just means something unexpected, like tripping and falling in the street. One might think that exotic phenomena from theories of pattern formation and self-organization may provide a sufficient explanation for the emergence of orderly (unsurprising) state transitions. However, they do not. These patterns certainly have beautiful and intrinsic structures that unfold over short periods of time, but self-organization per se cannot explain the ability of biological agents to avoid surprise indefinitely. However, there is a solution that is almost tautological in its simplicity:

The solution lies in noting that surprise in ensemble dynamics is exactly the same as the (negative log) evidence for a model in statistics: $\mathcal{L} = -\ln p(s \mid m)$ (see table 12.1). The conceptual link between surprise and log-evidence rests on assuming that every agent or person is a model of their environment or, more specifically, the sensory data to which they are exposed. This means that to minimize average surprise (entropy), each agent should maximize the evidence for its model of sensory exchanges with the world. Model optimization of this sort is a solved problem in statistics and machine learning (e.g., MacKay, 1995; Kropotov & Vetrov, 2009). In fact, most forms of statistical inference rest on comparing the evidence for one model relative to another, given some data. So what does this mean for our brains? It suggests that we are obliged to optimize our model of the world through evolution, neurodevelopment, and learning. In other words, we are statistical engines that make inferences about the world, given the (sensory) data available to us. The idea that we are *inference machines* is very old and was most clearly articulated by the renowned physicist Hermann von Helmholtz (1866). Indeed, perception has been explicitly equated with hypothesis testing (Gregory, 1980), and the brain has been referred to as a Helm-holtz machine (Dayan, Hinton, & Neal, 1995). More recent incarnations of this idea appear as the Bayesian brain hypothesis (Kersten, Mamassian, & Yuille, 2004; Knill & Pouget, 2004) as instantiated in schemes like predictive coding (Mumford, 1992; Rao & Ballard, 1998). All these explanations borrow from Helmholtz's idea that the brain makes inferences about its sensations. A large body of work in theoretical neuroscience provides a plausible and compelling account of perception and the architecture of the wet-ware (brain) required to make these inferences. The ensuing perspective on biological systems says something quite profound: It says that all biological organisms can be regarded as a model of the environmental niches (econiches) they inhabit. In this sense, each species represents the product of evolutionary model optimization, and each phenotype (including our brain) is a physical model or transcription of causal structure in its econiche. However, we have overlooked one small problem: Optimizing models is not easy and, in most situations, evaluating surprise or model evidence is an intractable problem. This is where the free energy comes in.

Free energy was introduced (in the context of quantum physics) by Richard Feynman (1972) to solve the sort of difficult integration problems inherent in computing model evidence. It has been exploited in statistics and machine learning (e.g., Neal & Hinton, 1998) as a very efficient way of measuring and maximizing model evidence (i.e., minimizing surprise). The idea is quite simple: Instead of trying to minimize something that cannot be measured, one simply creates a bound that can be measured, which is always bigger than the unknown quantity. One then minimizes the unknown quantity by minimizing the bound. So, what is this bound? In physics and statistics, it is free energy (recent statistical treatments of evolution consider a related quantity called free-fitness; Sella & Hirsh, 2005). Its construction is simple (see figure 12.1): The free-energy bound is constructed by adding a non-negative (Kullback–Leibler divergence) quantity to surprise. The clever thing is that adding this term renders the free energy easily measurable. This Kullback–Leibler divergence measures the difference between two probability distributions; the first is called a proposal density and is an arbitrary probability distribution used to create the bound. The second is the posterior or conditional density on the causes of our sensations (e.g., the presence of an object in our field of view). The posterior density is the probability of causes after seeing their consequences. Minimizing the bound reduces the difference between the proposal and the posterior

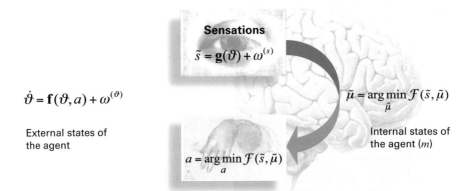

$$\dot{\vartheta} = \mathbf{f}(\vartheta, a) + \omega^{(\vartheta)}$$

External states of
the agent

Sensations

$$\tilde{s} = \mathbf{g}(\vartheta) + \omega^{(s)}$$

$$\tilde{\mu} = \arg\min_{\tilde{\mu}} \mathcal{F}(\tilde{s}, \tilde{\mu})$$

Internal states of
the agent (m)

$$a = \arg\min_{a} \mathcal{F}(\tilde{s}, \tilde{\mu})$$

Action to minimize a bound on surprise

$$\mathcal{F} = D(q(\vartheta) \| p(\vartheta)) - \left\langle \ln p(\tilde{s}(a) | \vartheta, m) \right\rangle_q$$

$$= Complexity - Accuracy$$

$$a = \arg\max Accuracy$$

Perception to optimize the bound

$$\mathcal{F} = D(q(\vartheta | \tilde{\mu}) \| p(\vartheta | \tilde{s})) - \ln p(\tilde{s} | m)$$

$$= Divergence + Surprise$$

$$\tilde{\mu} = \arg\min_{\tilde{\mu}} Divergence$$

Figure 12.1
The free-energy principle. This schematic shows the dependencies among the quantities that define the free energy of an agent or brain, denoted by m. These include its generalized internal states $\tilde{\mu}(t)$ and sensory signals $\tilde{s}(t)$ (generalized states include their generalized motion; i.e., velocity, acceleration, etc.). The environment is described by equations, which specify the motion of its states ϑ, which depend on action $a(t)$. Both internal brain states and action minimize free-energy $\mathcal{F}(\tilde{s}, \tilde{\mu})$, which is a function of sensory input and the internal states. Internal states encode a proposal density $q(\vartheta | \tilde{\mu})$ on the causes of sensory input. These comprise states of the world and the amplitude of random fluctuations $\omega(t)$. The lower panels provide the key equations behind the free-energy formulation. The right equality shows that optimizing brain states, with respect to the internal states, makes the proposal density an approximate conditional density on the causes of sensory input. Furthermore, it shows that free energy is an upper bound on surprise. This is because the first term of the equality is a divergence between the proposal density and the true conditional or posterior density. Because this divergence can never be less than zero, minimizing free energy renders it a proxy for surprise. At the same time, the proposal density becomes the posterior density. The left equality shows that action can only reduce free energy by selectively sampling sensory data that are predicted under the proposal density.

density. When they are identical, free energy becomes surprise or negative log-evidence. This means to evaluate surprise, we have to make
(Bayesian) inferences about what caused our sensations. This is the
Bayesian brain hypothesis, where minimizing free energy entails Bayes-
optimal perception. In short, free energy converts an intractable mathematical problem into a simple optimization problem. This statistical
device furnishes another important perspective on how we, as organisms,
work. It suggests that we minimize surprise by optimizing an upper
bound on surprise. In other words, everything we do can be cast in terms
of optimization. This is self-evidently true in many contexts, certainly in
fields like reinforcement learning and economics (Rescorla & Wagner,
1972; Sutton & Barto, 1981; Camerer, 2003; Daw & Doya, 2006) but also
in fields like evolutionary biology, where adaptive fitness is optimized.

12.2.1   The Bayesian Brain

The Bayesian brain hypothesis makes complete sense in this context. If
our imperative is to reduce surprise, then we need to have some reference
or expectations against which to measure surprise. These expectations
depend upon some model of the world and its current state. The probabilistic state of the world we infer is the proposal density described
earlier (figure 12.1) and, when things are working properly, corresponds
to the true but unknown posterior density. In the brain, this proposal
density (or, more precisely, its sufficient statistics like its mean or average)
may be encoded by neuronal activity or connection strengths among
different parts of the brain. This leads to an understanding of perceptual
inference and learning as changing synaptic activity and connectivity,
respectively, to minimize free energy. There are many schemes that have
been proposed to implement this optimization. Among the more popular
is predictive coding. Under some simplifying assumptions about the
shape of the probability densities involved, the free energy reduces to
the sum of squared prediction error (see figure 12.2). In short, minimizing
free energy corresponds to reducing prediction errors. The hierarchical
scheme depicted in figure 12.3 (plate 34) represents a fairly plausible
architecture that the brain might use to suppress prediction errors and
thereby reduce free energy. Crucially, this scheme is based on a gradient
descent of free energy (squared prediction error) and, as such, can be
cast as a set of ordinary differential equations. It is these equations of
motion that we suppose provide a model for neuronal dynamics that will
be used in the second part of this chapter.

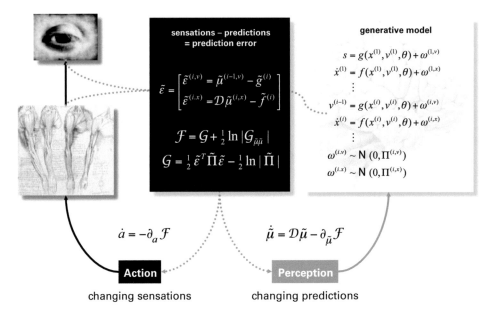

Figure 12.2
Action and perception. This schematic illustrates the bilateral role of free energy (i.e., prediction error) in driving action and perception: Action: Acting on the environment by minimizing free energy enforces a sampling of sensory data that is consistent with the current representation (i.e., changing sensations to minimize prediction error). This is because free energy is a mixture of complexity and accuracy (the first expression for free energy in figure 12.1). Crucially, action can only affect accuracy. This means the brain will reconfigure its sensory epithelia to sample inputs that are predicted by its representations; in other words, to minimize prediction errors. The equation above the label "Action" simply states that action performs a gradient descent on (i.e., minimizes) free energy. Perception: Optimizing free energy by changing the internal states that encode the proposal density makes it an approximate posterior or conditional density on the causes of sensations. This follows because free energy is surprise plus a Kullback–Leibler divergence between the proposal and conditional densities (the second expression for free energy in figure 12.1). Because this difference is non-negative, minimizing free energy makes the proposal density an approximate posterior probability. This means the agent implicitly infers or represents the causes of its sensory samples in a Bayes-optimal fashion. At the same time, the free energy becomes a tight bound on surprise that is minimized through action. The equation above the label "Perception" simply states that internal states perform a gradient descent on (i.e., minimize) free energy. This gradient descent is in a moving frame of reference for generalized states and accumulates gradients over time for the parameters. Prediction error: The equations show that the free energy comprises a (Gibbs) energy $\mathcal{G}(t)$, which is effectively the (precision weighted) sum of squared prediction error. This error contains the sensory prediction error and other differences that mediate empirical priors on the motion of hidden states. The predictions rest on a generative model of how sensations are caused. These models have to explain complicated dynamics on continuous states with hierarchical or deep causal structure. An example of one such generic model is shown on the right. Generative model: Here, $g^{(i)}$ and $f^{(i)}$ are continuous nonlinear functions of (hidden) causes and states, parameterized by $\theta \subset \vartheta$ at the ith level of a hierarchical dynamic model. The random fluctuations $\omega^{(i,u)}:u \in x,v$ play the role of observation noise at the sensory level and state noise at higher levels. Hidden causes $v^{(i)} \subset \vartheta$ link hierarchical levels, where the output of one level provides input to the next. Hidden states $x^{(i)} \subset \vartheta$ link dynamics over time and lend the model memory. Gaussian assumptions about the random fluctuations specify the likelihood of the model and furnish empirical priors in terms of predicted motion. These assumptions are encoded by the precision or inverse variance of the random fluctuations on hidden causes and the motion of hidden states; $\Pi^{(i,v)}$ and $\Pi^{(i,x)}$, respectively. These depend on precision parameters $\gamma \subset \vartheta$. The associated message-passing scheme implementing perception is shown in figure 12.3 (plate 34). Here, $\mathcal{D}$ is a temporal derivative operator that acts on generalized states.

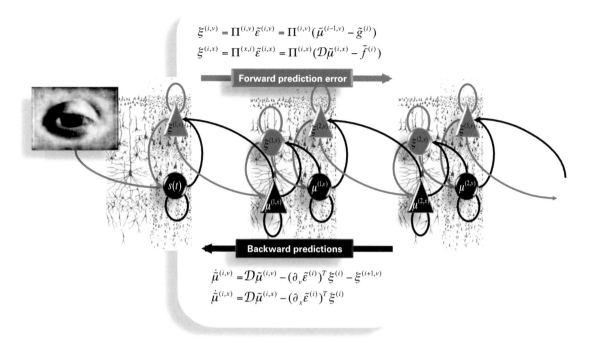

$$\xi^{(i,v)} = \Pi^{(i,v)} \tilde{\varepsilon}^{(i,v)} = \Pi^{(i,v)} (\tilde{\mu}^{(i-1,v)} - \tilde{g}^{(i)})$$
$$\xi^{(i,x)} = \Pi^{(x,i)} \tilde{\varepsilon}^{(i,x)} = \Pi^{(i,x)} (\mathcal{D}\tilde{\mu}^{(i,x)} - \tilde{f}^{(i)})$$

Forward prediction error

Backward predictions

$$\dot{\tilde{\mu}}^{(i,v)} = \mathcal{D}\tilde{\mu}^{(i,v)} - (\partial_v \tilde{\varepsilon}^{(i)})^T \xi^{(i)} - \xi^{(i+1,v)}$$
$$\dot{\tilde{\mu}}^{(i,x)} = \mathcal{D}\tilde{\mu}^{(i,x)} - (\partial_x \tilde{\varepsilon}^{(i)})^T \xi^{(i)}$$

Figure 12.3 (plate 34)
Hierarchical message-passing in the brain. The schematic details a neuronal architecture that optimizes the conditional expectations of causes in hierarchical models of sensory input of the sort illustrated in figure 12.2. It shows the putative cells of origin of forward-driving connections that convey prediction error from a lower area to a higher area (red arrows) and nonlinear backward connections (black arrows) that construct predictions (Mumford, 1992; Friston, 2005). These predictions try to explain away (inhibit) prediction error in lower levels. In this scheme, the sources of forward and backward connections are superficial and deep pyramidal cells (triangles), respectively, where state units are black and error units are red. The equations represent a generalized gradient descent on free energy using the generative model of the previous figure. Predictions and prediction error: If we assume that synaptic activity encodes the conditional expectation of states, then recognition can be formulated as a gradient descent on free energy. Under Gaussian assumptions, these recognition dynamics can be expressed compactly in terms of precision-weighted prediction errors $\xi^{(i,u)}:u \in x,v$ on the causal states and motion of hidden states (at level i of the hierarchy). The ensuing equations suggest two neuronal populations that exchange messages: causal or hidden state-units encoding expected states, and error units encoding prediction error. Under hierarchical models, error units receive messages from the state units in the same level and the level above, whereas state units are driven by error units in the same level and the level below. These provide bottom-up messages that drive conditional expectations $\mu^{(i,u)}:u \in x,v$ toward better predictions to explain away prediction error. These top-down predictions correspond to $g(\tilde{\mu}^{(i,u)})$ that are specified by the generative model. This scheme suggests the only connections that link levels are forward connections conveying prediction error to state units and reciprocal backward connections that mediate predictions. Note that the prediction errors that are passed forward are weighted by their precision. This tells us that precision may be encoded by the postsynaptic gain or sensitivity or error units, which also has to be optimized: see Friston (2010) for further details.

In summary, surprise cannot be measured directly, but we can induce a bound on surprise called free energy and reduce this bound by optimizing the activity and connectivity in our brains. This renders free energy approximately the same as surprise and obliges us to make Bayesian inferences about the state of our world. The implementation of this optimization may rest upon the minimization of prediction errors of the sort considered by predictive coding. In this context, the gradient descent on free energy (prediction errors) provides a plausible account of the dynamics that underlie synaptic activity (perceptual inference) and synaptic efficacy (perceptual learning). An important aspect of this optimization is the proper estimation of the precision (inverse variance or uncertainty) associated with prediction errors. In the generalized predictive coding scheme of figure 12.3 (plate 34), we consider this precision to be encoded by synaptic gain, which has to be optimized in exactly the same way as synaptic activity (encoding expected states of the world) and synaptic efficacy (encoding the coupling among these states). The role of precision or synaptic gain will become important later when we consider the difference between action and action–observation. The scheme described in figure 12.3 (plate 34) has been used to explain many different aspects of perceptual learning and inference in psychophysics and psychology. Figure 12.4 shows an example of perceptual categorization using simulated bird songs. However, perceptual inference and learning does not itself reduce surprise; it just reduces the difference between free energy and surprise. To understand how surprise per se is reduced, we have to consider action and the active sampling of sensory data:

12.2.2   Active Inference

So far, we have seen that perception can be understood as furnishing a proxy for surprise, in the sense that perception reduces the divergence between the proposal density and the true conditional density over hidden states causing sensations. In doing this, it makes free energy a tighter bound or better approximation to surprise. Next, we consider how action can actually reduce surprise. In brief, we can minimize prediction error in one of two ways: We can either change our expectations or predictions (perception) or we can change the things that are predicted (action). This perspective suggests that we should selectively sample data (or place ourselves in relation to the world) so that we experience what we expect to experience. In other words, we will act upon the world to ensure that our predictions come true (Friston, Daunizeau, Kilner, & Kiebel, 2010). This is exactly the sort of behavior that we were trying to

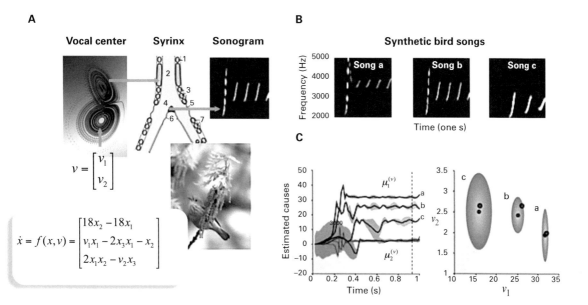

A

Vocal center   Syrinx   Sonogram

$$v = \begin{bmatrix} v_1 \\ v_2 \end{bmatrix}$$

$$\dot{x} = f(x, v) = \begin{bmatrix} 18x_2 - 18x_1 \\ v_1 x_1 - 2x_3 x_1 - x_2 \\ 2x_1 x_2 - v_2 x_3 \end{bmatrix}$$

B   Synthetic bird songs

Frequency (Hz)

Song a   Song b   Song c

Time (one s)

C

Estimated causes

$\mu_1^{(v)}$

$\mu_2^{(v)}$

Time (s)

v_2

v_1

Figure 12.4
Birdsongs and perceptual categorization. (A) The generative model of birdsong used in this simulation comprises a Lorenz attractor with two control parameters (or hidden causes) (v_1, v_2), which, in turn, delivers two control parameters to a synthetic syrinx to produce "chirps" that were modulated in amplitude and frequency (an example is shown as a sonogram). Simulated chirps were presented to a synthetic bird to see if it could infer the hidden causes and thereby categorize the song. This entails minimizing free energy by changing the conditional expectations of the control parameters. Examples of this perceptual inference or categorization are shown on the right. (B) Three simulated songs are shown in sonogram format. Each comprises a series of chirps whose frequency and number fall progressively from song **a** to song **c** as a causal state (known as the Raleigh number; μ_{v_1} in the left panel) is decreased. (C) The graph on the left depicts the conditional expectations of the hidden causes, shown as a function of peristimulus time for the three songs. It shows that the causes are identified after about 600 ms with high conditional precision (90% confidence intervals are shown in gray). The graph on the right shows the conditional density on the causes shortly before the end of peristimulus time (i.e., the dotted line in the left panel). The small dots correspond to conditional expectations, and the gray areas correspond to the 90% conditional confidence regions. Note that these encompass the true values (large dots) that were used to generate the songs. These results illustrate the nature of perceptual categorization under the inference scheme in figure 12.3 (plate 34): Here, recognition corresponds to mapping from a continuously changing and chaotic sensory input to a fixed point in perceptual space.

explain at the beginning; namely, how do biological systems avoid surprising exchanges with the environment?

It is fairly easy to show that the only part of free energy that can be changed by action is sensory prediction error. This simple fact provides a nice explanation for how we interact with the world at a number of levels. First, in biological terms, it suggests that our muscles are wired to cancel sensory prediction errors. We are all familiar with this as a reflex: If I stretched the muscles in your leg by tapping the tendons below your knee, then they respond by contracting to cancel the unpredicted stretch-receptor signals. This reflects a basic functional architecture in movement (motor) control; whereby movements are elicited by prediction errors about the position of limbs: At its simplest, this is the classical motor reflex. If we generalize this view of how the brain controls our bodies, then peripheral motor or muscle systems are enslaved to fulfill predictions. This means we only have to expect or predict an action, and it will be executed automatically. The resulting perspective implies a curious yet compelling relationship between action and perception: On the one hand, perception optimizes predictions so that actions can minimize surprise, whereas, on the other hand, our motor behavior is prescribed entirely by perceptual predictions. If action and perception work in synergy, we will navigate our econiche, never straying from well-trodden paths, eluding surprise (and potential danger).

At a more abstract level, the selective sampling of sensory data we expect to encounter may provide a metaphor for the way we live. This is particularly true of scientists, who spend most of their lives designing experiments to gather data they hope will confirm their predictions (hypotheses). Indeed, one could regard any phenotype as garnering evidence for its own existence. This brings us back to the notion that each individual is a model of its environment, which has to be continually affirmed by actively sampling from that environment. So far, we have only considered action as supplying further evidence for internal models of how the world works. Is this sufficient to explain behaviors such as goal-seeking, exploration, and innovation? Not quite. To conclude this summary, we will look at the fundamental role of prior expectations in shaping predictions and behavior.

12.2.3 Policies and Priors

Clearly, if each individual is adapted or optimized to their own environment, either at an evolutionary level or on a day-to-day basis in terms of learning and inference, the expectations of each individual must differ. Furthermore, we must inherit some aspect of these expectations, such that the physical form encoding each generation's model of its econiche is conserved (e.g., the way that the brain is wired). This speaks to the important role of innate or prior expectations about how and what we will sample from the world. For example, the fact we have eyes belies the fact our environment is bathed in light; and we avoid the dark because we expect to see things. This perspective touches on situated and embodied cognition (Ziemke, 2002) and the notion that we adapt environment to fulfill our expectations (Kirsh, 1996; Buason, Bergfeldt, & Ziemke, 2005).

In the free-energy formulation, prior expectations are a key determinant of behavior and are an integral part of an individual's model. These priors may not be very complicated but can have a profound effect on what we expose ourselves to. For example, one could cast innately rewarding states (e.g., being sated or warm) as states we expect to encounter and that we are least likely to avoid. In brief, if an agent expects to move when, and only when, it is not in a rewarding state, then action will fulfill this prior and remove it from costly (nonrewarding states). This means that the probability of finding an agent in a nonrewarding state is much smaller than finding it in a rewarding state. This is precisely the low-entropy distribution of states we want to explain and can be accounted for by one prior belief: "I will move unless rewarded." Simulations of this implicit policy produce remarkably intentional and adaptive behaviors that can solve benchmark problems in optimal control theory (like the mountain car problem: see figure 12.5 for an example). Heuristically, agents in these simulations move through the space of their states as if they were in a medium with negative viscosity or friction. This means that in most parts of state space they speed up, until they find states they, *a priori*, believe they should occupy. At this point, the viscosity becomes positive, and the agent slows down to exploit the state it expects to be in. The trick here is to formulate prior expectations about movement through state space in terms of cost, or loss, functions of the sort considered in reinforcement and value learning. In this example, cost (negative reward) controls the viscosity the agent believes it will encounter at different points in state space. Viscosity is positive only in low-cost, or rewarding, regions, and it is these regions that agents populate. This is one example of a generic link between active inference and optimal decision theory. Briefly, the complete class theorem shows that all admissible decision rules are equivalent to a Bayesian decision policy given

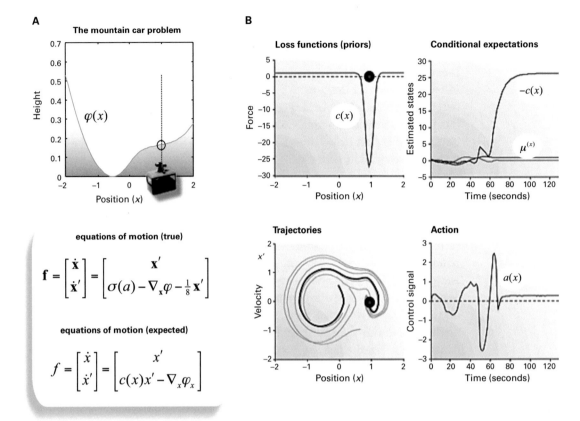

A

The mountain car problem

$\varphi(x)$

Height / Position (x)

equations of motion (true)

$$\mathbf{f} = \begin{bmatrix} \dot{\mathbf{x}} \\ \dot{\mathbf{x}}' \end{bmatrix} = \begin{bmatrix} \mathbf{x}' \\ \sigma(a) - \nabla_{\mathbf{x}}\varphi - \frac{1}{8}\mathbf{x}' \end{bmatrix}$$

equations of motion (expected)

$$f = \begin{bmatrix} \dot{x} \\ \dot{x}' \end{bmatrix} = \begin{bmatrix} x' \\ c(x)x' - \nabla_x\varphi_x \end{bmatrix}$$

B

Loss functions (priors)

Force / Position (x)

$c(x)$

Conditional expectations

Estimated states / Time (seconds)

$-c(x)$

$\mu^{(x)}$

Trajectories

Velocity / Position (x)

Action

Control signal / Time (seconds)

$a(x)$

Figure 12.5

Solving the mountain car problem with prior expectations. (A) This illustration shows how paradoxical but adaptive behavior (e.g., moving away from a target to ensure it is secured later) emerges from simple priors on the motion of hidden states in the world. The illustration shows the landscape or potential energy function (with a minimum at position $x = -0.5$) that exerts forces on a mountain car. The car is shown at the target position on the hill at $x = 1$, indicated by the ball. The true and expected equations of motion of the car are shown in the lower panel. Crucially, at $x = 0$ the force on the car cannot be overcome by the agent, because a squashing function $-1 \leq \sigma(a) \leq 1$ is applied to action to prevent it being greater than one. This means that the agent can only access the target by starting halfway up the left hill to gain enough momentum to carry it up the other side. (B) The results of active inference under priors that destroy fixed points outside the target domain. The priors are encoded in a loss, or cost, function $c(x)$ (upper-left panel), which acts like negative friction. When "friction" is negative, the car expects to go faster. The inferred hidden states (upper-right panel) show that the car explores its landscape until it encounters the target, when friction increases (i.e., cost decreases) dramatically to prevent the car from escaping the target (by falling down the hill). The ensuing trajectory is shown in the lower-left panel. The paler lines provide exemplar trajectories from different trials, with different starting positions. In the real world, friction is constant. However, the car "expects" friction to change as it changes position, thus enforcing exploration or exploitation. These expectations are fulfilled by action (lower-right panel).

some prior beliefs and a cost function (North, 1968). This means that any decision is optimal for a Bayesian generative model and cost function or it is not rational. In fact, the implicit equivalence between priors and cost functions means that we can recast any cost function as a prior belief.

The example in figure 12.5 illustrates this by incorporating the cost function into prior beliefs about motion through state space. It also illustrates a potentially ubiquitous dynamical mechanism for generating itinerant or wandering exploration of state space. The basic idea is that unattractive or surprising fixed points destroy themselves by being rendered unstable. We have referred to this as autovitiation (for details, see Friston, 2010). We will pursue this theme later in the context of winnerless competition among unstable fixed points that prescribe visual and proprioceptive predictions, which action fulfills. This sort of prior on state-transitions (a policy) provides a simple explanation for foraging behavior in ethology and, to a certain extent, addresses the exploitation–exploration trade-off in game theory and economics (Ishii, Yoshida, & Yoshimoto, 2002; Cohen, McClure, & Yu, 2007). One might ask: Where do these innate priors come from?

The answer is implicit in their evolutionary motivation; in that they can be specified genetically and elaborated through (Bayes-optimal) learning. This would explain how one generation can tell the next what is valuable (expected), without having to prescribe the details of how to attain valuable states. This is a nice aspect of the free-energy formulation because it connects dynamics at different levels or scales. For example, the same free energy is minimized by inferring things about someone on the phone and by the evolution of our ancestors. The only difference is that the long-term average of free energy is optimized by evolution, development, and learning, whereas perception minimizes free energy over short timescales. Notably, the long-term average or path-integral of energy is called "action" in physics. This means the free-energy principle is formally identical to Hamilton's principle of least *action*: Hamilton's principle of least action describes classical mechanics, when energy is concerned. The free-energy principle appeals to the same idea to explain conservative ensemble dynamics in self-organizing systems.

12.2.4   Summary

In conclusion, we have reviewed the motivation for the free-energy principle in terms of explaining how self-organizing adaptive and biological systems manage to resist a tendency to disorder. When we unpack this principle, we see that it accommodates both perception and action while embedding the action–perception cycle in an evolutionary context. We have seen that the underlying imperative of all biological systems is to minimize (a free-energy bound) on surprise; and that surprise, self-evidently, depends upon predictions. These predictions can be constrained by prior expectations, which allow our behavior to be optimized by evolution and neurodevelopment (learning). In the next section, we will apply these ideas to understand how agents emit sequences of movements or action. We will focus on handwriting, noting that the basic principles should apply to any structured and sequential pattern of behavior. This example has been chosen to highlight the central role of itinerant dynamics in furnishing prior expectations about action and concomitant perception.

12.3   Action and Its Observation

In this section, we describe a generative model of handwriting and then apply the fee-energy scheme of the previous section to simulate emergent neuronal dynamics and behavior. To create these simulations, all we have to do is specify a generative model. This model and (generalized) sensations define the free energy, which determines the dynamics of action and neuronal states encoding the conditional expectations of hidden states in the world. Action and perception are prescribed by the following two equations that appear in figure 12.2, which simulate neuronal and behavioral responses, respectively.

$$\dot{\mu} = \mathcal{D}\tilde{\mu} - \partial_{\tilde{\mu}}\mathcal{F}(\tilde{s}(a),\mu)$$

$$\dot{a} = -\partial_a \mathcal{F}(\tilde{s}(a),\mu). \tag{12.1}$$

The first equation represents a generalized or instantaneous gradient descent on free energy for the conditional expectations of hidden states causing sensory input (i.e., neuronal activity). The first term represents their expected generalized motion, and the second is simply the gradient of the free energy with respect to the expectations. The reason that this is a generalized descent is that it is formulated in generalized coordinates of motion, such that the first term augments and anticipates the descent so that it becomes effectively instantaneous. The second equality is the equivalent gradient descent for action. Both of these equations rest upon the free energy, which is a function of sensory information and current expectations. This function depends upon a generative model, which is specified completely by equations of motion of the hidden states and a function mapping hidden states to sensory signals (see figure 12.2). This means all we have to do to simulate action and perception is to specify the equations of the generative model and then solve or integrate equation (12.1) over time. In what follows, we describe the generative model that will be used for the remainder of this chapter. We have chosen this model because it embodies the sort of itinerant dynamics considered in previous chapters. In particular, we focus on stable heteroclinic channels and how they prescribe expectations about movements.

12.3.1   Itinerant Dynamics and Attractors

Our agent was equipped with a simple hierarchical model of its sensorium based on a Lotka–Volterra system. The particular form of this model has been discussed previously as the basis of putative speech decoding (Kiebel, Daunizeau, & Friston, 2009). Here, it is used to model a stable heteroclinic channel (Rabinovich, Huerta, & Laurent, 2008) encoding successive locations to which the agent expects its arm to move. The resulting trajectory was contrived to simulate synthetic handwriting.

  A stable heteroclinic channel is a particular form of (stable) itinerant trajectory or orbit that revisits a sequence of (unstable) fixed points. In our model, there are two sets of hidden states, which we will associate with two levels of a hierarchical model. The first set $x^{(2)} \in \mathbb{R}^{6 \times 1}$ corresponds to the state space of a Lotka–Volterra system. This is an abstract (attractor) state space, in which a series of attracting points are visited in succession. The second set $x^{(1)} = \{x_1, x_2, x_1', x_2'\}$ corresponds to the (angular) positions and velocities of two joints in (two-dimensional) physical space. The dynamics of hidden states at the first level embody the agent's prior expectation that the arm will be drawn to a particular location, $v^{(1)} = g(x^{(2)})$ specified by the attractor states of the second level. This is implemented simply by placing a (virtual) elastic band between the tip of the arm and the attracting location. The hidden states basically draw the arm's extremity (finger) to a succession of locations to produce an orbit or trajectory, under classical Newtonian mechanics. We chose the locations so that the resulting trajectory looked like handwriting. These hidden states generate both proprioceptive and visual (extroceptive) sensory data: The proprioceptive data are the angular positions and velocities of the two joints $x^{(1)}$, and the visual information was the location of the arm in physical (Cartesian) space $\{\ell_1, \ell_1 + \ell_2\}$, where $\ell_2(x^{(1)})$

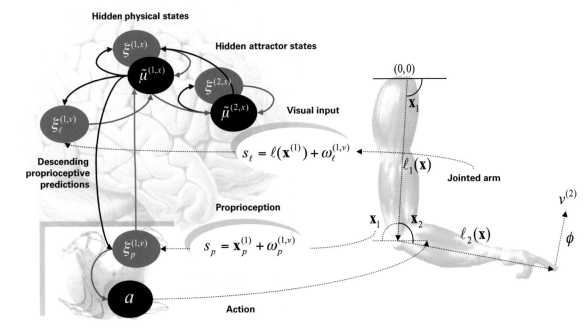

Figure 12.6 (plate 35)
Simulating self-generated movement. This schematic details a simulated (mirror neuron) system and the motor plant that it controls (left and right, respectively). The right panel depicts the functional architecture of the supposed neural circuits underlying active inference. The red ovals represent prediction error-units (neurons or populations), whereas the black ovals denote state units encoding conditional expectations about hidden states of the world (for simplicity, we have omitted hidden causes). The hidden states are split into two hierarchical levels: the higher abstract attractor states (that support stable heteroclinic orbits) and lower physical states of the arm (angular positions and velocities of the two joints). Red arrows are forward connections conveying prediction errors, and black arrows are backward connections mediating predictions. Motor commands are emitted by the black units in the ventral horn of the spinal cord. Note that these just receive prediction errors about proprioceptive states. These, in turn, are the difference between sensed proprioceptive input from the two joints and descending predictions from optimized representations in the motor cortex. The two-jointed arm has a state space that is characterized by two angles, which control the position of the finger that will be used for writing in subsequent figures.

Table 12.2
Variables and quantities specific to the writing example of active inference (see main text for details).

Variable	Description
$x^{(2)} \in \mathbb{R}^{6 \times 1}$	**Hidden attractor states:** A vector of hidden states that specify the current location toward which the agent expects its arm to be pulled.
$x^{(1)} \in \mathbb{R}^{4 \times 1}$	**Hidden effector states:** Hidden states that specify the angular position and velocity of the ith joint of a two-jointed arm.
$\ell_1(x^{(1)}) \in \mathbb{R}^{2 \times 1}$ $\ell_2(x^{(1)}) \in \mathbb{R}^{2 \times 1}$	**Joint locations:** Locations of the end of the two arm parts in Cartesian space. These are functions of the angular positions of the joints.
$v^{(1)} = g(x^{(2)}) \in \mathbb{R}^{2 \times 1}$	**Attracting location:** The location toward which the arm is drawn. This is specified by the hidden attractor states.
$\phi(x^{(1)}, v^{(1)}) \in \mathbb{R}^{2 \times 1}$	**Newtonian force:** This is the angular force on the joints exerted by the attracting location.
$A \in \mathbb{R}^{6 \times 6} \subset \theta$	**Attractor parameters:** A matrix of parameters that govern the (sequential Lotka–Volterra) dynamics of the hidden attractor states.
$L \in \mathbb{R}^{2 \times 6} \subset \theta$	**Cartesian parameters:** A matrix of parameters that specify the attracting locations associated with each hidden attractor state.

is the displacement of the finger from the location of the second joint $\ell_1(x^{(1)})$ [see figure 12.6 (plate 35) and table 12.2].

Crucially, because this generative model generates two (proprioceptive and visual) sensory modalities, the solutions to equation (12.1) implement Bayes-optimal multisensory integration. However, because action is also trying to reduce prediction errors, it will move the arm to reproduce the expected trajectory (under the constraints of the motor plant). In other words, the arm will trace out a trajectory prescribed by the itinerant priors (to cancel proprioceptive prediction errors). This closes the loop, producing autonomous self-generated sequences of behavior of the sort described below. Note that the real world does not contain any attracting locations or elastic bands: The only causes of observed movement are the self-fulfilling expectations encoded by the itinerant dynamics of the generative model. In short, hidden attractor states essentially prescribe the intended movement trajectory, because they generate predictions that action fulfills. This means expected states encode conditional percepts (concepts) about latent abstract states (that do not exist in the absence of action), which play the role of intentions. We now describe the model formally.

12.3.2 The Generative Model

The model used in this section concerns the movements of a two-joint arm. When simulating active inference, it is important to distinguish between the agent's generative model and the actual dynamics generating sensory data. To make this distinction clear, we will use boldface for true equations and states, and those of the generative model will be written in italics. Proprioceptive input corresponds to the angular position and velocity of both joints, whereas the visual input corresponds to the location of the extremities of both parts of the arm. This means the mapping from hidden states to sensory consequences is

$$\mathbf{g}^{(1)} = g^{(1)} = \begin{bmatrix} x^{(1)} \\ \ell_1(x^{(1)}) \\ \ell_1(x^{(1)}) + \ell_2(x^{(1)}) \end{bmatrix}. \tag{12.2}$$

We will ignore the complexities of inference on retinotopically mapped visual input and assume the agent has direct access to the locations of the arm in visual space. The kinetics of the arm conforms to Newtonian laws, under which action forces the angular position of each joint. Both joints have an equilibrium position at 90 degrees; with inertia $m_i \in 8,4$ and viscosity $\kappa_i \in 4,2$, giving the following equations of motion for the hidden states:

$$\mathbf{x}^{(1)} = \begin{bmatrix} \mathbf{x}_1 \\ \mathbf{x}_2 \\ \mathbf{x}_1' \\ \mathbf{x}_2' \end{bmatrix} \quad \mathbf{f}^{(1)} = \begin{bmatrix} \mathbf{x}_1' \\ \mathbf{x}_2' \\ (a_1 + \mathbf{v}_1 - \frac{1}{4}(\mathbf{x}_1 - \frac{\pi}{2}) - \kappa_1\mathbf{x}_1')/m_1 \\ (a_2 + \mathbf{v}_2 - \frac{1}{4}(\mathbf{x}_2 - \frac{\pi}{2}) - \kappa_2\mathbf{x}_2')/m_2 \end{bmatrix}. \tag{12.3}$$

However, the agent's empirical priors on this motion have a very different form. Its generative model assumes the finger is pulled to a (goal) location $v^{(1)}$ by a force $\phi(t)$, which implements the virtual elastic band above:

$$x^{(1)} = \begin{bmatrix} x_1 \\ x_2 \\ x_1' \\ x_2' \end{bmatrix} \quad f^{(1)} = \begin{bmatrix} x_1' \\ x_2' \\ (\phi^T \ell_2 \ell_2^T O \ell_1 - \frac{1}{16}(x_1 - \frac{\pi}{2}) - \kappa_1 x_1')/m_1 \\ (\phi^T O \ell_2 - \frac{1}{16}(x_2 - \frac{\pi}{2}) - \kappa_2 x_2')/m_2 \end{bmatrix}$$

$$\ell_1 = \begin{bmatrix} \cos(x_1) \\ \sin(x_1) \end{bmatrix} \quad \ell_2 = \begin{bmatrix} -\cos(-x_2 - x_1) \\ \sin(-x_2 - x_1) \end{bmatrix} \quad O = \begin{bmatrix} 0 & -1 \\ 1 & 0 \end{bmatrix}$$

$$\phi = \tfrac{1}{2}(v^{(1)} - \ell_1 - \ell_2). \tag{12.4}$$

The (moving) target location is specified by the second level of the hierarchy as a nonlinear (softmax) function of the hidden attractor states:

$$v^{(1)} = g(x^{(2)}) = Ls(x^{(2)})$$

$$f^{(2)} = A\sigma(x^{(2)}) - \tfrac{1}{8}x^{(2)} + \begin{bmatrix} 1 \\ \vdots \\ 1 \end{bmatrix}$$

$$\sigma(x_i) = \frac{1}{1+e^{2x_i}} \quad s(x_i) = \frac{e^{2\alpha_i}}{\sum_j e^{2x_j}}.$$

(12.5)

Heuristically, these equations of motion mean that the agent thinks that changes in its world are caused by the dynamics of attractor states on an abstract (conceptual) space. The currently active state selects a location $v^{(1)}$ in the agent's physical (Cartesian) space, which exerts a force $\phi(t)$ on its finger. The equations of motion in equation (12.4) pertain to the resulting motion of the arm in Cartesian space, whereas equation (12.5) mediates the attractor dynamics driving these movements.

The (Lotka–Volterra) form of the equations of motion for the hidden attractor states ensures that only one has a high value at any one time and imposes a particular sequence on the underlying states. Lotka–Volterra dynamics basically induce competition among states that no state can win. The resulting winnerless competition rests on the (logistic) function $\sigma(x^{(2)})$, whereas the sequence order is determined by the elements of the matrix

$$A = \begin{bmatrix} 0 & -\tfrac{1}{2} & -1 & -1 & \cdots \\ -\tfrac{3}{2} & 0 & -\tfrac{1}{2} & -1 & \\ -1 & -\tfrac{3}{2} & 0 & -\tfrac{1}{2} & \ddots \\ -1 & -1 & -\tfrac{3}{2} & 0 & \\ \vdots & & \ddots & & \ddots \end{bmatrix}.$$

(12.6)

Each attractor state has an associated location in Cartesian space, which draws the arm toward it. The attracting location is specified by a mapping from attractor space to Cartesian space, which weights different locations

$$L = \begin{bmatrix} 1 & 1.1 & 1.0 & 1 & 1.4 & 0.9 \\ 1 & 1.2 & 0.4 & 1 & 0.9 & 1.0 \end{bmatrix}$$

(12.7)

with a softmax function $s(x^{(2)})$ of the attractor states. The location parameters were specified by hand but could, in principle, be learned as described in Friston et al. (2009, 2010). The inertia and viscosity of the arm were chosen somewhat arbitrarily to reproduce realistic writing movements over 256 time bins, each corresponding to roughly 8 ms (i.e., a second). Unless stated otherwise, we used a log-precision of 4 for sensory noise and 8 for random fluctuations in the motion of hidden states.

Figure 12.7 shows the results of integrating equation (12.1) using the generative model above. Figure 12.7B shows the hidden states embodying Lotka–Volterra dynamics (the hidden joint states are smaller in amplitude). These generate predictions about the position of the joints (figure 12.7A) and consequent prediction errors that drive action. Action is shown on figure 12.7D and displays intermittent forces that move the joint to produce a motor trajectory. This trajectory is shown on figure 12.7C in visual space over time. This trajectory or orbit is translated as a function of time to reproduce handwriting. Although this is a pleasingly simple way of simulating an extremely complicated motor trajectory, it should be noted that this agent has a very limited repertoire of behaviors; it can only reproduce this sequence of graphemes and will do so *ad infinitum*.

In summary, we have covered the functional architecture of a generative model whose autonomous (itinerant) expectations prescribe complicated motor sequences through active inference. This rests upon itinerant dynamics (stable heteroclinic channels) that can be regarded as a formal prior on abstract causes in the world. These are translated into physical movement through classical Newtonian mechanics, which correspond to the physical states of the model. Action tries to fulfill predictions about proprioceptive inputs and is enslaved by autonomous predictions, producing realistic behavior. These trajectories are both caused by neuronal representations of abstract (attractor) states and cause those states in the sense that they are conditional expectations. Closing the loop in this way ensures a synchrony between internal expectations and external outcomes.

In the next section, we will make a simple change that means that movements are no longer caused by the agent. However, we will see that the conditional expectations about attractor states are relatively unaffected, which means that they still anticipate observed movements. We conclude with this example because it illustrates nicely the potential role of itinerant dynamics in explaining some of the higher cognitive aspects of brain function. Our focus here is on emulating the electrophysiologic phenomenology of the mirror neuron system; in particular, the fact that certain neurons in the ventral premotor cortex and inferior parietal cortex respond not only to the execution of particular movement

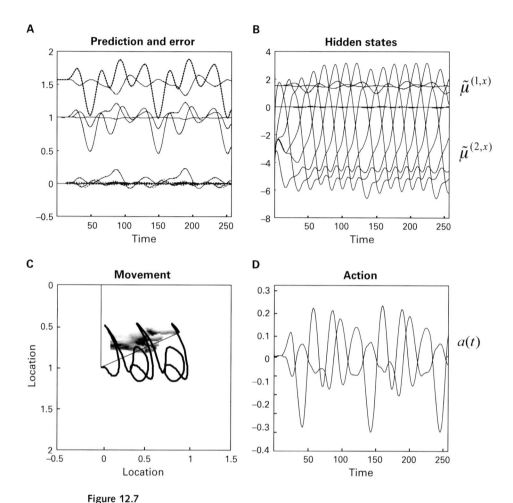

Figure 12.7

Itinerant dynamics and active inference. This illustration shows the results of simulated action (writing), under active inference, in terms of conditional expectations about hidden states of the world (B), consequent predictions about sensory input (A), and the ensuing behavior (C) that is caused by action (D). The autonomous dynamics that underlie this behavior rest upon the expected hidden states that follow Lotka–Volterra dynamics. These are the thinner lines in (B). The hidden physical states (thicker lines) have smaller amplitudes and map directly onto the predicted proprioceptive and visual signals (shown in panel A). The visual locations of the two joints are shown above the predicted joint positions and angular velocities that fluctuate around zero. The dotted lines correspond to prediction error, which shows small fluctuations about the prediction. Action tries to suppress this error by "matching" expected changes in angular velocity through exerting forces on the joints. These forces are shown on (D). The subsequent movement of the arm is traced out in (C); this trajectory has been plotted in a moving frame of reference so that it looks like synthetic handwriting (e.g., a succession of letters j and a). The straight lines on (C) denote the final position of the two-jointed arm, and the hand icon shows the final position of its finger.

primitives but also when these movements are observed in other agents (Di Pellegrino, Fadiga, Fogassi, Gallese, & Rizzolatti, 1992; Gallese & Goldman, 1998; Rizzolatti & Craighero, 2004; Fogassi et al., 2005).

12.3.3 Action–Observation

The simulations above were repeated but with one small but important change. Basically, we reproduced the same movements, but the proprioceptive consequences of action were removed, so that the agent could see but not feel the arm moving. From the agent's perspective, this is like seeing an arm that looks like its own arm but does not generate proprioceptive input (i.e., the arm of another agent). However, the agent still expects the arm to move with a particular itinerant structure and will try to predict the trajectory with its generative model. In this instance, the hidden states still represent itinerant dynamics (intentions) that govern the motor trajectory, but these states do not produce any proprioceptive prediction errors and therefore do not result in action. Crucially, the perceptual representation still retains its anticipatory or prospective aspect and can therefore be taken as a perceptual representation of intention, not of self, but of another. We will see later that this representation is almost exactly the same under action–observation as it is during action.

Practically speaking, to perform these simulations, we simply recorded the forces produced by action in the previous simulation and replayed them as exogenous forces (real causes in equation 12.2) to move the arm. This change in context (agency) was modeled by down-weighting the precision of proprioceptive signals. This is exactly the same mechanism that we have used previously to model attention (Feldman & Friston, 2010). In this setting, reducing the precision of proprioceptive prediction errors prevents them from having any influence on perceptual inference (i.e., the agent cannot feel changes in its joints). Furthermore, action is not compelled to reduce these prediction errors because they have no precision. In these simulations, we reduced the log-precision of proprioceptive prediction errors from 8 to –8. To illustrate the key results of these simulations of action–observation, in relation to simulated action, we recorded the activity of units encoding hidden attractor states and examined their relationship to observed movements.

12.3.4 Place-Cells, Itinerancy, and Oscillations

It is interesting to think about the attractor states as representing trajectories through abstract representational spaces (cf., the activity of place cells; O'Keefe, 1999; Tsodyks, 1999; Burgess, Barry, & O'Keefe, 2007). Figure 12.8 illustrates the sensory or perceptual correlates of units representing expected attractor states. The left-hand panels (figure 12.8A, C) show the activity of one (the fourth) hidden state unit under action, whereas the right-hand panels (figure 12.8B, 12.8D) show exactly the same unit under action–observation. The upper panels (figure 12.8A, B) show the trajectories in visual space, in terms of horizontal and vertical displacements (gray lines). The black dots correspond to the time bins in which the activity of the hidden state unit exceeded an amplitude threshold of two arbitrary units. The key thing to take from these results is that the activity of this unit is very specific to a limited part of Cartesian space and, crucially, a particular trajectory through this space. The analogy here is between directionally selective place-cells of the sort studied in hippocampal recordings: In tasks involving goal-directed, stereotyped trajectories, the spatially selective activity of hippocampal cells depends on the animal's direction of motion (Battaglia, Sutherland, & McNaughton, 2004). A further interesting connection with hippocampal dynamics is the prevalence of theta rhythms during action: "Driven either by external landmarks or by internal dynamics, hippocampal neurons form sequences of cell assemblies. The coordinated firing of these active cells is organized by the prominent 'theta' oscillations in the local field potential (LFP): place cells discharge at progressively earlier theta phases as the rat crosses the respective place field (phase precession)" (Geisler et al., 2010). Quantitatively, the dynamics of the hidden state-units in figure 12.7A show quasi-periodic oscillations in the (low) theta range. The notion that quasi-periodic oscillations may reflect stable heteroclinic channels is implicit in many treatments of episodic memory and spatial navigation, which "require temporal encoding of the relationships between events or locations" (Dragoi & Buzsáki, 2006), and may be usefully pursued in the context of active inference under itinerant priors.

Notice that the same "place" and "directional" selectivity is seen under action and observation (figure 12.8). The direction selectivity can be seen more clearly in the lower panels (figure 12.8C, D), in which the same data are displayed but in a moving frame of reference (to simulate writing). They key thing to note here is that this unit responds preferentially when, and only when, the motor trajectory produces a downstroke, but not an upstroke. There is an interesting dissociation in the firing of this unit under action and action–observation: During observation, the unit only starts responding to downstrokes *after* it has been observed once. This reflects the finite amount of time required for visual information to entrain the perceptual dynamics and establish veridical predictions.

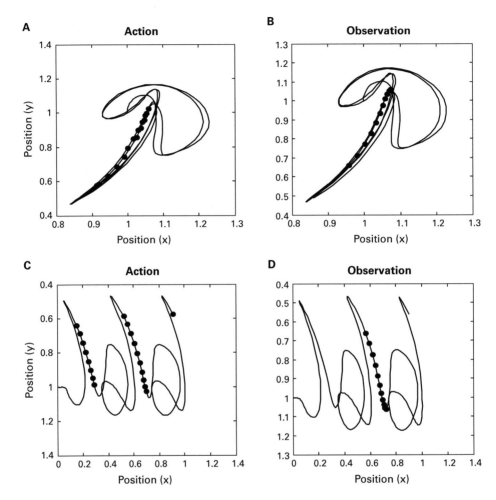

Figure 12.8
Simulating action–observation. These results illustrate the sensory or perceptual correlates of units encoding expected hidden (attractor) states. The left-hand panels (A, C) show the activity of one (the fourth attractor) hidden state-unit under action, whereas the right-hand panels (B, D) show exactly the same unit under action–observation. The upper panels (A, B) show the trajectory in visual space in terms of horizontal and vertical position (gray lines). The dots correspond to the time bins during which the activity of the state unit exceeded an amplitude threshold of two arbitrary units. The key thing to take from these results is that the activity of this unit is very specific to a limited part of visual space and, crucially, a particular trajectory through this space. Notice that the same selectivity is seen under action and observation. The implicit direction selectivity can be seen more clearly in the lower panels (C, D), in which the same data are displayed but in a moving frame of reference to simulate writing. They key thing to note here is that this unit responds preferentially when, and only when, the motor trajectory produces a downstroke, but not an upstroke.

12.4   Conclusion

In this chapter, we have tried to show that some aspects of action, perception, and high-level (cognitive) inference are consistent with (Bayesoptimal) active inference under the free-energy principle. Put simply, the brain does not represent intended motor acts or the perceptual consequences of those acts separately. The constructs represented in the brain are both intentional and perceptual: They are amodal inferences about the states of the world generating sensory data that have both sensory and motor correlates, depending upon the context in which they are made. The predictions generated by these representations are modality specific, prescribing both exteroceptive (e.g., visual) and interoceptive (e.g., proprioceptive) predictions, which action fulfills. The functional segregation of motor and sensory cortex could be regarded as a hierarchical decomposition, in the brain's model of its world, which provides predictions that are primarily sensory (e.g., visual cortex) or proprioceptive (motor cortex). If true, this means that high-level representations can be used to furnish predictions in either visual or proprioceptive modalities, depending upon the context in which those predictions are called upon.

In one sense, this conclusion takes us back to very early ideas concerning the nature of movements and intentions. The notion of an ideomotor reflex or response was introduced in the 1840s by the Victorian physiologist and psychologist William Benjamin Carpenter. The ideomotor response (reflex) refers to the process whereby a thought or mental image induces reflexive or automatic movements, often very small and potentially outside awareness. Active inference formalizes this idea and suggests that all movements are prescribed by mental images that correspond to prior beliefs about what will happen next. These priors are inherently dynamic and itinerant. This suggests that our exchanges with our environment are constrained to an exquisite degree by local and global brain dynamics and that these dynamics have been carefully crafted by evolution, neurodevelopment, and experience to optimize behavior.

Acknowledgments

The Wellcome Trust funded this work. I am grateful to Tony Dickinson for highlighting the connections with ideomotor theory.

References

Ashby, W. R. (1947). Principles of the self-organizing dynamic system. *Journal of General Psychology*, *37*, 125–128.

Battaglia, F. P., Sutherland, G. R., & McNaughton, B. L. (2004). Local sensory cues and place cell directionality: additional evidence of prospective coding in the hippocampus. *Journal of Neuroscience*, *24*(19), 4541–4550.

Bernard, C. (1974). *Lectures on the Phenomena Common to Animals and Plants*. Trans. H. E. Hoff, R. Guillemin, & L. Guillemin. Springfield, IL: Charles C. Thomas.

Buason, G., Bergfeldt, N., & Ziemke, T. (2005). Brains, bodies, and beyond: competitive co-evolution of robot controllers, morphologies, and environments. *Genetic Programming and Evolvable Machines*, *6*(1), 25–51.

Burgess, N., Barry, C., & O'Keefe, J. (2007). An oscillatory interference model of grid cell firing. *Hippocampus*, *17*(9), 801–812.

Carhart-Harris, R. L., & Friston, K. J. (2010). The default-mode, ego-functions and free-energy: a neurobiological account of Freudian ideas. *Brain*, *133*(Pt 4), 1265–1283.

Camerer, C. F. (2003). Behavioural studies of strategic thinking in games. *Trends in Cognitive Sciences*, *7*(5), 225–231.

Cohen, J. D., McClure, S. M., & Yu, A. J. (2007). Should I stay or should I go? How the human brain manages the trade-off between exploitation and exploration. *Philosophical Transactions of the Royal Society of London. Series B, Biological Sciences*, *362*(1481), 933–942.

Daw, N. D., & Doya, K. (2006). The computational neurobiology of learning and reward. *Current Opinion in Neurobiology*, *16*(2), 199–204.

Dayan, P., Hinton, G. E., & Neal, R. M. (1995). The Helmholtz machine. *Neural Computation*, *7*, 889–904.

Di Pellegrino, G., Fadiga, L., Fogassi, L., Gallese, V., & Rizzolatti, G. (1992). Understanding motor events: a neurophysiological study. *Experimental Brain Research*, *91*, 176–180.

Dragoi, G., & Buzsáki, G. (2006). Temporal encoding of place sequences by hippocampal cell assemblies. *Neuron*, *50*(1), 145–157.

Evans, D. J. (2003). A non-equilibrium free-energy theorem for deterministic systems. *Molecular Physics*, *101*, 1551–1554.

Feldman, H., & Friston, K. J. (2010). Attention, uncertainty, and free-energy. *Frontiers in Human Neuroscience*, *2*(4), 215.

Feynman, R. P. (1972). *Statistical Mechanics*. Reading, MA: Benjamin.

Fogassi, L., Ferrari, P. F., Gesierich, B., Rozzi, S., Chersi, F., & Rizzolatti, G. (2005). Parietal lobe: from action organization to intention understanding. *Science*, *308*, 662–667.

Friston, K. J. (2005). A theory of cortical responses. *Philosophical Transactions of the Royal Society of London. Series B, Biological Sciences*, *360*, 815–836.

Friston, K. (2010). The free-energy principle: a unified brain theory? *Nature Reviews. Neuroscience*, *11*(2), 127–138.

Friston, K., Daunizeau, J., & Kiebel, S. (2009). Active inference or reinforcement learning? *PLoS ONE*, *4*(7), e6421.

Friston, K. J., Daunizeau, J., Kilner, J., & Kiebel, S. J. (2010). Action and behavior: a free-energy formulation. *Biological Cybernetics*, *102*(3), 227–260.

Gallese, V., & Goldman, A. (1998). Mirror-neurons and the simulation theory of mind reading. *Trends in Cognitive Sciences*, *2*, 493–501.

Geisler, C., Diba, K., Pastalkova, E., Mizuseki, K., Royer, S., & Buzsáki, G. (2010). Temporal delays among place cells determine the frequency of population theta oscillations in the hippocampus. *Proceedings of the National Academy of Science USA*, *107*(17), 7957–7962.

Gregory, R. L. (1980). Perceptions as hypotheses. *Philosophical Transactions of the Royal Society of London. Series B, Biological Sciences*, *290*, 181–197.

Grist, M. (2010) Changing the Subject. RSA. Available at: www.thesocialbrain.wordpress.com pp. 74–80. http://www.thersa.org/projects/reports/changing-the-subject

Haken, H. (1983). *Synergetics: An Introduction. Non-equilibrium Phase Transition and Self-organization in Physics, Chemistry and Biology* (3rd ed.). Berlin: Springer-Verlag.

Hinton, G. E., & van Camp, D. (1993). Keeping neural networks simple by minimizing the description length of weights. In Proceedings of COLT-93 (pp. 5–13).

Huang, G. (2008). Is this a unified theory of the brain? *New Scientist*, May 23 (2658), 30–33.

Ishii, S., Yoshida, W., & Yoshimoto, J. (2002). Control of exploitation-exploration meta-parameter in reinforcement learning. *Neural Networks*, *15*(4–6), 665–687.

Kauffman, S. (1993). *The Origins of Order: Self-Organization and Selection in Evolution*. Oxford, UK: Oxford University Press.

Kersten, D., Mamassian, P., & Yuille, A. (2004). Object perception as Bayesian inference. *Annual Review of Psychology*, *55*, 271–304.

Kiebel, S. J., Daunizeau, J., & Friston, K. J. (2009). Perception and hierarchical dynamics. *Frontiers in Neuroinformatics*, *3*, 20.

Kirsh, D. (1996). Adapting the environment instead of oneself. *Adaptive Behavior*, *4*(3/4), 415–452.

Knill, D. C., & Pouget, A. (2004). The Bayesian brain: the role of uncertainty in neural coding and computation. *Trends in Neurosciences*, *27*(12), 712–719.

Kropotov, D., & Vetrov, D. (2009). General solutions for information-based and Bayesian approaches to model selection in linear regression and their equivalence. *Pattern Recognition and Image Analysis*, *19*(3), 447–455.

Lifshitz, E. M., & Pitaevskii, L. P. (1981). *Physical Kinetics* (Course of Theoretical Physics, Vol. 10, 3rd ed.). London: Pergamon.

MacKay, D. J. C. (1995). Free-energy minimization algorithm for decoding and cryptoanalysis. *Electronics Letters*, *31*, 445–447.

Mumford, D. (1992). On the computational architecture of the neocortex. II. The role of cortico-cortical loops. *Biological Cybernetics*, *66*, 241–251.

Neal, R. M., & Hinton, G. E. (1998). A view of the EM algorithm that justifies incremental, sparse, and other variants. In M. I. Jordan (Ed.), *Learning in Graphical Models* (pp. 355–368). Dordrecht: Kluwer Academic Publishers.

Nicolis, G., & Prigogine, I. (1977). *Self-organization in Non-equilibrium Systems* (p. 24). New York: John Wiley.

North, D. W. (1968). A tutorial introduction to decision theory. *IEEE Trans. Systems Science and Cybernetics*, *4*(3), 200–210.

O'Keefe, J. (1999). Do hippocampal pyramidal cells signal non-spatial as well as spatial information? *Hippocampus*, *9*(4), 352–364.

Rabinovich, M., Huerta, R., & Laurent, G. (2008). Neuroscience: Transient dynamics for neural processing. *Science*, *321*(5885), 48–50.

Rao, R. P., & Ballard, D. H. (1998). Predictive coding in the visual cortex: a functional interpretation of some extra-classical receptive field effects. *Nature Neuroscience*, *2*, 79–87.

Rescorla, R. A., & Wagner, A. R. (1972). A theory of Pavlovian conditioning: variations in the effectiveness of reinforcement and nonreinforcement. In A. H. Black & W. F. Prokasy (Eds.), *Classical Conditioning II: Current Research and Theory* (pp. 64–99). New York: Appleton Century Crofts.

Rizzolatti, G., & Craighero, L. (2004). The mirror-neuron system. *Annual Review of Neuroscience*, *27*, 169–192.

Sella, G., & Hirsh, A. E. (2005). The application of statistical physics to evolutionary biology. *Proceedings of the National Academy of Sciences of the United States of America, 102*(27), 9541–9546.

Sutton, R. S., & Barto, A. G. (1981). Toward a modern theory of adaptive networks: expectation and prediction. *Psychological Review, 88*(2), 135–170.

Thornton, C. (2010). Some puzzles relating to the free-energy principle: comment on Friston. *Trends in Cognitive Sciences, 14*(2), 53–54, author reply 54–55.

Tsodyks, M. (1999). Attractor neural network models of spatial maps in hippocampus. *Hippocampus, 9*(4), 481–489.

von Helmholtz, H. (1866). Concerning the perceptions in general. In *Treatise on Physiological Optics* (Vol. III, 3rd ed.). (Trans. J. P. C. Southall, *Opt. Soc. Am.*, Section 26, 1925; reprinted by Dover, New York, 1962.)

Ziemke, T. (2002). Introduction to the special issue on situated and embodied cognition. *Cognitive Systems Research, 3*(3), 271–274.

13 Perception, Action, and Utility: The Tangled Skein

Samuel J. Gershman and Nathaniel D. Daw

Summary

Statistical decision theory seems to offer a clear framework for the integration of perception and action. In particular, it defines the problem of maximizing the utility of one's decisions in terms of two subtasks: inferring the likely state of the world, and tracking the utility that would result from different candidate actions in different states. This computational-level description underpins more process-level research in neuroscience about the brain's dynamic mechanisms for, on the one hand, inferring states and, on the other hand, learning action values. However, a number of different strands of recent work on this more algorithmic level have cast doubt on the basic shape of the decision-theoretic formulation, specifically the clean separation between states' probabilities and utilities. We consider the complex interrelationship between perception, action, and utility implied by these accounts.

13.1 Introduction

Normative theories of learning and decision making are motivated by a computational-level analysis of the task facing an organism: *What* should the animal do to maximize future reward? However, much of the recent excitement in this field concerns ideas about *how* the organism arrives at its decisions and reward predictions: implementational and algorithmic questions about which the computational-level analysis is more or less silent. Answers to these algorithmic questions are essentially claims about *dynamics*: how the decision variables that support behavior are learned across trials from experience, and how they are transformed within a trial to effect a decision. Thus, these theories offer a somewhat unique intersection of dynamical and information processing content: The transformations of decision variables in these theories characterize the within- or between-trial dynamics of learning and choice, but, as decision variables, they also map onto computational-level descriptions. This chapter focuses on this interplay between computational quantities and the more process-level questions of how they are manipulated algorithmically.

At the computational level, statistical decision theory—and its relatives utility theory and reinforcement learning—seems to offer a clear framework for the integration of perception and action. Actions are chosen to optimize expected future utility. These expectations are with respect to latent states of the task, and the role of perception is to analyze stimuli so as to form probabilistic beliefs about these states. This framework supports a sequentially staged view of the problem—perception guiding evaluation—which has more or less implicitly licensed two influential streams of work in neuroscience, studying either stage in isolation.

The question of this chapter is what becomes of this seemingly clean computational separation at the algorithmic and implementational levels. The computations mandated by decision theory are, in general, intractable, and many different approximations replace them in practice, with underappreciated consequences for the interdependency of perception and action. Work in approximate inference, for instance, considers realizable (e.g., variational or Monte Carlo) approximations to the expected value computation and involves trading off the relative cost of approximations in the action and sensory stages or even entirely collapsing the two in various ways. These approximations induce a variety of dynamic patterns (in learning, inference, and decision stages) that are not anticipated by a purely computational-level analysis, and we present evidence that many behavioral and neural phenomena are naturally explained in terms of the dynamics of approximate algorithms. In the following, we first review the classical view before attempting to unravel the tangled skein of perception, action, and utility that arises in practice.

13.2 The Classical View

We begin by formalizing mathematically the problem of decision under uncertainty.[1] Consider a utility function $U(s,a)$ (or more pessimistically, its negation, the loss function) that depends on the agent's action a and a hidden state of the task s, which may be continuous and high-dimensional. For an agent seeking to maximize expected utility (or minimize loss), the optimal action is given by

$$a^* = \operatorname{argmax}_a \mathbb{E}_\pi [U(s,a)]$$

$$= \operatorname{argmax}_a \int_s \pi(s \mid x) U(s,a) ds,$$

(13.1)

where $\pi(s|x)$ is the agent's posterior belief about the hidden state conditional on observing sense data x, given by Bayes' rule:

$$\pi(s \mid x) = \frac{p(x \mid s)p(s)}{\int_s p(x \mid s)p(s)ds}.$$

(13.2)

In other words, the agent posits a generative model of the hidden and observed task variables in the form of a joint distribution $p(s,x)$, and then uses Bayes' rule to "invert" the generative model and infer the hidden state. The agent then considers what utility it can expect to achieve for an action, which is an average of utilities for taking the action in each state, weighted by the state's posterior probability. The generic role commonly imputed to the perceptual system is the computation of this posterior belief (Lee & Mumford, 2003; Knill & Pouget, 2004; Friston, 2005).

The assumptions of statistical decision theory are, in various forms, pervasive throughout psychology, neuroscience, economics, and ecology (not to mention statistics and engineering; see, e.g., Berger, 1985). They are the basis of signal detection theory and drift-diffusion models in perceptual psychology (Green & Swets, 1966; Bogacz, Brown, Moehlis, Holmes, & Cohen, 2006); of optimal control theory in sensorimotor control (Kording & Wolpert, 2006; Trommershäuser, Maloney, & Landy, 2008); of Bellman's equation in reinforcement learning (Sutton & Barto, 1998; Dayan & Daw, 2008); of subjective expected utility theory in economics (Von Neumann & Morgenstern, 1947; Savage, 1954); and of foraging theory in behavioral ecology (McNamara & Houston, 1980; Stephens & Krebs, 1986). More recently, neuroscientists have begun to probe the brain for signatures of these assumptions, in particular the neural computations of utilities and posterior probabilities (Glimcher, 2003).

We focus on two aspects of decision theory that have important implications for its implementation in the brain:

1. Decision theory implies a strong distinction or separation between probabilities and utilities. In particular, the posterior must be computed *independently* of the expected utility. This assumption is sometimes known as probabilistic sophistication (Machina & Schmeidler, 1992; Bossaerts, Preuschoff, & Hsu, 2008). It means that I can state how much

enjoyment I would derive from having a picnic in sunny weather, independently of my belief that it will be sunny tomorrow.

2. The integral over s in equations (13.1) and (13.2) is generally intractable. Although most investigations of decision theory in psychology and economics make Gaussian or multinomial assumptions about $\pi(s|x)$, these assumptions are not generally applicable to real-world decision-making tasks, where distributions may not take any convenient parametric form. Even if they do, the integrals may still resist closed-form solutions. This means that if the brain is to perform the necessary calculations, it must use some form of approximation.

Although statistical decision theory has been criticized on many other grounds (see, e.g., Kahneman & Tversky, 1979; Camerer, 1998), we focus on these aspects because they highlight the algorithmic and implementational commitments of the theory. Statistical decision theory, to be directly implemented in the brain, requires segregated representations of probability and utility and a mechanism for performing approximate inference. We discuss each of these requirements in turn. Then, in section 13.5, we suggest how these requirements may in fact be intimately connected.

13.3   Segregation of Probability and Utility in the Brain?

In this section, we discuss evidence in favor of the classical view that perception (state inference) and utility are computed and represented independently. We then describe several challenges to this view based on behavioral and neural data.

13.3.1   State Inference

The basic sequential staging of state inference to action, via utility, seems to be in accord with the gross organization of at least the posterior half of cortex. Visual information arrives in occipital cortex and progresses anteriorly through the dorsal visual stream on the way toward neurons with direct control of effectors in primary motor cortex, just in front of the central sulcus. Progressions of this sort are thought to instantiate a hierarchically staged inference process: For example, in the influential architecture for the ventral stream proposed by Riesenhuber and Poggio (1999), object representations are built up through a hierarchy of receptive fields, with orientation- and position-tuned simple cells (in V1) at the bottom of the hierarchy view-tuned cells (in inferotemporal cortex) at the top of the hierarchy. Contemporary probabilistic models (e.g., Lee & Mumford, 2003; Friston, 2005) recapitulate this framework in the language of statistical inference: Visual cortex is inverting an internal "image model" to recover the latent objects that generated the sensory inputs. These models have in common an essentially inferential characterization of visual cortex.

Theories of this sort, if they consider utility at all, view it as entering at a fairly late stage of the processing stream, and experiments on vision throughout the hierarchy tend to consider perceptual variables in isolation from affective ones. All this is licensed, or indeed mandated, by the segregation of probability and utility in statistical decision theory (Bossaerts et al., 2008).

If the role of visual perception is ultimately to estimate a distribution over states, does this estimate have a discrete neural correlate? Perhaps the most detailed and compelling answer comes from studies of motion perception. Here, the state being inferred is the direction of dot motion given noisy sensory information. Newsome, Britten, and Movshon (1989) recorded from direction-selective neurons in visual area MT while monkeys performed what is now known as the "random dots" task: Monkeys view a display of randomly and coherently moving dots intermixed and must report the direction of the coherent motion to earn a juice reward. Neurons in MT appear to report instantaneous motion energy; aggregating their spikes over time allows estimating the state (i.e., the motion direction). Indeed, varying the coherence of motion energy, the experimenters showed a remarkable correspondence between physiologic discrimination curves from aggregated spikes and psychophysical discrimination curves from monkeys' behavioral reports. A follow-up study by Salzman, Britten, and Newsome (1990) established the causal nature of this relationship by showing that microstimulation of these neurons systematically biased the reported direction of motion.

The brain appears to perform an analogous integration of instantaneous motion energy into an aggregate state estimate one synapse downstream from MT, in the lateral intraparietal area (LIP). There, Shadlen and Newsome (2001) observed direction-selective neurons that appeared to integrate motion evidence over time in a manner that predicted the timing of behavioral responses. These and other data were interpreted in terms of classical signal detection concepts (Gold & Shadlen, 2002), with LIP neurons reporting a log-likelihood ratio for motion direction (the "weight of evidence") based on sensory evidence provided by inputs from MT.[2] It is worth noting here that while these signal detection variables are computational-level quantities, it is principally their process-level dynamics (e.g., the accumulation of log-likelihood and its equivalence to a bounded diffusion process) that are the objects of study. Indeed, the dynamical content of these theories has been studied in isolation (Bogacz et al., 2006).

So far so good. On this view, the visual system (areas V1 and MT) furnishes LIP with sensory evidence, which in turn computes a quantity (the weight of evidence) directly related to the posterior distribution over motion direction. Note, however, that the utility function in the dots task is essentially trivial (e.g., one for a correct report of motion direction, and zero for an incorrect one). As mentioned, statistical decision theory licenses the search for state estimation while ignoring utility; in contrast, because of the simple form of the utility function, the overall expected utility is just proportional to the likelihood in the random dots task, and so these functions cannot be distinguished.

13.3.2   Utility

What about utility? A mostly separate body of work studies the mapping from states and actions to their utilities. Although there are a number of neural players involved in valuation, the most detailed work concerns the putative involvement of the midbrain dopamine system and its targets in learning the utilities that follow different states and actions. In this work, in a sort of mirror image of the simplistic utility function used in perceptual investigations such as the random dots task, the state is typically taken as unitary and wholly observed, posing no difficulties of ambiguous or uncertain perception.

Even given perceptual certainty, research on valuation generally assumes—both theoretically and in its experimental designs—that there is additional, irreducible stochasticity in the consequences subsequent to a state: For instance, a particular (wholly identifiable) picture might be followed by juice on half of trials, chosen randomly. In equation (1), this stochasticity might be characterized by folding it into the state (e.g., defining two states for the picture, differentially rewarded albeit perceptually indistinguishable). However, in the interest of separating perceptual uncertainty from stochasticity in state and outcome dynamics, outcome stochasticity can equivalently be characterized by introducing a nested level of averaging in equation (1), over the outcomes according to their probability given the state.[3] Much work concerns incremental learning rules for taking a running average over experienced outcomes' utilities, so as to learn an estimate of their expectation; this is the purview of reinforcement learning (for a recent review, see Niv, 2009). In particular, prominent accounts of the responses of dopamine neurons suggest that they carry a "reward prediction error" signal for updating such a running average (Schultz, Dayan, & Montague, 1997). The targets of these neurons, notably in the striatum and prefrontal cortex, are believed to be involved in valuation and action selection (Montague, King-Casas, & Cohen, 2006).

Insofar as this strategy already suggests an alternative to the staged representation of probabilities and utilities—because it directly learns utilities in expectation over outcome stochasticity and so forgoes representing their decomposition into separate outcome probabilities and utilities—these theories suggest an alternative to the simple, two-stage mapping of decision theory onto the brain. However, again distinguishing uncertainty about the perceptual state from stochasticity in its consequences, these mechanisms do seem to fit the bill as the complement to the perceptual state inference systems discussed earlier: They map a given (assumed known) perceptual state and action to its utility (the latter in expectation over outcome stochasticity).

Indeed, numerous authors (Daw, Courville, & Touretzky, 2006; Dayan & Daw, 2008; Braun, Mehring, & Wolpert, 2010; Gershman & Niv, 2010; Rao, 2010) have argued that the full problem of decision making under perceptual uncertainty—when both the perceptual state and the utilities are unknown and nontrivial—can essentially be treated by the composition of these two mechanisms: a perceptual state inference mechanism along the lines of Gold and Shadlen (2002), and a state utility learning mechanism of the sort described by Schultz et al. (1997). These ideas recapitulate the two-stage probability-utility architecture envisioned by statistical decision theory.

13.3.3 Challenges

The full story, however, is not so simple. First, abundant evidence indicates that reward modulation occurs at all levels of the visual hierarchy, including V1 (Shuler & Bear, 2006; Serences, 2008) and even before that in the lateral geniculate nucleus (Komura et al., 2001; O'Connor, Fukui, Pinsk, & Kastner, 2002). For example, Shuler and Bear (2006) trained rats to associate monocular stimulation with liquid reward and found that V1 neurons altered their firing patterns to predict the timing of reward. Second, the visual system appears to sacrifice probabilistic fidelity increased sensitivity to behaviorally relevant (i.e., highly rewarding) stimuli. Machens, Gollisch, Kolesnikova, and Herz (2005) measured the sound ensembles that are preferentially encoded by grasshopper auditory receptor neurons and found that the distribution of optimal stimulus ensembles diverged from the distribution of natural sounds. Specifically, the ensembles were concentrated in a region of stimulus space occupied by mating signals. This finding also has important implications for approximate inference schemes, which we revisit in section 13.5.2.

More specific to the particular ideas and areas discussed here, if visual responses in the lateral geniculate nucleus are already reward-modulated, the idea of far-downstream LIP as a pure representation of posterior state probability is dubious. Indeed, other work varying rewarding outcomes for actions (Platt & Glimcher, 1999; Sugrue, Corrado, & Newsome, 2004) shows that neurons in LIP are indeed modulated by the probability and amount of reward expected for an action—probably better thought of as related to expected utility rather than state probability per se. (Recall that the dots task essentially confounds these two quantities.) Moreover, area LIP is a poor candidate for a purely perceptual representation of perceived state, as it is a transitional area involved not just in visual perception but also action, specifically saccade control. (Monkeys in these experiments use saccades to signal their motion judgments.) But recall that area LIP is only one synapse downstream from the instantaneous motion energy representation in MT. If it already represents expected utility of saccades, there seems to be no candidate for an intermediate stage of pure probability representation over states.

A different source of contrary evidence comes from behavioral economics. The classic Ellsberg paradox (Ellsberg, 1961) revealed preferences in human choice behavior that are *not* probabilistically sophisticated. The example given by Ellsberg involves drawing a ball from an urn containing 30 red balls and 60 black or yellow balls in an unknown proportion. Subjects are asked to choose between pairs of gambles (A versus B or C versus D) drawn from the following set:

	Red	Yellow	Black
A	$100	$0	$0
B	$0	$100	$0
C	$100	$0	$100
D	$0	$100	$100

Experimentally, subjects prefer A over B and D over C. The intuitive reasoning is that in gambles A and D, the probability of winning $100 is known (unambiguous), whereas in B and C it is unknown (ambiguous). Hence, this pattern of preferences is sometimes known as *ambiguity aversion* and has been repeatedly demonstrated in a variety of paradigms (for a recent review, see Loewenstein, Rick, & Cohen, 2008). Crucially, there is *no* subjective probability distribution that can produce this pattern of preferences. This is widely regarded as violating the assumption of probability-utility segregation in statistical decision theory. In summary, despite the fact that researchers have worked separately on perception and utility, data from both physiology and behavior speak against a clean separation of systems. Addressing these discrepancies theoretically is a major task. The data appear to demand algorithms with richer dynamical interactions between perceptual and motivational systems. In section 13.5, we discuss several possible approaches.

13.4 Approximate Inference

In this section, we discuss a key algorithmic challenge for decision theory: calculating expectations under the posterior. When the hidden state s is high-dimensional and continuous, analytical tractability is elusive, and some form of approximation must be used. As we discuss later, such methods preserve an (approximate) mapping to the ideal decision variables, but they make different claims about the series of steps used to (approximately) compute them. Often, the signatures of these different approximation steps have been argued to be reflected in the dynamics of behavior (e.g., of learning or perception).

Computing posterior distributions approximately is a common problem in statistics and machine learning, where the approaches tend to fall into one of two classes:

- *Monte Carlo approximations* (Robert & Casella, 2004), where the posterior is approximated by a set of samples $s^{1:M}$. The law of large numbers guarantees that as M gets larger, the approximation converges to the true posterior. Generally, one cannot draw samples directly from the posterior, so two variations of the method are typically used. In *importance sampling*, samples are drawn from a proposal distribution $g(s)$ and then weighted according to:

$$w^m \propto \frac{p(x \mid s^m)p(s^m)}{g(s^m)}. \tag{13.3}$$

The Monte Carlo approximation of expected utility is then given by

$$\mathbb{E}_\pi[U(s,a)] \approx \sum_{m=1}^{M} w^m U(s^m, a). \qquad (13.4)$$

For certain generative models, an online version of importance sampling, known as *particle filtering*, is also possible, where the weights are updated after each observation. The second variation is known as *Markov chain Monte Carlo* and involves drawing the samples from a Markov chain whose stationary distribution is the posterior. Thus, sampling from the chain for long enough will eventually produce (unweighted) samples from the posterior.

· *Variational approximations* (Jordan, Ghahramani, Jaakkola, & Saul, 1999), where the posterior is approximated by a more tractable distribution q chosen from a family of distributions $\mathcal{Q}$ so as to minimize the Kullback–Leibler (KL) divergence between q and π:

$$q^* = \mathrm{argmin}_{q \in \mathcal{Q}} \ \mathrm{KL}(q \,\|\, \pi), \qquad (13.5)$$

where the KL divergence is defined as

$$\mathrm{KL}(q \,\|\, \pi) = \int_s q(s) \log \frac{q(s)}{\pi(s \mid x)} \, ds. \qquad (13.6)$$

The KL divergence is minimized (to zero) when $q = \pi$, but generally π is not in $\mathcal{Q}$. The expected utility can then be approximated by $\mathbb{E}_q[U(s,a)]$, which by design should be tractable.

All of these variations have recently been explored in different contexts. Sanborn, Griffiths, Navarro, To, and Sanborn (2010) suggested that human categorization phenomena are well described by a version of particle filtering, and Daw and Courville (2008) have made a similar argument in the context of animal conditioning. Markov chain Monte Carlo approximations have been suggested as explanations for the dynamics of perceptual multistability (Gershman, Vul, & Tenenbaum, 2009). Variational methods, while underappreciated, have begun to be considered as possible explanation for various associative learning phenomena (Daw, Courville, & Dayan, 2008; Sanborn & Silva, 2009).

None of these algorithmic models has yet been explored systematically in the context of decision theory. However, several experimental findings are suggestive. Most Bayesian models assume that the posterior changes gradually as more information is acquired, and consequently the expected utility should change gradually as well. In a choice task, for example, the animal is tasked with estimating the expected utility associated with each choice, where the hidden state represents a scalar association parameter governing the relationship between choice and reward (Kruschke, 2008). Assuming humans and animals are "soft" maximizers, gradual changes in expected utility imply gradual changes in choice behavior. However, careful analysis reveals that, at the individual subject level, the dynamics of choice behavior are quite different: Responses appear to change abruptly over the course of learning and never to reach stable asymptote (Gallistel, Fairhurst, & Balsam, 2004). One explanation, proposed by Daw and Courville (2008), is that subjects use a Monte Carlo approximation like particle filtering to approximate the posterior, and abrupt changes arise from the stochastic nature of the sampling process when only a small number of samples are used.

Another suggestive experimental finding is an effect known as *highlighting* (Medin & Bettger, 1991; Kruschke, 1996), which concerns the trial order–dependent dynamics of the learning of predictions about cues. In the balanced version of the experimental design, subjects are presented with three cues (A, B, and C) and two outcomes (R and S). In the first phase, subjects observe $AB \rightarrow R$ three times as often as $AC \rightarrow S$. In the second phase, the same contingencies are preserved, but the proportions are reversed: now $AC \rightarrow S$ occurs three times as often as $AB \rightarrow R$. When tested with A alone, subjects predict R (a primacy effect), whereas when tested with the novel compound BC, subjects predict S (a recency effect). As shown by Kruschke (2006), this combination of primacy and recency effects is very difficult to explain by normative Bayesian models. Instead, Kruschke showed that an approximate learning algorithm, which he named "locally Bayesian learning," could explain these effects by propagating sufficient statistics (rather than full posterior distributions) between layers in a neural network. The basic insight was that the local propagation induces sequential dependencies even when the underlying generative model lacks such dependencies. Later work by Sanborn and Silva (2009) showed that locally Bayesian learning could be interpreted as a variational message-passing algorithm and suggested other elaborations in the same family of algorithms (see also Daw et al., 2008).

13.5   New Vistas

We have so far treated approximate inference as an inherently probabilistic computation, consistent with the decision-theoretic framework.

However, what is mainly interesting about these inference schemes is that they suggest ways of weakening or abandoning the separation between probabilities and utilities. We discuss two possible versions of this revision. The first answer attempts to reframe decision theory purely in terms of inference; that is, to dispense with a privileged concept of utility and deal entirely with probabilities. In this setting, utilities influence probabilistic approximations in the same manner as other variables. The second answer attempts to stay within the decision-theoretic framework but ups the ante by treating the approximations themselves as decisions, with costs determined by the computational effort required by the approximations.

13.5.1 Decision Making as Probabilistic Inference

A rich vein of recent work in machine learning has explored the idea that decision problems can be reframed as inference problems (Dayan & Hinton, 1997; Toussaint & Storkey, 2006; Hoffman, de Freitas, Doucet, & Peters, 2009; Vlassis & Toussaint, 2009; Theodorou, Buchli, & Schaal, 2010). Although these approaches differ in their precise mathematical formulation, the common idea is that by transforming the utility function appropriately, one can treat it as a probability density function parameterized by the action and hidden state. Consequently, maximizing the "probability" of utility with respect to action, while marginalizing the hidden state, is formally equivalent to maximizing the expected utility. That is, sensory inference is optimization—of the posterior probability of the causes, given the data—and the optimization underlying utility maximization can be framed in parallel terms.

Although this is more or less an algebraic maneuver, it has profound implications for the organization of decision-making circuitry in the brain. In machine learning, the importance of this insight has been that the stable of approximations and tricks that have been developed to tame difficult problems of probabilistic inference can also be applied to action optimization. The neuroscientific version of this insight is that what appear to be dedicated motivational and valuation circuits may instead be regarded as parallel applications of the same underlying computational mechanisms over effectively different likelihood functions.

One version of this idea has been explored by Botvinick and An (2009). Building on earlier work in computer science (Cooper, 1988; Tatman & Shachter, 1990), Botvinick and An argued that the dorsolateral prefrontal cortex (DLPFC) could be thought of as computing action policies by iteratively updating probabilistic beliefs over action nodes in a kind of directed graphical model known as an "influence diagram." They proved that this algorithm converges to the optimal policy and then went on to show that it could reproduce several behavioral signatures of goal-directed behavior commonly associated with the DLPFC (see also Daw, Niv, & Dayan, 2005).

The most detailed articulation of common mechanisms for inference and decision, however, has come from the work of Karl Friston and his colleagues (for a recent review, see Friston, 2010). Friston has argued that many aspects of neural computation can be subsumed under a single "free-energy principle." To understand this principle, let us return briefly to the variational approximation described in section 13.4. A basic identity from probability theory defines the relationship between the KL divergence and the marginal likelihood $p(x) = \int_s p(x \mid s)p(s)ds$:

$$\mathrm{KL}(q \parallel \pi) = \log p(x) + \mathcal{F}(x,s), \tag{13.7}$$

where $\mathcal{F}(x,s)$ is known as the *free energy* in statistical physics. In the context of perceptual inference in neuroscience, the marginal likelihood can be understood as a measure of how well the brain's internal model explains its sensory inputs, after integrating out the causes of the inputs. Because the KL divergence is always non-negative, the negative free-energy is a lower bound on the log marginal likelihood. Thus, optimizing an internal model by minimizing free energy (with respect to the model parameters) is equivalent to maximizing a lower bound on the log marginal likelihood.

Friston and colleagues (Friston, Daunizeau, & Kiebel, 2009; Friston, Daunizeau, Kilner, & Kiebel, 2010) formulate the decision optimization problem in these terms. There are at least two separable claims here. The technical thrust of the work is similar to the ideas discussed earlier: If one specifies a desired equilibrium state distribution (here playing the role of the utility function), then this can be optimized by free-energy minimization with respect to actions. However, the authors build on this foundation to assert a much more provocative concept: that for biologically evolved organisms, the desired equilibrium is by definition just the species' evolved equilibrium state distribution, and so minimizing free energy with respect to actions is, in effect, equivalent to maximizing expected utility. What makes this claim provocative is that it rejects decision theory's core distinction between a state's likelihood and its utility: Nowhere in the definition of free energy is utility mentioned. The mathematical equivalence rests on the evolutionary argument that hidden states with high prior probability also tend to have high utility. This situation arises through a combination of evolution and ontogenetic development, whereby the brain is immersed in a "statistical bath" that prescribes the landscape of its prior distribution. Because agents who find themselves more often in congenial states are more likely to survive, they inherit (or develop) priors with modes located at the states of highest congeniality. Conversely, states that are surprising given your evolutionary niche—like being out of water, for a fish—are maladaptive and should be avoided.

Although the free-energy principle appears at the least to be a very useful formulation for exposing the computational parallelism between perceptual and decision problems, the more radical maneuver of treating them both as literally optimizing a single objective function is harder to swallow. A state's equilibrium likelihood and its utility are, on the classical view, not the same thing; rare events might be either unusually bad (being out of water, for a fish), good (being elected president, for an African American), or indeed neither. The idea that the two are united within a biological niche seems in one sense to appeal to evolutionary considerations to the end of substituting equilibrium for evolution and risks precluding adaption or learning. Should the first amphibian out of water dive back in? If a wolf eats deer not because he is hungry but because he is attracted to the equilibrium state of his ancestors, would a sudden bonanza of deer inspire him to eat only the amount to which he is accustomed? How can he adapt his diet if an ice age arises, or a new competitive deer-eating predator? Should a person immersed in the "statistical bath" of poverty her entire life refuse a winning lottery ticket, as this would necessitate transitioning from a state of high equilibrium probability to a rare one? In all these cases, the possibility of upward mobility, within the individual, seems to rest on at least some role for traditional notions of utility or fitness in guiding their decisions. However, the idea remains intriguing that in the ethological setting, these have more in common with probability than a decision theorist might expect.

13.5.2 The Costs of Representation and Computation

Probabilistic computations make exorbitant demands on a limited resource, and in a real physiological and psychological sense, these demands incur a cost that debits the utility of action. As shown in recent experiments by Kool, McGuire, Rosen, and Botvinick (2010), humans are "cognitive misers" who seek to avoid effortful thought at every opportunity, and this effort diminishes the same neural signals that are excited by reward (Botvinick, Huffstetler, & McGuire, 2009).

One example of this issue arises in representing probability distributions over future states. We have mentioned already that predominant accounts of the dopamine system suggest that this system learns utilities in expectation over stochastic future states, rather than adopting the full decision-theoretically motivated representation of learning the probabilities of outcomes, and their utilities, separately, and computing utilities by integrating over them. (In reinforcement learning, the latter approach is known as "model-based.") These representations can actually be distinguished by clever experiments probing how behavior reacts to abrupt changes in circumstances. For instance, one can study whether a rat who has learned to lever-press for food while hungry will continue to do so when full: A full probabilistic representation over outcomes will adjust its expected utilities to the changed outcome value, whereas representing utilities only in expectation can preclude this and so predicts hapless working for unwanted food. The upshot of many such experiments is that the brain adopts both approaches, depending on circumstances. As suggested by Daw et al. (2005) and Keramati, Dezfouli, and Piray (2011), which circumstances elicit which approach can be explained by a sort of meta-optimization over the costs (e.g., extra computation) of maintaining the full representation relative to its benefits (better statistical accuracy).

Thus, whether to represent a probability distribution over states, altogether, may itself be subject to (meta) decision-theoretic analysis. Assuming the agent does represent probabilities, a finer question is how these should be approximated. Making the natural assumption that more accurate approximations of the posterior incur larger costs, it would make sense for the brain to seek an approximation that balanced the costs of computation against the utility of accuracy. However, this principle appears to make a strict segregation of probability and reward not only impossible but foolhardy.

Consider a simple Monte Carlo scheme for approximating expected utilities by drawing samples from the state distribution. Vul, Goodman, Griffiths, and Tenenbaum (2009) analyzed the effects of imposing sampling costs on an such an agent. They showed, using a simple two-alternative forced-choice example and levels of sampling cost, that maximal total expected utility (gains minus costs) is achieved with remarkably few samples (of the order 1–50), which was argued to capture phenomena such as probability matching observed in humans playing similar tasks. A key feature of this cost–benefit analysis of approximation is that it crosscuts probability and utility: The costs of adopting more or less faithful approximation to the probability must be weighed against the utility foregone by making worse decisions.

A more general analysis of this problem was recently undertaken by Gershman and Wilson (2010), exploring the idea that the brain might adopt approximate forms of the probability distribution over states and treat its choice of which approximation to use as a "meta-decision." They incorporated a neurally motivated approximation cost into the utility function and then derived a variational lower bound on the log expected utility (closely related to the free-energy bound on the log marginal likelihood). By maximizing this bound with respect to the choice of approximate distribution, the agent can near-optimally balance the costs and benefits of accurately approximating the state distribution. They showed that this model could account for the finding by Machens et al. (2005) that auditory representations seem to overrepresent behaviorally relevant signals (like mating calls). The basic idea is that approximate distributions that represent the entire auditory spectrum with high fidelity are metabolically costly and that accurately representing low-utility auditory signals is metabolically wasteful. Thus, approximations that concentrate their density in regions of high utility will achieve a higher utility lower bound. Finally, then, choosing appropriate approximations at the sensory level pushes utility considerations back to this level, perhaps explaining why the brain seems not to respect this basic decision-theoretic distinction.

13.6 Conclusion

This chapter has attempted to demonstrate that although statistical decision theory provides a tantalizingly simple framework for decision making, the neural reality is not so simple: Perception, action, and utility are ensnared in a tangled skein. To unravel this skein—or at least to motivate its tangle—we have pointed to new ideas that reconfigure the relationships between these variables and that suggest novel organizations for the underlying neural systems. These novel organizations involve a richer ensemble of dynamical interactions between perceptual and motivational systems than that which is anticipated by statistical decision theory, and some of the signatures of these processes appear to coincide with the dynamics of behavior and neural signals.

The ideas discussed in this chapter borrow from recent as well as old computational concepts from artificial intelligence, engineering, statistics, and physics. There still remain many ideas from these sources that have yet to percolate into the consciousness of neuroscientists. For example, an extremely rich research tradition in artificial intelligence has examined how to incorporate computational costs into decision-making systems (e.g., Horvitz, 1988; Russell & Wefald, 1991; Zilberstein, 1995). We hope that contact with these ideas will reinvigorate thinking about the organizational principles of the brain.

Acknowledgments

S.J.G. was supported by a graduate research fellowship from the National Science Foundation. N.D.D. was supported by a Scholar Award from the McKnight Foundation, a Young Investigator Award from NARSAD, and NIH grant MH087882.

Notes

1. Our treatment is more precisely characterized as Bayesian decision theory, which is the most widely used special case of statistical decision theory. For discussion of alternatives to Bayesian decision theory, see Berger (1985). Some of these alternatives are considered in the context of vision by Maloney and Zhang (2010) and in the context of two-alternative forced choice tasks by Zacksenhouse, Bogacz, and Holmes (2010).

2. The log-likelihood ratio is equivalent to the log-posterior odds ratio under a uniform prior.

3. More generally, states may occur in sequence, and the aggregate value will depend on a series of nested expectations over each successive state, as in the Bellman equation defining utility in a Markov decision process (Sutton & Barto, 1998).

References

Berger, J. (1985). *Statistical Decision Theory and Bayesian Analysis*. Berlin: Springer.

Bogacz, R., Brown, E., Moehlis, J., Holmes, P., & Cohen, J. (2006). The physics of optimal decision making: a formal analysis of models of performance in two-alternative forced-choice tasks. *Psychological Review*, *113*(4), 700–765.

Bossaerts, P., Preuschoff, K., & Hsu, M. (2008). The neurobiological foundations of valuation in human decision making under uncertainty. In P. W. Glimcher, C. F. Camerer, E. Fehr, & R. A. Poldrack (Eds.), *Neuroeconomics: Decision Making and the Brain* (pp. 351–364). New York: Elsevier Press.

Botvinick, M., & An, J. (2009). Goal-directed decision making in prefrontal cortex: a computational framework. *Advances in Neural Information Processing Systems*, *21*, 169–176.

Botvinick, M., Huffstetler, S., & McGuire, J. (2009). Effort discounting in human nucleus accumbens. *Cognitive, Affective & Behavioral Neuroscience*, *9*(1), 16.

Braun, D., Mehring, C., & Wolpert, D. (2010). Structure learning in action. *Behavioural Brain Research*, *206*(2), 157–165.

Camerer, C. (1998). Bounded rationality in individual decision making. *Experimental Economics*, *1*(2), 163–183.

Cooper, G. (1988). A method for using belief networks as influence diagrams. In Workshop on Uncertainty in Artificial Intelligence (pp. 55–63). Minneapolis: Association for Uncertainty in AI.

Daw, N., & Courville, A. (2008). The pigeon as particle filter. *Advances in Neural Information Processing Systems, 20*, 369–376.

Daw, N., Courville, A., & Dayan, P. (2008). Semi-rational models of conditioning: The case of trial order. In N. Chater & M. Oaksford (Eds.), *The Probabilistic Mind: Prospects for Bayesian Cognitive Science* (pp. 431–452). Oxford: Oxford University Press.

Daw, N., Courville, A., & Touretzky, D. (2006). Representation and timing in theories of the dopamine system. *Neural Computation, 18*(7), 1637–1677.

Daw, N., Niv, Y., & Dayan, P. (2005). Uncertainty-based competition between prefrontal and dorsolateral striatal systems for behavioral control. *Nature Neuroscience, 8*(12), 1704–1711.

Dayan, P., & Daw, N. (2008). Decision theory, reinforcement learning, and the brain. *Cognitive, Affective & Behavioral Neuroscience, 8*(4), 429–453.

Dayan, P., & Hinton, G. (1997). Using expectation-maximization for reinforcement learning. *Neural Computation, 9*(2), 271–278.

Ellsberg, D. (1961). Risk, ambiguity, and the Savage axioms. *Quarterly Journal of Economics, 75*(4), 643–669.

Friston, K. (2005). A theory of cortical responses. *Philosophical Transactions of the Royal Society B. Biological Sciences, 360*(1456), 815.

Friston, K. (2010). The free-energy principle: a unified brain theory? *Nature Reviews. Neuroscience, 11*(2), 127–138.

Friston, K., Daunizeau, J., & Kiebel, S. (2009). Reinforcement learning or active inference. *PLoS One, 4*(7), e6421.

Friston, K., Daunizeau, J., Kilner, J., & Kiebel, S. (2010). Action and behavior: a free-energy formulation. *Biological Cybernetics, 102*(3), 227–260.

Gallistel, C., Fairhurst, S., & Balsam, P. (2004). The learning curve: implications of a quantitative analysis. *Proceedings of the National Academy of Sciences of the United States of America, 101*(36), 13124.

Gershman, S., & Niv, Y. (2010). Learning latent structure: carving nature at its joints. *Current Opinion in Neurobiology, 20*(2), 251–256.

Gershman, S., & Wilson, R. (2010). The neural costs of optimal control. In J. Lafferty, C. K. I. Williams, J. Shawe-Taylor, R.S. Zemel, & A. Culotta (Eds.), Advances in Neural Information Processing Systems 23 (pp. 712–720). Vancouver, Canada.

Gershman, S., Vul, E., & Tenenbaum, J. (2009). Perceptual multistability as Markov chain Monte Carlo inference. In Y. Bengio, D. Schuurmans, J. Lafferty, C. K. I. Williams, & A. Culotta (Eds.), Advances in Neural Information Processing Systems 22 (pp. 611–619.) Vancouver, Canada.

Glimcher, P. (2003). *Decisions, Uncertainty, and the Brain: The Science of Neuroeconomics.* Cambridge, MA: MIT Press.

Gold, J., & Shadlen, M. (2002). Banburismus and the brain: decoding the relationship between sensory stimuli, decisions, and reward. *Neuron, 36*(2), 299–308.

Green, D., & Swets, J. (1966). *Signal Detection Theory and Psychophysics.* New York: Wiley.

Hoffman, M., de Freitas, N., Doucet, A., & Peters, J. (2009). An expectation maximization algorithm for continuous Markov decision processes with arbitrary rewards. In D. von Dyk & M. Welling (Eds.), Twelfth International Conference on Artificial Intelligence and Statistics. Citeseer (pp. 232–239). Clearwater Beach, FL.

Horvitz, E. (1988). Reasoning about beliefs and actions under computational resource constraints. *International Journal of Approximate Reasoning, 2*(3), 337–338.

Jordan, M., Ghahramani, Z., Jaakkola, T., & Saul, L. (1999). An introduction to variational methods for graphical models. *Machine Learning*, *37*(2), 183–233.

Kahneman, D., & Tversky, A. (1979). Prospect theory: an analysis of decision under risk. *Econometrica*, *47*, 263–291.

Keramati, M., Dezfouli, A., & Piray, P. (2011). Speed/accuracy trade-off between the habitual and the goal-directed processes. *PLoS Computational Biology*, *7*(5), e1002055.

Knill, D., & Pouget, A. (2004). The Bayesian brain: the role of uncertainty in neural coding and computation. *Trends in Neurosciences*, *27*(12), 712–719.

Komura, Y., Tamura, R., Uwano, T., Nishijo, H., Kaga, K., & Ono, T. (2001). Retrospective and prospective coding for predicted reward in the sensory thalamus. *Nature*, *412*(6846), 546–549.

Kool, W., McGuire, J., Rosen, Z., & Botvinick, M. (2010). Decision making and the avoidance of cognitive demand. *Journal of Experimental Psychology. General*, *139*, 665–682.

Kording, K., & Wolpert, D. (2006). Bayesian decision theory in sensorimotor control. *Trends in Cognitive Sciences*, *10*(7), 319–326.

Kruschke, J. (1996). Base rates in category learning. *Journal of Experimental Psychology. Learning, Memory, and Cognition*, *22*(1), 3–26.

Kruschke, J. (2006). Locally Bayesian learning with applications to retrospective revaluation and highlighting. *Psychological Review*, *113*(4), 677–698.

Kruschke, J. (2008). Bayesian approaches to associative learning: from passive to active learning. *Learning & Behavior*, *36*(3), 210.

Lee, T., & Mumford, D. (2003). Hierarchical Bayesian inference in the visual cortex. *JOSA A*, *20*(7), 1434–1448.

Loewenstein, G., Rick, S., & Cohen, J. (2008). Neuroeconomics. *Annual Review of Psychology*, *59*, 647–672.

Machens, C., Gollisch, T., Kolesnikova, O., & Herz, A. (2005). Testing the efficiency of sensory coding with optimal stimulus ensembles. *Neuron*, *47*(3), 447–456.

Machina, M., & Schmeidler, D. (1992). A more robust definition of subjective probability. *Econometrica*, *60*(4), 745–780.

Maloney, L., & Zhang, H. (2010). Decision-theoretic models of visual perception and action. *Vision Research*, *50*, 2362–2374.

McNamara, J., & Houston, A. (1980). The application of statistical decision theory to animal behaviour. *Journal of Theoretical Biology*, *85*(4), 673–690.

Medin, D., & Bettger, J. (1991). Sensitivity to changes in base-rate information. *American Journal of Psychology*, *104*(3), 311–332.

Montague, P., King-Casas, B., & Cohen, J. (2006). Imaging valuation models in human choice. *Annual Review of Neuroscience*, *29*, 417–448.

Newsome, W., Britten, K., & Movshon, J. (1989). Neuronal correlates of a perceptual decision. *Nature*, *341*(6237), 52–54.

Niv, Y. (2009). Reinforcement learning in the brain. *Journal of Mathematical Psychology*, *53*(3), 139–154.

O'Connor, D., Fukui, M., Pinsk, M., & Kastner, S. (2002). Attention modulates responses in the human lateral geniculate nucleus. *Nature Neuroscience*, *5*(11), 1203–1209.

Platt, M., & Glimcher, P. (1999). Neural correlates of decision variables in parietal cortex. *Nature*, *400*(6741), 233–238.

Rao, R. (2010). Decision making under uncertainty: a neural model based on partially observable Markov decision processes. *Frontiers in Computational Neuroscience*, *4*, 1–18.

Riesenhuber, M., & Poggio, T. (1999). Hierarchical models of object recognition in cortex. *Nature Neuroscience*, *2*, 1019–1025.

Robert, C., & Casella, G. (2004). *Monte Carlo Statistical Methods*. Berlin: Springer-Verlag.

Russell, S., & Wefald, E. (1991). Principles of metareasoning. *Artificial Intelligence*, *49*(1–3), 361–395.

Salzman, C., Britten, K., & Newsome, W. (1990). Cortical microstimulation influences perceptual judgements of motion direction. *Nature*, *346*(6280), 174–177.

Sanborn, A., & Silva, R. (2009). Belief propagation and locally Bayesian learning. In N. Taatgen & H. van Rijn (Eds.), Proceedings of the 31st Annual Conference of the Cognitive Science Society. Vol. 31. Edinburgh, Scotland

Sanborn, A., Griffiths, T., Navarro, D., To, S., & Sanborn, A. (2010). Rational approximations to rational models: Alternative algorithms for category learning. *Psychological Review*, *117*(4), 1144–1167.

Savage, L. (1954). *The Foundations of Statistics*. New York: John Wiley & Sons.

Schultz, W., Dayan, P., & Montague, P. (1997). A neural substrate of prediction and reward. *Science*, *275*(5306), 1593.

Serences, J. (2008). Value-based modulations in human visual cortex. *Neuron*, *60*(6), 1169–1181.

Shadlen, M., & Newsome, W. (2001). Neural basis of a perceptual decision in the parietal cortex (area LIP) of the rhesus monkey. *Journal of Neurophysiology*, *86*(4), 1916.

Shuler, M., & Bear, M. (2006). Reward timing in the primary visual cortex. *Science*, *311*(5767), 1606.

Stephens, D., & Krebs, J. (1986). *Foraging Theory*. Princeton, NJ: Princeton University Press.

Sugrue, L., Corrado, G., & Newsome, W. (2004). Matching behavior and the representation of value in the parietal cortex. *Science*, *304*(5678), 1782.

Sutton, R., & Barto, A. (1998). *Reinforcement Learning: An Introduction*. Cambridge, MA: MIT Press.

Tatman, J., & Shachter, R. (1990). Dynamic programming and influence diagrams. *IEEE Transactions on Systems, Man, and Cybernetics*, *20*(2), 365–379.

Theodorou, E., Buchli, J., & Schaal, S. (2010). Learning policy improvements with path integrals. In International Conference on Artificial Intelligence and Statistics. Editors: Y.W. Teh & M. Titterington. 9, 828:835.

Toussaint, M., & Storkey, A. (2006). Probabilistic inference for solving discrete and continuous state Markov decision processes. In W. Cohen & A. Moore (Eds.), Proceedings of the 23rd International Conference on Machine Learning (pp. 945–952). New York: ACM.

Trommershäuser, J., Maloney, L., & Landy, M. (2008). Decision making, movement planning and statistical decision theory. *Trends in Cognitive Sciences*, *12*(8), 291–297.

Vlassis, N., & Toussaint, M. (2009). Model-free reinforcement learning as mixture learning. In L. Bottou & M. Littman (Eds.), Proceedings of the 26th Annual International Conference on Machine Learning (pp. 1081–1088). New York: ACM.

Von Neumann, J., & Morgenstern, O. (1947). *Theory of Games and Economic Behavior*. Princeton, NJ: Princeton University Press.

Vul, E., Goodman, N., Griffiths, T., & Tenenbaum, J. (2009). One and done? Optimal decisions from very few samples. In N. Taatgen & H. van Rijn (Eds.), Proceedings of the 31st Annual Conference of the Cognitive Science Society (pp. 66–72). Edinburgh, Scotland

Zacksenhouse, M., Bogacz, R., & Holmes, P. (2010). Robust versus optimal strategies for two-alternative forced choice tasks. *Journal of Mathematical Psychology*, *54*(2), 230–246.

Zilberstein, S. (1995). Operational rationality through compilation of anytime algorithms. *AI Magazine*, *16*(2), 79.

14   Short Guide to Modern Nonlinear Dynamics

Valentin S. Afraimovich, Mikhail I. Rabinovich, and Pablo Varona

Summary

In this chapter we describe important concepts of modern nonlinear dynamics that contribute to understand different aspects of neural activity. We also provide comments on specific topics and experiments discussed throughout this book.

14.1   Dynamical Systems

14.1.1   Basic Notions

Processes in nature can roughly be divided into random or deterministic processes. Two realizations of a random process with identical initial conditions can be completely different, whereas they are the same for a deterministic process (Lichtenberg & Lieberman, 1992; Ott, 1992; Katok & Hasselblatt, 1995; Afraimovich & Hsu, 2002). Dynamical systems (DSs) are mathematical models of deterministic processes. In other words, a DS is a mathematical model of the evolution of a real system (physical, biological, economic, etc.) whose state at any instant of time $t > 0$ is uniquely determined by its initial state. A state of a DS is described by a collection of variables x that are chosen according to their capability for intrinsic interpretation and primality of description of data, symmetry, and so forth.

The set of the states forms the *phase space* of the DS. The definition of the DS includes also a collection of *evolution operators* $\varphi^t, t > 0$, that realize the law under which the system that starts at an initial point x_0 comes to a point x_t at the instant of time t.

The operators satisfy the "group identity"

$$\phi^{t_1+t_2} x_0 = \phi^{t_1} \left(\phi^{t_2} x_0 \right) = \phi^{t_2} \left(\phi^{t_1} x_0 \right)$$

valid for all initial points x_0 and all non-negative values of t_1, t_2. This reflects the simple fact that the DS arrives to the state $x_{t_1+t_2}$ successively spending first the amount t_1 of time and then t_2. Usually, the phase space $X = \{x\}$ is endowed with some structure—it is either a topological or metric space or even a differential manifold, and the operators (mappings) $\varphi^t : X \to X$ are continuous (piece-wise continuous) or smooth (piece-wise smooth). One distinguishes a DS with discrete and continuous times. A DS with continuous time is usually determined by ordinary differential equations (ODEs) $\dot{x} = F(x)$ where the evolution operators are given by solutions: $\phi^t x_0 := x(t, x_0)$. A DS with discrete time is generated by a map $f : X \to X$, so that $f^0 x = x, f^1 x = f(x), f^2 x = f[f(x)]$, and so forth.

A *trajectory* (an orbit) $\Gamma(x_0) := \bigcup_{t \geq 0} f^t x_0$ is a geometric image of a motion of the DS: the motion of the DS corresponds to the movement of a representative point under the action of the evolution operators along the trajectory. Such idea comes from French mathematicians of the nineteenth century (mainly, Henri Poincaré) and switches the attention from formulas to geometry, which has proved to be extremely helpful in the building of the DS theory.

For a DS with continuous time, a trajectory is usually a curve embedded into X, whereas for a DS with discrete time, a trajectory is a discrete set. For a DS with continuous time, an equilibrium state corresponds to a "degenerate curve," a point; a periodic motion corresponds to a closed curve; and a quasi-periodic motion with m basic frequencies corresponds to a curve on an m-dimensional torus embedded into the phase space. Motions in a DS with dissipation are divided into established regimes and transient processes.

In the phase space of a DS, an *attractor* corresponds to an established regime, an invariant set attracting all trajectories close to it. An established periodic oscillation corresponds to a *limit cycle*, an isolated closed curve. An established chaotic oscillation is related, generally, to a *strange attractor* consisting of unstable trajectories.

Different types of attractors are reflected in the form of the corresponding signals (observables) generated by a DS; see figure 14.1.

14.1.2 Types of Dynamical Systems

According to the type of equations and methods used for their study, DSs are partitioned into *finite dimensional* (DS with finite-dimensional phase space) and *infinite dimensional* (distributed). Conversely,

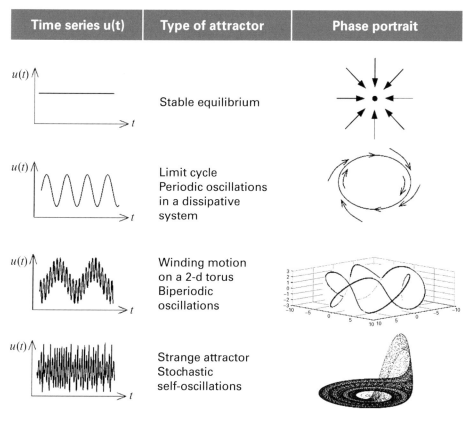

Time series u(t)	Type of attractor	Phase portrait

Figure 14.1
Illustration of different attractors.

finite-dimensional DSs are divided into *conservative* and *dissipative*. Conservative DSs preserve the phase volume. A very important class of conservative DSs consists of *Hamiltonian systems* with time-independent Hamiltonian functions.

In the phase space of a dissipative DS, there is an absorbing region (a ball of dissipation) such that each trajectory eventually comes to this region and does not leave it after that.

The motion of *structural stability* is very important for the theory of dissipative DS. A structurally stable DS is nonsensitive to small changes of parameters. Its motions before and after changing parameters are topologically identical (equivalent). Structurally stable DSs form open regions in a functional space of all DSs. Non–structurally stable DSs are situated outside these regions. The passage through a boundary of a region of a structurally stable DS is accompanied by a bifurcation—a shift in behavior of a DS (Arnold, Afraimovich, Ilyashenko, & Shilnikov, 1986; Kuznetsov, 1998). For a one-parameter family of DS, if one knows the structure of the DS for an initial value of the parameter and all bifurcations, one may predict its structure for the final value of the parameter. This is important because small changes in certain parameters of a nonlinear DS can cause, for instance, equilibria to appear or disappear or to change from attracting to repelling and vice versa, leading to large and sudden changes of the behavior of the system.

14.1.3 Equilibrium Points

An equilibrium point x_0 satisfies the equation $F(x_0) = 0$. The behavior of the trajectories in a neighborhood of x_0 depends on the roots $\lambda_1, \ldots, \lambda_n$

COMMENT 14.1
Limit Cycle and Strange Attractor in Neuronal Systems

There are several reports of demonstrated rhythmic (limit cycle) and chaotic (strange attractor) spontaneous activity of individual neurons in vitro (for a review, see Rabinovich & Abarbanel, 1998 and Korn & Faure, 2003). We present here several examples: Figure 14.C1 illustrates a limit cycle, the dynamical image of rhythmic spontaneous activity of an individual neuron; Figure 14.C2 illustrates the transformation of a limit cycle to a strange attractor in a bursting neuron by changing the control parameter; and figure 14.C3 displays the visualization of a chaotic attractor from averaged EEG data.

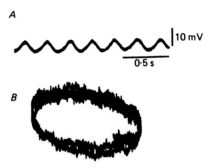

A

10 mV

0·5 s

B

Figure 14.C1
Spontaneous oscillations of an individual neuron (A) and its phase portrait (B). Adapted with permission from Llinas and Yarom (1986), copyright © Wiley, 1986.

COMMENT 14.1
(continued)

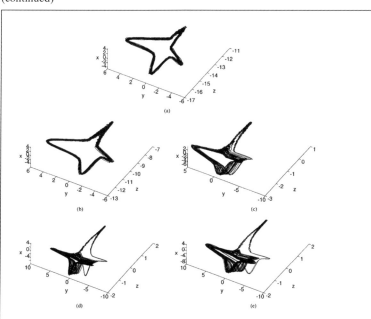

Figure 14.C2
State-space reconstructions from an isolated stomatogastric neuron for different values of the DC current injected as a stimulus: (a) I = 2 nA, (b) I = 1nA, (c) I = 0 nA, (d) I = –1 nA, (e) I = –2 nA. These phase portraits have been obtained applying singular value decomposition to a time-delay state-space reconstruction using a time delay of 5 ms (see Abarbanel et al., 1996).

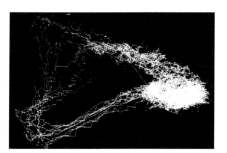

Figure 14.C3
Visualization of a chaotic attractor from averaged EEG data. Adapted with permission from Freeman (1988), copyright © IEEE, 1998.

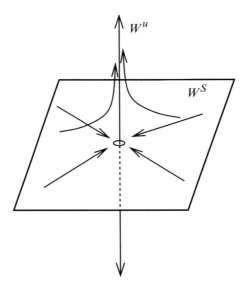

Figure 14.2
A phase portrait in the vicinity of a saddle equilibrium point.

of the characteristic equation $\det[DF(x_0) - \lambda \mathrm{Id}] = 0$. Let the real part Re $\lambda_i < 0, i = 1,\ldots,p$, and Re $\lambda_j > 0, j = p+1,\ldots,n$. If $p = n$ ($p = 0$), the point x_0 is called the stable (unstable) *node*. All trajectories going through points close to x_0 tend to x_0 as time $t \to +\infty$ for a stable node (and $t \to -\infty$ for an unstable node). If $p \neq n$ and $p \neq 0$, the point x_0 is said to be a *saddle*. It lies in the intersection of two surfaces: the p-dimensional stable *separatrix* $W^s_{x_0}$ and $(n - p)$-dimensional unstable separatrix $W^u_{x_0}$. They consist of trajectories that tend to x_0 as $t \to +\infty$ for $W^s_{x_0}$ and $t \to -\infty$ for $W^u_{x_0}$. Other trajectories leave the vicinity of the saddle as $t \to \pm\infty$ (figure 14.2). A trajectory belonging to the intersection $W^s_{x_0} \cap W^u_{x_0}$ different from x_0 is said to be *homoclinic*. If x_0 and x_1 are two saddles, then a trajectory belonging to $W^u_{x_0} \cap W^s_{x_1}$ is said to be *heteroclinic*.

14.1.4 Limit Cycles

A solution $x = \varphi(t)$ of the system $\dot{x} = F(x)$ is periodic if $p(t + T) = p(t)$ for each t where $T > 0$ is a period. A closed trajectory L in the phase space corresponds to such a solution. An isolated periodic trajectory is called a *limit cycle*. The behavior of the trajectories in the vicinity of L depends on the numbers $\gamma_1, \gamma_2,\ldots,\gamma_n$, called multipliers, which can be found

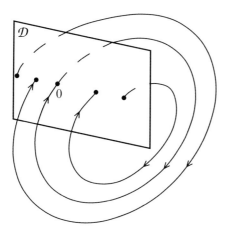

Figure 14.3
Trajectories in the neighborhood of a saddle limit cycle.

by solving the system linearized at L. One of the multipliers, say γ_n, is always 1. If $|\gamma_i| < 1$ ($|\gamma_i| > 1$) for $i = 1,2,\ldots,n-1$, then the trajectory L is stable (unstable). If p multipliers belong to the open disk of radius 1 centered at the origin of the complex plane, $p < n - 1$, and $n - 1 - p$ multipliers are greater than 1 by absolute value then L is a saddle-type trajectory. It belongs to the intersection of the $(p + 1)$-dimensional stable separatrix W_L^s and the $(n - p)$-dimensional unstable separatrix W_L^u. The surface W_L^s (W_L^u) consists of trajectories that tend to L as $t \to +\infty$ ($t \to -\infty$). If $n = 3, p = 1$, and $\gamma_1 > 1, 0 < \gamma_2 < 1$, then W_L^s (W_L^u) is a topological cylinder (figure 14.3).

One can study the behavior of trajectories in the vicinity of L by considering their traces on an $(n - 1)$-dimensional surface $\mathcal{D}$ (*Poincaré section*) that intersects transversally L and all trajectories close to L. If a point $m_0 \in \mathcal{D}$ is close enough to L, then a trajectory that goes through m_0 intersects $\mathcal{D}$ at another point m_1 so that a map $f : \mathcal{D}_1 \to \mathcal{D}$ (*Poincaré map*) is well defined where $\mathcal{D}_1 \subset \mathcal{D}$ is a small neighborhood of the point $\mathcal{O} := L \cap \mathcal{D}$ (see figure 14.4). The Poincaré map generates in fact a DS with discrete time. The map f is differentiable, and the eigenvalues of its differential (Jacobian matrix) at $\mathcal{O}$ are exactly multipliers $\gamma_1,\ldots,\gamma_{n-1}$ of L. If $|\gamma_i| \neq 1$ $i = 1,\ldots,n-1$, then $L(\mathcal{O})$ is called hyperbolic, and the behavior of the trajectories is completely determined by the system linearized at L (at $\mathcal{O}$). Only hyperbolic periodic trajectories are realized in a structurally stable DS. Changes of parameters of a DS may lead to the occurrence

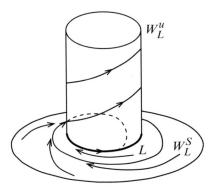

Figure 14.4
Schematic representation of a Poincaré map.

of the equality $|\gamma_i| = 1$ for some i, $1 \le i \le n-1$, and, thus, to some bifurcation. The main bifurcations of limit cycles are presented in figure 14.5; some of them lead to the appearance of dynamical chaos.

Stable and unstable manifolds (separatrices) of periodic trajectories can intersect each other. A trajectory belonging to the intersection $\Gamma := W_L^s \cap W_L^u$ is called *homoclinic* if $\Gamma \ne L$.

If this intersection occurs without tangency (i.e., transversally), then an infinite set of saddle-type closed trajectories lies in a neighborhood of $\Gamma \cup L$. Thus, the existence of a homoclinic trajectory is an indicator of chaotic behavior of the trajectories.

There are systems with continuous time for which the Poincaré map is globally defined. These are DSs of the form $\dot{x} = F(x,\theta)$, $\dot{\theta} = \omega$ (where F is 2π-periodic in θ vector-function) that describe an action of a periodic perturbation on a system of ODEs. Here, the global Poincaré section is $\theta = 0$; each trajectory intersects it infinitely many times. Here, the behavior of the trajectories in the original system is completely defined by the DS with discrete time.

14.2   Chaotic Dynamics

When we say "chaos," we usually imagine a very complex picture with many different elements that move in different directions, collide with each other, and appear and disappear randomly. Thus, according to everyday intuition, a large number of degrees of freedom is an important attribute of chaos. It seems reasonable to think that in the opposite case, for systems with only a few degrees of freedom, the dynamical behavior

Type of bifurcation	Notes	Examples and references
Local bifurcations		
Period-doubling	Below the period doubling bifurcation, a stable periodic orbit exists. As the control parameter μ is increased, the original periodic orbit becomes unstable, and the orbit with double period appears.	Cerebellar Purkinje cells (Mandelblat et al., 2001) Pacemaker neurons (Maeda et al., 1998)
Saddle-node 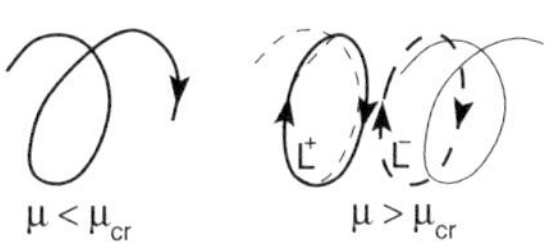	A pair of periodic orbits is created out of nothing. One of the of the orbits is unstable (the saddle L^-), while the other is stable (the node L^+). The saddle–node bifurcation is fundamental to the study of neural systems since it is one of the most basic processes by which periodic rhythms are created.	AB neuron from the crustacean pyrloric CPG (Guckenheimer et al., 1993)
Period-adding cascade 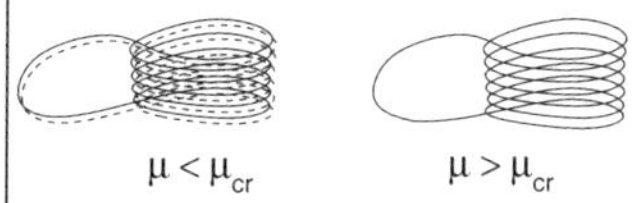	This bifurcation consists of several saddle-node bifurcations in which a (n+1)–spike bursting behavior is born and the n-spike bursting behavior dissapears.	Burst flexibility in coupled chaotic neurons (Huerta et al., 1997) Neural relaxation oscillators (Coombes and Osbaldestin, 2000) Chay neuron model (Chay 1985, Gu et al., 2003) Bursting electronic neuron (Maeda and Makino, 2000)
Global bifurcations		
Period-doubling cascade	This diagram shows not one, but rather an infinite number of period doubling bifurcations. As μ is increased a period two orbit becomes a period four orbit, etc. This process converges at a finite value of μ, beyond which a chaotic motion and an infinite number of unstable periodic orbits appear to exist.	Thermosensitive neurons (Feudel et al., 2000) Aplysia R15 neuron (Canavier et al., 1990) Salamander visual system (Crevier and Meister, 1998)
Saddle-node homoclinic 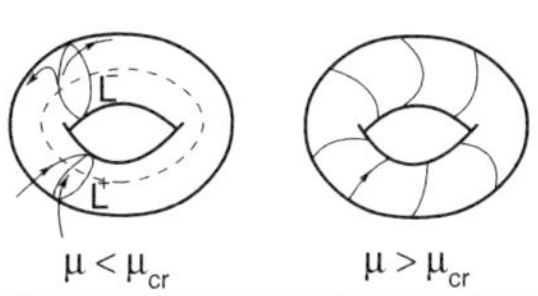	This bifurcation is characterized by the transition from the synchronization regime (stable limit cycle L^+ on an invariant torus) to the quasiperiodic regime (beating). The stable and unstable L^- limit cycles collide and disappear.	Periodic modulation of tonic spiking activity VLSI neuron model (Bondarenko et al., 2003)
Blue-sky catastrophe 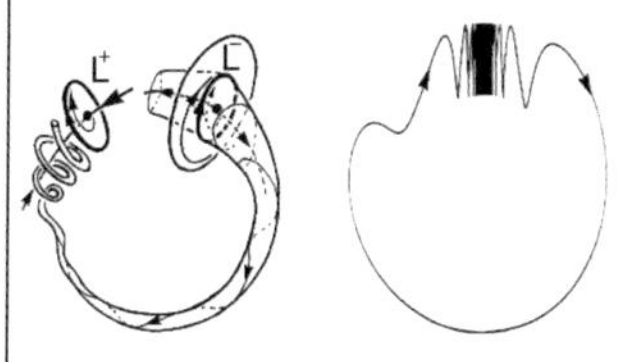	At control parameter values smaller than the critical one, the system has two periodic orbits: a stable orbit L^+ and a saddle orbit L^-. The orbits, which do not lie in the stable manifold of L^- tend to L^+ as time increases. This is one of the basic processes by which periodic bursts are created.	Leach heart interneuron model (Shilnikov and Cymbalyuk, 2005) (Gavrilov and Shilnikov, 2000) Pacemaker neuron model (Soto-Trevino et al., 2005)

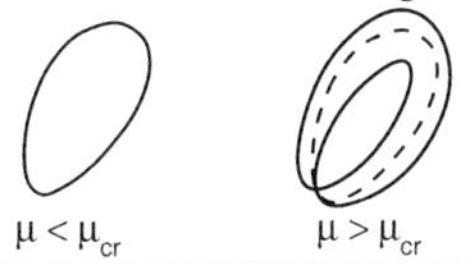

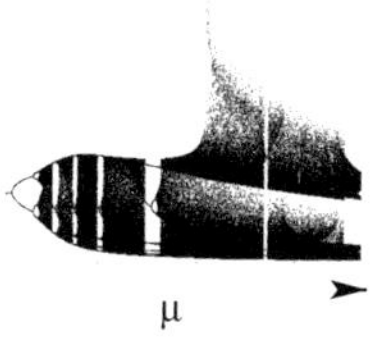

Figure 14.5
Six examples of limit cycle bifurcations observed in living and model neural systems.

must be simple and predictable. The discovery of dynamical chaos destroyed this traditional view. Systems evolving in time according to deterministic rules may demonstrate capricious and seemingly unpredictable behavior independently of the number of degrees of freedom that they possess. The reason for such behavior is the instability of their trajectories and, as the consequence, the sensitive dependence on initial conditions. Authors have proposed several quantities to measure the amount of instability that a system possesses. We begin with the description of metric complexity (see Takens, 1981, 1983 and Afraimovich and Hsu, 2002).

14.2.1 Metric Complexity Function and Related Notions

Consider a DS with discrete time generated by a map f of a phase space M. We assume that M is a metric space; that is, for every two points x and y in M, a distance $d(x,y)$ is defined. Fix an arbitrary set A of initial points and denote by

$$\Gamma_n(x) = \bigcup_{k=0}^{n-1} f^k x$$

a piece of trajectory going through $x \in A$ of temporal length n. Two such pieces $\Gamma_n(x)$ and $\Gamma_n(y)$ are said to be (ε, n)-separated if $d(f^k x, f^k y) \geq \varepsilon$ for some $0 \leq k \leq n-1$. The maximally possible number different up to ε of such pieces is denoted as

$$C_{\varepsilon,n}(A) = \max\{\text{number of } (\varepsilon, n)\text{-separated pieces}\}$$

and is called the (ε, n)-complexity of A. One can define the complexity in a slightly different way. Introduce a sequence of distances $d_n(x,y)$ as follows:

$$d_n(x,y) = \max_{0 \leq j \leq n-1} d(f^j x, f^j y).$$

Given $\varepsilon > 0, n > 0, A \subset M$, the set $Y \subset A$ is called (ε, n)-separated if $d_n(x,y) \geq \varepsilon$ for each pair $(x,y) \in Y$. The number

$$C_{\varepsilon,n}(A) = \max\{ |Y|, \ Y \subset A \text{ is } (\varepsilon, n)\text{-separated}\}$$

is called the (ε, n)-complexity of A. Here, $|Y|$ is the number of elements (the cardinality) in Y. It is easy to see that these two definitions determine the same quantity.

The complexity function contains information not only about the asymptotic behavior ($n \rightarrow \infty$) but also about fluctuation during the process of evolution. Its asymptotic behavior is characterized by two main quantities: the *topological entropy*,

$$h = h_{\text{top}}(A) := \lim_{\varepsilon \to 0} \overline{\lim_{n \to \infty}} \frac{\ln C_{\varepsilon,n}(A)}{n},$$

and the *fractal dimension*,

$$b := \lim_{n \to \infty} \overline{\lim_{\varepsilon \to 0}} \frac{1}{-\ln \varepsilon} \ln C_{\varepsilon,n}(A),$$

of the set A. Thus, if $0 < b < \infty, 0 < h < \infty$, the complexity function can be represented as follows:

$$C_{\varepsilon,n}(A) = \varepsilon^{-b} e^{hn} S(\varepsilon,n),$$

where $S(\varepsilon,n)$ is a slow changing function; that is,

$$\lim_{\varepsilon \to 0} \frac{\ln S(\varepsilon,n)}{-\ln \varepsilon} = 0, \quad \lim_{n \to \infty} \frac{\ln S(\varepsilon,n)}{n} = 0.$$

To illustrate these notions, consider a system generated by a map of the interval $[0,L]$ with exponential divergence of trajectories (e.g., $x \rightarrow 2x_1 \bmod 1$). If δx_0 is an initial displacement (the distance between two points) and $\delta x_n \geq \varepsilon$ is the displacement at the instant n of time, then $\varepsilon \leq \delta x_0 e^{hn}$; that is, the points are ε-separated. Their number is

$$C_{\varepsilon,n}(A) \cong l_A \frac{1}{\delta x_0} \cong \frac{l_A}{\varepsilon} e^{hn},$$

where l_A is the length of an initial interval A. Thus, $b = 1, S(\varepsilon,n) = l_A$. If A is not an interval but a fractal set of dimension b, then from the inequality

$$\left(\varepsilon / \delta x_0 \right)^b \leq e^{hn}$$

we obtain

$$C_{\varepsilon,n} \cong \left(\frac{l_A}{\varepsilon} \right)^b e^{hn}.$$

COMMENT 14.2
Dimension and Lyapunov Exponents in EEG Experiments

Many pathologic states have been examined, ranging from seizures, toxic states, and psychiatric disorders to Alzheimer's, Parkinson's, and other neurodegenerative diseases. The interpretation of these results in terms of "functional sources" and "functional networks" allows identification of different basic patterns of brain dynamics: (1) normal, ongoing dynamics during a task or resting state in healthy subjects; this state is characterized by a high complexity and a relatively low and fluctuating level of synchronization of the neuronal networks; (2) hypersynchrony of epileptic seizures; (3) dynamics of degenerative encephalopathies with an abnormally low level of synchronization between areas. Only intermediate levels of rapidly fluctuating synchronization are associated with normal information processing (Stam, 2005).

In experiments published by Tomberg (1999), nonaveraged scalp-recorded brain potentials were analyzed in humans while they were either silently reading a book or in idle alert conditions. The dimension of the strange attractors was estimated from the EEG at each of 14 scalp electrodes. When the subject was fully alert but not engaged in any specific task, the dimension ranged between 5.2 and 5.9. When the subject was silently reading a book, the dimension was higher in the left lateral anterior extrasylvian temporal cortex, but did not change in the adjacent left perisylvian cortex or over the right side of the brain. The increase of dimension in the left lateral extrasylvian temporal cortex during reading, as the author supposes, reflects enhanced processing operations in the semantic (Wernicke) areas. These results provide some evidence that increasing a fractal dimension is related to specific cognitive brain processing.

In the study by Osowski, Swiderski, Cichocki, and Rysz (2007), the authors developed a method of estimation of the short-term largest Lyapunov exponent of EEG time-series segments for the detection and prediction of the epileptic seizure. The analysis of the data showed that the change of the largest Lyapunov exponent provides plenty of information regarding the epileptic seizure. In particular, the minimum value of Lyapunov exponent indicates fairly well the seizure moment.

For systems with continuous time, the complexity function, the topological entropy, and the fractal dimension are defined in the same way.

14.2.2 Dynamical Chaos

We define now dynamical chaos. In practice, scientists deal with a signal (an observable). Very often, they do not know which system generates the observable. We say that an observable $\alpha(t)$ is generated by a dynamical system (φ, M) if there exists an initial point $x_0 \in M$ such that $\alpha(t) = \beta(\varphi x_0)$, where $\beta : M \to \mathbf{R}$ is a function. For the sake of simplicity, we can assume that time is discrete, $t \in \mathbf{Z}$, so that $\alpha(t) = \alpha(n) =: \alpha_n$. We introduce the space of all bounded observables $B = \{\boldsymbol{\alpha} = (\alpha_0, \alpha_1, \alpha_2, \ldots)\}$ endowed with the norm

$$\|\boldsymbol{\alpha}\| = \sum_{k=0}^{\infty} |\alpha_k| \Big/ 2^k$$

(i.e., B is a Banach space). The shift map $T\boldsymbol{\alpha} = (\alpha_1, \alpha_2, \ldots)$ generates a "universal" DS containing all bounded observables.

We say that an observable $\boldsymbol{\alpha}$ is deterministically generated if the fractal dimension $b = b(A) < \infty$ and the topological entropy $h_{\text{top}}(A) < \infty$, where A is the set of all points of accumulation of the trajectory $\{T^i\boldsymbol{\alpha}\}$ in the space B. Because of the Mane theorem (Stark, 2001), it follows that the DS (T^k, A) is topologically identical with the DS generated by the map

$$(\alpha_k, \ldots, \alpha_{k+n-1}) \to (\alpha_{k+1}, \ldots, \alpha_{k+n})$$

on the finite-dimensional phase space where n is an arbitrary number such that $n > 2b+1$. In other words, deterministically generated observables are generated by finite-dimensional DSs with finite entropy. Furthermore, if the topological entropy is positive, then an exponential growth of the complexity function is guaranteed.

Summarizing, one can say that a system (φ^t, M) *possesses dynamical chaos if $0 \leq b(M) < \infty, 0 < h < \infty$.*

To realize an exponential growth of the complexity function on an attractor, the DS performs a sequential stretching and folding in a neighborhood of the attractor [see figure 14.6, Rabinovich–Fabrikant attractor (Rabinovich & Fabrikant, 1979)].

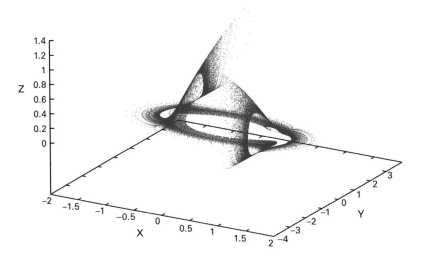

Figure 14.6
Rabinovich–Fabrikant attractor.

Lyapunov Exponents

An average of characteristic values of an attractor A can be found by analyzing the motion of a trajectory dense in it. Let $x = x_0(t)$ be a solution of the ODE $\dot{x} = F(x)$, $x \in \mathbf{R}^n$, representing such a trajectory. We shall consider the deformation of the "spherical" volume element along the trajectory. The deformation is determined by the difference $x(t) - x_0(t) = \xi(t)$, where $x(t)$ represents a trajectory close to the original one. The difference is governed by the ODE

$$\xi_j = \sum_{k=1}^{n} a_{ik}(t)\xi_k, \ j = 1,\ldots,n, \ \dot{a}_{ik}(t) = \frac{\partial F_i[x_0(t)]}{\partial x_k}.$$

In its motion along the trajectory, the volume element decreases in some directions and increases in others, so the sphere is transformed into an ellipsoid; moreover, the directions of the semi-axes of the ellipsoid change as well as their lengths $l_j(t), j = 1,\ldots,n$. The limits

$$\lambda_j = \lim_{t \to \infty} \frac{1}{t} \ln {l_j(t)} \big/ {l(0)}$$

[where $l(0)$ is the radius of the sphere at $t = 0$] are referred to as the Lyapunov characteristic exponents. They are real numbers. The one corresponding to the direction tangent to the trajectory equals 0. If $\lambda_j > 0$

for some $j \in \{1,...,n\}$, then the system will manifest sensitive dependence on initial points (at least, in the jth direction) and exponential growth of the complexity function (i.e., the positiveness of the topological entropy). In other words, the positiveness of a Lyapunov exponent indicates the occurrence of dynamical chaos in the DS (Ott, 1992; Katok & Hasselblatt, 1995).

For any ergodic invariant measure μ with the support on the attractor, the Lyapunov characteristic exponents are the same for each trajectory going through a typical initial point with respect to the measure μ. So, the Lyapunov characteristic exponents $\{\lambda_j\}$ can be treated as characteristic of an ergodic measure: $\lambda_1 = \lambda_1(\mu),...,\lambda_n = \lambda_n(\mu)$.

Typical points with respect to μ form a subset A_μ of the attractor A (sometimes, much smaller than A). The growth of the complexity function $C_{\varepsilon,n}(A_\mu)$ is determined therefore not by the topological entropy $h_{\text{top}}(A)$ but by the quantity

$$h_\mu := \lim_{\varepsilon \to 0} \overline{\lim_{n \to \infty}} \frac{1}{n} \ln C_{\varepsilon,n}(A_\mu),$$

which is called the Kolmogorov–Sinai (KS; or measure-theoretical) entropy. Generally, $h_\mu < h_{\text{top}}(A)$.

For some measures that are called physical, natural (or Sinai–Ruelle–Bowen) measures, there exists a remarkable relation (Pesin equality) between Lyapunov exponents and the KS entropy,

$$h_\mu = \sum{}^+ \lambda_j(\mu),$$

where the sum is taken over positive Lyapunov exponents.

14.2.3 Synchronization

Synchronization is a phenomenon that can be observed in two or more dissipative DSs coupled by a dissipative coupling (Rabinovich, Varona, & Abarbanel, 2000; Pikovsky et al., 2001; Mosekilde, Maistrenko, Postnov, & Maistrenko, 2002). It is realized as an adjustment of rhythms of their oscillations. If oscillations are periodic, then a very weak coupling may cause synchronization. If they are chaotic, then synchronization appears if the coupling is strong enough. Synchronized regimes for periodic oscillations correspond to stable limit cycles situated on two-dimensional invariant tori in the full phase space. The rotation number of such a limit cycle is m/n, where $n(m)$ is the number of turns around the parallel

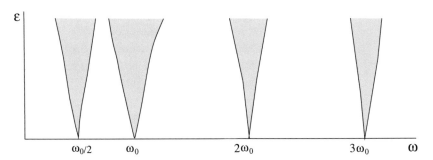

Figure 14.7
Illustration of Arnold tongues as a function of the forcing amplitude ε.

(meridian) of the limit cycle on the torus. It corresponds to the relation $n\omega_1 = m\omega_2$ between frequencies of individual oscillations and the equality

$$\lim_{t \to \infty} \frac{\phi_1(t)}{\phi_2(t)} = \frac{m}{n}$$

for their phases $\varphi_1(t)$ and $\varphi_2(t)$. In this case, one says that $m : n$-synchronization occurs. The region in the space of parameters for which such a limit cycle exists is called an Arnold tongue, and it is illustrated in figure 14.7 (for two-parameter systems).

For the case of chaotic individual oscillations, it is possible sometimes to introduce for them instantaneous phases and mean frequencies. Then relations similar to those for periodic cases hold, so phases and mean frequencies are adjusted while amplitudes are noncorrelated (or weakly correlated). Such a phenomenon is called the $m : n$ phase synchronization (Pikovsky et al., 2001), but in a general situation it is unclear how to introduce the phase variables, so the phase synchronization notion is applicable only for specific cases.

Another case where theory and applications of chaotic synchronization phenomenon are well developed is the master–slave synchronization (Pecora, Carroll, Johnson, Mar, & Heagy, 1997). It reflects the situation where the coupling is one-directional: One system (master) acts onto another (slave) and forces it to behave in time according to itself. Mathematically, it means that in the synchronized regime there is a functional relation between the solution $x(t)$ of the master system and $y(t)$ of the slave system: $y(t) = g[x(t)]$. The smoothness of the function g depends on the rate of coupling: If the coupling is very strong, then g is differentiable; for a weaker case, it could be Lipschitz-continuous and even only Hölder-continuous. But always an attractor corresponding to the synchronized regime belongs to the graph of g in the joint phase space. There is not a clear mathematical picture in the case of bidirectional coupling of different systems; the situation is still in the process of study.

14.3 Homoclinic and Heteroclinic Dynamics

Homoclinic and heteroclinic trajectories are very special orbits of DSs mainly because of two reasons: (1) they can cause birth (and death) of

COMMENT 14.3
Simple and Complex Dynamics in EEG Experiments

EEGs in epilepsy, Parkinson's disease, and some other diseases show limit-cycle dynamics due to coherent collective behavior synchrony of neurons. However, healthy EEGs are mostly unsynchronized. A comprehensive review of nonlinear dynamical analyses of EEG and magnetoencephalography data was published by Stam (2005). In spite of many promising results and reasonable predictions, the idea of considering EEG activity as low-dimensional chaos (limit cycle or low-dimensional strange attractor) does not look now as exciting as it did 20 years ago. EEG time series of healthy people usually represent nonstationary transient brain dynamics with metastable states (EEG microstate; see Van de Ville, Britz, & Michel, 2010) and is characterized by many degrees of freedom. In other words, information in the brain is embedded in many different temporal scales of electrophysiologic activity and is lost when the activity is averaged over larger intervals of time. Most cognitive EEG studies report event-related potentials. The event-related potential is simply the time-domain average of EEG traces locked to the onset of some experimental event such as stimulus onset or button press. The reasoning behind this approach is that background noise in the EEG is averaged out over many trials, and the remaining fluctuations reflect activation of different cognitive systems. The dependent variable is usually the peak amplitude of some component (e.g., the P300), the average voltage over some larger time window, or a peak-to-peak or base-to-peak amplitude difference. To the extent that neuroelectric dynamics are oscillatory and non-phase-locked to the event, a considerable amount of cognitively relevant information in EEG may be lost in time-domain averaging (Makeig, Debener, Onton, & Delorme, 2004). This is illustrated in figure 14.C4. Thus, event-related potentials are useful for providing a glimpse of the global neural processing but may be of limited use for elucidating complex electrophysiologic dynamics.

COMMENT 14.3
(continued)

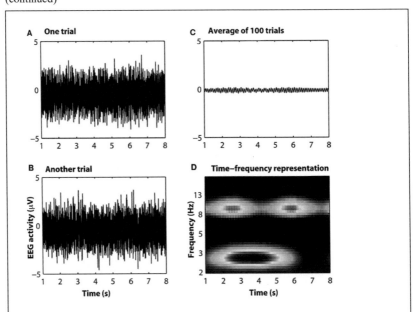

Figure 14.C4
Simulated data showing how information contained in raw EEG data (A and B: single "trials") is not apparent in the event-related potential (C) but is readily observable in the time–frequency representation (D). Adapted with permission from Cohen (2011).

Nevertheless in some cases low-dimensional models of EEG are still very useful. For example, Kim and Robinson (2008) studied epileptic limit cycles, and their model includes key physiologic features such as cortico-cortical propagation and delayed feedbacks via subcortical pathways. When driven by noise, the model reproduced and unified many properties of EEGs like spectral peaks that correspond to the frequency of the epileptic limit cycle.

periodic attractors and (2) they may serve as indicators of chaotic behavior in DSs.

14.3.1 Homoclinic Situation

Let Γ be a homoclinic trajectory belonging to the intersection $W_L^u \cap W_L^s$ of the stable and unstable manifolds of a saddle periodic orbit L. If this intersection occurs without tangency, then (as it is known from Poincaré times) the behavior of trajectories around Γ is very complex. In particular, there are infinitely many saddle limit cycles in a neighborhood of Γ. If W_L^s and W_L^u are tangent to each other along Γ, the situation is even more complex—there is a deep mathematical theory describing systems with homoclinic tangencies and their perturbations (Gonchenko, Turaev, & Shilnikov, 1996).

If x_0 is a saddle equilibrium point of a system $\dot{x} = F(x)$ and $\lambda_1,\dots,\lambda_n$ are roots of the characteristic equations ordered in such a way that

$$\lambda_1 > \dots \geq \operatorname{Re} \lambda_m > 0 > \operatorname{Re} \lambda_{m+1} \geq \dots \geq \operatorname{Re} \lambda_n,$$

then the quantity

$$v = -\frac{\operatorname{Re} \lambda_{m+1}}{\lambda_1}$$

is called the saddle value. It describes how the displacement from the manifold is changing while a trajectory is going through a neighborhood of x_0 (figure 14.8). If $v > 1$, the saddle x_0 is called dissipative. A Shilnikov theorem tells us that the disappearance of a homoclinic trajectory of a dissipative saddle can be accompanied by the birth of a stable limit cycle provided that dim $W^u = 1$ ($m = 1$) (Shilnikov, Shilnikov, Turaev, & Chua, 1998, 2001).

If $n = 3$, $\lambda_{2,3} = \alpha \pm i\omega$, $\omega \neq 0$, then x_0 is called the saddle-focus. It follows from another Shilnikov theorem (Shilnikov et al., 1998, 2001) that if $v < 1$, the existence of a homoclinic trajectory Γ implies a very complex dynamics around it; in particular, an infinite collection of saddle limit cycles exists in a neighborhood of Γ. Similar results are obtained for $n > 3$. This kind of chaotic dynamics (which is sometimes called Shilnikov chaos) is realized in some mathematical models of neurons and other biological systems.

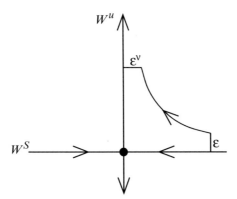

Figure 14.8
An initial displacement of order ε becomes of order ε^{v} after the orbits pass through a neighborhood of a stable equilibrium point.

14.3.2   Heteroclinic Cycles and Sequences

Recent work in a number of areas has highlighted ways in which heteroclinic connections within attractors can be responsible for intermittent and twisting behavior in nonlinear DSs (see, for instance, Afraimovich, Ashwin, & Kirk, 2010). Moreover, heteroclinic dynamics may serve as an appropriate mathematical framework for transient processes that can be treated as an itinerary through metastable states (see chapter 4). We consider the case where metastable states are just saddle equilibrium points $S_1,\ldots,S_N$ of a system $\dot{x} = F(x)$, $x \in \mathbf{R}^n$. Let the eigenvalues $\lambda_1^{(i)}, \ldots, \lambda_n^{(i)}$ of the matrix of the system linearized at S_i be ordered in such a way that

$$\lambda_1^{(i)} > \ldots \geq \operatorname{Re} \lambda_{m_i}^{(i)} > 0 > \operatorname{Re} \lambda_{m_i+1}^{(i)} \geq \ldots \geq \operatorname{Re} \lambda_n^{(i)},$$

then on the m_i-dimensional unstable manifold W_i^u, there is a strongly unstable one-dimensional manifold W_i^{uu} tangent to the eigenvector corresponding to $\lambda_1^{(i)}$. It consists of S_i and two trajectories Γ^+ and Γ^- (see figure 14.9); that is, $W_i^{uu} = \Gamma_i^+ \cup S_i \cup \Gamma_i^-$. If $\Gamma_i^+ \subset W_{i+1}^s$, $i = 1,\ldots,N-1$, then the set $\Gamma := \bigcup_{i=1}^{N} S_i \bigcup_{i=1}^{N-1} \Gamma_i^+$ is said to be a heteroclinic sequence. If $S_N = S_1$, then Γ is called the heteroclinic cycle (contour), see figure 14.10. Heteroclinic cycles can serve as attractors provided that the saddle values

$$-\frac{\operatorname{Re} \lambda_{m_i+1}^{(i)}}{\lambda_1^{(i)}} = v_i > 1$$

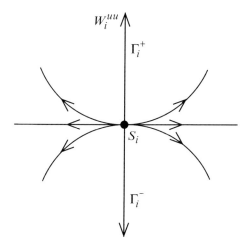

Figure 14.9
A strongly unstable manifold on the unstable manifold of the saddle S_i.

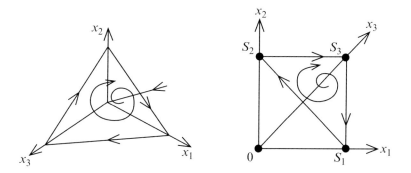

Figure 14.10
A heteroclinic cycle serving as an attractor in the winnerless situation.

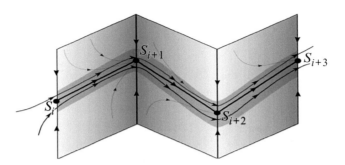

Figure 14.11
Schematic representation of a stable heteroclinic sequence.

and Γ is characterized by $\dim W_i^u = 1$, $i = 1,\ldots,N$. Such a situation is realized in systems for which the winnerless competition principle takes place (Rabinovich, Varona, Selverston, & Abarbanel, 2006).

If $S_N \neq S_1$, then one deals with a heteroclinic sequence (figure 14.11). If $v_i > 1, i = 1,\ldots,N$, and $\dim W_i^u = 1$, then still some kind of stability holds: Any orbit going through an initial point in a vicinity of S_1 stays in a neighborhood of Γ until it reaches a neighborhood of S_N. If $\dim W_i^u > 1$ for some i, then most such orbits still do not leave a neighborhood of Γ, but some of them $[\cong 20\%$ if $\dim W_i^u = 2$ (Tristan & Rabinovich, 2011)] leave a vicinity of Γ and go to other attracting sets in the phase space.

Some results exist where metastable sets are represented by saddle limit cycles (Komarov, Osipov, Suykens, & Rabinovich, 2009), but the situation needs to be studied more carefully.

14.4   Conclusion

About 60 years ago, the French mathematician Jacques Hadamard asked the following question: Will it ever happen that mathematicians will know enough about the physiology of the brain, and neurophysiologists enough of mathematical discovery, for efficient cooperation to be possible?

Today we can say that this is happening, and we are witnesses of and participants in these ongoing efforts, as has been shown in this book. To conclude, we wish to make a brief remark about two pending subjects: one relates to the dynamical theory of complex systems, and the other relates to map models as an effective method to describe intrinsic neuron dynamics to model complex neuronal systems.

The main "complexity question" is not "What are the constituents of the brain (neurons, synapses, networks, etc.)?" anymore, but rather "How does the brain work with these different elements in different temporal and spatial scales?" The dynamics of complex systems is not a solid mathematical theory yet. It is an approach that integrates a wide variety of studies on dynamics of hierarchical multiagent systems that puts together key concepts such as the following: (1) *Functionality*, a concept related to the dependence of the interconnections between parts with a common temporal goal. When studying the parts in isolation does not work, the nature of complex systems can be probed by investigating how changes in one part affect the dynamics of the whole. (2) *Metastability*: The riddles of the macroscopic and the microscopic generate complex neuronal patterns—modes that are usually metastable and controlled by synchronization and long-range inhibition. (3) *Behavior complexity*: To describe the behavior of a system, we try to describe the response function (i.e., actions as a function of the environment). However, unless simplifying assumptions are made in complex systems, this requires an amount of information that grows exponentially with the complexity of the environment, which makes the problem unsolvable. This list of concepts, of course, can continue. For example, a researcher of complex system often emphasizes the concept of "contrasts"; that is, complex systems often simultaneously exhibit opposing characteristics such as simplicity and complexity, order and disorder, random and predictable behavior, repeating patterns and transients (for a review, see Bar-Yam, 2004). The success of a computational approach for the analysis of complex cortex models is possible if the researchers have formulated a reasonable set of specific questions and hypotheses that can be addressed to a large extent with these models. One can find examples of such success in the papers of Izhikevich and Edelman (2008), Bazhenov, Rulkov, and Timofeev (2008), and Rulkov and Bazhenov (2008).

Regarding the description of individual neural dynamics, since the classical work of Hodgkin and Huxley, biological neuron models have consisted of ordinary differential equations representing the evolution of the transmembrane voltage and the dynamics of ionic conductances. Recently, discrete dynamical systems—also known as map models—have begun to receive attention as convenient and valid phenomenological neuron models. Such simple and computationally inexpensive models often keep several properties and the appearance of complex biophysical models and are compatible with many of the existing plasticity and learning paradigms of more complex theoretical approaches (Cazelles,

Courbage, & Rabinovich, 2001; Rulkov, 2002; Ibarz, Casado, & Sanjuán, 2011). These models are especially important for the description of many agent systems (Bazhenov et al., 2008; Rulkov & Bazhenov, 2008) and provide a way to explore complex network behavior including theoretical analysis using the dynamical entities that we have described in this chapter.

Acknowledgments

V.S.A. was partially supported by PROMEP grant UASLP-CA21. M.R. acknowledges support from ONR grant N00014–07–1-074. P.V. was supported by MICINN BFU2009–08473.

References

Abarbanel, H. D. I., Huerta, R., Rabinovich, M. I., Rulkov, N. F., Rowat, P. F., & Selverston, A. (1996). Synchronized action of synaptically coupled chaotic model neurons. *Neural Computation*, 8(8), 1567–1602.

Afraimovich, V. S. & Hsu, S-B. (2002). *Lectures on Chaotic Dynamical Systems*. Providence, RI: American Mathematical Society.

Afraimovich, V., Ashwin, P., & Kirk, V. (Eds) (2010). Robust heteroclinic and switching dynamics. *Dynamical Systems*, 25(3), 285–286.

Arnold, V., Afraimovich, V., Ilyashenko, Yu., & Shilnikov, L. (1986). Bifurcation theory. In V .I. Arnold (Ed.), *Encyclopedia of Mathematical Sciences* (Vol. 5, pp. 7–205). Moscow: Springer.

Bar-Yam, Y. (2004). *Making Things Work: Solving Complex Problems in a Complex World*. Boston, MA: NECSI Knowledge Press.

Bazhenov, M., Rulkov, N. F., & Timofeev, I. (2008). Effect of synaptic connectivity on long-range synchronization of fast cortical oscillations. *Journal of Neurophysiology*, *100*, 1562–1575.

Bondarenko, V. E., Cymbalyuk, G. S., Patel, G., DeWeerth, S. P., & Calabrese, R. L. (2003). A bifurcation of a synchronous oscillations into a torus in a system of two mutually inhibitory VLSI neurons: experimental observation. *Neurocomputing*, *52–54*, 691–698.

Canavier, C. C., Clark, J. W., & Byrne, J. H. (1990). Routes to chaos in a model of a bursting neuron. *Biophys. J.*, 57, 1245-1251.

Cazelles, B., Courbage, M., & Rabinovich, M. (2001). Anti-phase regularization of coupled chaotic maps modelling bursting neurons. *Europhysics Letters*, *56*, 504–509.

Chay, T. R. (1985). Chaos in a three-variable model of an excitable cell. *Physica D*, *16*, 233–242.

Cohen, M.X. (2011). It's about time. *Frontiers in Human Neuroscience*, 5(2).

Coombes, S., & Osbaldestin, A. H. (2000). Period-adding bifurcations and chaos in a periodically stimulated excitable neural relaxation oscillator. *Physical Review E*, *62*, 4057–4066.

Crevier, D. W., & Meister, M. (1998). Synchronous period-doubling in flicker vision of salamander and man. *Journal of Neurophysiology*, *79*, 1869–1878.

Feudel, U., Neiman, A., Pei, X., Wojtenek, W., Braun, H., Huber, M., & Moss, F. (2000). Homoclinic bifurcation in a Hodgkin-Huxley model of thermally sensitive neurons. *Chaos*, *10*, 231–239.

Freeman, W. (1988). Strange attractors that govern mammalian brain dynamics shown by trajectories of electroencephalographic (EEG) potential. *IEEE Transactions on Circuits and Systems, 35*(7), 781–783.

Gavrilov, N., & Shilnikov, A. (2000). Example of a Blue Sky catastrophe. *American Mathematical Society Transactions, 200*, 99–105.

Gonchenko, S. V., Turaev, D. V., & Shilnikov, L. P. (1996). Dynamical phenomena in systems with structurally unstable Poincare homoclinic orbits. *Interdisc. J. Chaos, 6*(1), 1–17.

Guckenheimer, J., Gueron, S., & Harris-Warrick, R. M. (1993). Mapping the dynamics of a bursting neuron. *Philosophical Transactions of the Royal Society of London, B Biological Sciences, 341*, 345–359.

Huerta, R., Rabinovich, M. I., Abarbanel, H. D. I., & Bazhenov, M. (1997). Spike-train bifurcation scaling in two coupled chaotic neurons. *Physical Review E, 55*, R2108–R2110.

Ibarz, B., Casado, J. M., & Sanjuán, M. A. F. (2011). Map-based models in neuronal dynamics. *Physics Reports, 501*, 1–74.

Izhikevich, E. M., & Edelman, G. M. (2008). Large-scale model of mammalian thalamocortical systems. *Proceedings of the National Academy of Sciences of the United States of America, 105*, 3593–3598.

Katok, A., & Hasselblatt, B. (1995). Introduction to the modern theory of dynamical systems. *Encyclopedia of Mathematics and its Applications 54*. Cambridge, UK: Cambridge University Press.

Kim, J. W., & Robinson, P. A. (2008). Controlling limit-cycle behaviors of brain activity. *Physical Review E: Statistical, Nonlinear, and Soft Matter Physics, 77*, 051914.

Komarov, M. A., Osipov, G. V., Suykens, J. A. K., & Rabinovich, M. I. (2009). Numerical studies of slow rhythms emergence in neural microcircuits: Bifurcations and stability. *Chaos (Woodbury, N.Y.), 19*(1), 015107.

Korn, H., & Faure, P. (2003). Is there chaos in the brain? II. Experimental evidence and related models. *Comptes Rendus de l Academie des Sciences. Serie II, 326*(9), 787–840.

Kuznetsov, Yu. A. (1998). *Elements of Applied Bifurcation Theory*. Berlin: Springer-Verlag.

Lichtenberg, A. J., & Lieberman, M. A. (1992). *Regular and Chaotic Dynamics*, 2nd ed. (Applied Mathematical Sciences, Vol. 38). New York: Springer-Verlag.

Llinas, R., & Yarom, Y. (1986). Oscillatory properties of guinea-pig inferior olivary neurons and their pharmacological modulation: an in vitro study. *Journal of Physiology, 376*, 163–182.

Makeig, S., Debener, S., Onton, J., & Delorme, A. (2004). Mining event-related brain dynamics. *Trends in Cognitive Sciences, 8*, 204–210.

Maeda, Y., & Makino, H. (2000). A pulse-type hardware neuron model with beating, bursting excitation and plateau potential. *BioSystems, 58*, 93–100.

Maeda, Y., Pakdaman, K., Nomura, T., Doi, S., & Sato, S. (1998). Reduction of a model for an Onchidium pacemaker neuron. *Biological Cybernetics, 78*, 265–276.

Mandelblat, Y., Etzion, Y., Grossman, Y., & Golomb, D. (2001). Period doubling of calcium spike firing in a model of a Purkinje cell dendrite. *Journal of Computational Neuroscience, 11*, 43–62.

Mosekilde, E., Maistrenko, Y., Postnov, D., & Maistrenko, Iu. (2002). *Chaotic Synchronization: Applications to Living Systems*. Singapore: World Scientific.

Osowski, S., Swiderski, B., Cichocki, A., & Rysz, A. (2007). Epileptic seizure characterization by Lyapunov exponent of EEG signal. *COMPEL: The International Journal for Computation and Mathematics in Electrical and Electronic Engineering, 26*(5), 1276.

Ott, E. (2002). *Chaos in Dynamical Systems*. Cambridge, UK: Cambridge University Press.

Pecora, L. M., Carroll, T. L., Johnson, J. A., Mar, D. J., & Heagy, G. F. (1997). Fundamentals of synchronization in chaotic systems, concepts, and applications. *Chaos (Woodbury, N.Y.)*, 7, 520.

Pikovsky, A., Rosenblum, M., & Kurths, J. (2001). *Synchronization: A Universal Concept in Nonlinear Science*. Cambridge, UK: Cambridge University Press.

Rabinovich, M. I., & Abarbanel, H. D. I. (1998). The role of chaos in neural systems. *Neuroscience, 87*(1), 5–14.

Rabinovich, M. I., & Fabrikant, A. L. (1979). Stochastic self-modulation of waves in nonequilibrium media. *Soviet Physics, JETP, 50*, 311.

Rabinovich, M. I., Varona, P., & Abarbanel, H. D. I. (2000). Nonlinear cooperative dynamics of living neurons. *International Journal of Bifurcation and Chaos in Applied Sciences and Engineering, 10*(5), 913–933.

Rabinovich, M. I., Varona, P., Selverston, A. I., & Abarbanel, H. D. I. (2006). Dynamical principles in neurosciense. *Reviews of Modern Physics, 78*, 1213–1265.

Rulkov, N. F. (2002). Modeling of spiking-bursting neural behavior using two-dimensional map. *Physical Review E: Statistical, Nonlinear, and Soft Matter Physics, 65*, 041922.

Rulkov, N. F., & Bazhenov, M. (2008). Oscillations and synchrony in large-scale cortical network models. *Journal of Biological Physics, 34*, 279–299.

Shilnikov, A., & Cymbalyuk, G. (2005). Transition between tonic spiking and bursting in a neuron model via the blue-sky catastrophe. *Physical Review Letters, 94*, 4101.

Shilnikov, L. P., Shilnikov, A., Turaev, D., & Chua, L. (1998). *Methods of Qualitative Theory in Nonlinear Dynamics. Part I*. Singapore: World Scientific.

Shilnikov, L. P., Shilnikov, A., Turaev, D., & Chua, L. (2001). *Methods of Qualitative Theory in Nonlinear Dynamics. Part II*. Singapore: World Scientific.

Soto-Trevino, C., Rabbah, P., Marder, E., & Nadim, F. (2005). Computational model of electrically coupled, intrinsically distinct pacemaker neurons. *Journal of Neurophysiology, 94*, 590–604.

Stam, C. J. (2005). Nonlinear dynamical analysis of EEG and MEG: Review of an emerging field. *Clinical Neurophysiology, 116*, 2266–2301.

Stark, J. (2001). Delay reconstruction: dynamics versus statistics. In A. I. Mees (Ed.), *Nonlinear Dynamics and Statistics* (pp. 81–103). Cambridge, MA: Birkhauser.

Takens, F. (1981). Detecting strange attractors in turbulence. In D. A. Rand & L.-S. Young (Eds.), *Dynamical Systems and Turbulence* (pp. 366–381). Lecture Notes in Mathematics, Vol. 898. Berlin: Springer-Verlag.

Takens, F. (1983). Distinguishing deterministic and random systems. In G. I. Barenblatt, G. Iooss, & D. D. Joseph (Eds.), *Nonlinear Dynamics and Turbulence* (pp. 314–333). Boston, MA: Pittman.

Tomberg, C. (1999). Focal enhancement of chaotic strange attractor dimension in the left semantic (Wernicke) human cortex during reading without concomitant change in vigilance level. *Neuroscience Letters, 263*, 177–180.

Tristan, I., & Rabinovich, M. I. (2012). Transient dynamics on the edge of stability. In G. Liu (Ed.), *Nonlinear Dynamics: New Directions*. In press.

Van de Ville, D., Britz, J., & Michel, C. M. (2010). EEG microstate sequences in healthy humans at rest reveal scale-free dynamics. *Proceedings of the National Academy of Sciences of the United States of America, 107*(42), 18179–18184.

Contributors

Valentin S. Afraimovich Instituto de Investigación en Comunicación Óptica, Universidad Autónoma de San Luis Potosí, San Luis Potosí, Mexico

Maxim Bazhenov Department of Cell Biology and Neuroscience, University of California, Riverside, Riverside, California, and Institute for Neural Computation, University of California, San Diego, La Jolla, California

Peter beim Graben Institut für deutsche Sprache und Linguistik, Humboldt-Universität zu Berlin, Berlin, Germany

Christian Bick Network Dynamics Group, Max Planck Institute for Dynamics and Self-Organization, Göttingen, Germany

Andreas Daffertshofer Faculty of Human Movement Sciences, VU University Amsterdam, Amsterdam, The Netherlands

Nathaniel D. Daw Center for Neural Science and Department of Psychology, New York University, New York, New York

Gustavo Deco Center for Brain and Cognition, Computational Neuroscience Group, and Institució Catalana de la Recerca i Estudis Avançats, Universitat Pompeu Fabra, Barcelona, Spain

Karl J. Friston The Wellcome Trust Centre for Neuroimaging, Institute of Neurology, University College of London, London, United Kingdom

Samuel J. Gershman Neuroscience Institute and Department of Psychology Princeton University, Princeton, New Jersey

John-Dylan Haynes Charité — Universitätsmedizin Berlin, Bernstein Center for Computational Neuroscience, Berlin, Germany

Raoul Huys Theoretical Neuroscience Group, Unité Mixte de Recherche 6233, Institut des Sciences du Mouvement, Centre National de la Recherche Scientifique, Marseille, France

Viktor Jirsa   Theoretical Neuroscience Group, Unité Mixte de Recherche 6233, Institut des Sciences du Mouvement, Centre National de la Recherche Scientifique, Marseille, France

Stefan J. Kiebel   Max Planck Institute for Human Cognitive and Brain Sciences, Leipzig, Germany

Scott Makeig   Institute for Neural Computation and Department of Neurosciences, University of California, San Diego, San Diego, California

Anthony R. McIntosh   The Rotman Research Institute, Baycrest Centre, Toronto, Canada

Vinod Menon   Cognitive and Systems Neuroscience Lab, Stanford University, Stanford, California

Dionysios Perdikis   Theoretical Neuroscience Group, Unité Mixte de Recherche 6233, Institut des Sciences du Mouvement, Centre National de la Recherche Scientifique, Marseille, France

Ajay Pillai   Brain Imaging and Modeling Section, National Institute on Deafness and Other Communication Disorders, National Institutes of Health, Bethesda, Maryland

Roland Potthast   Department of Mathematics and Statistics, University of Reading, Reading, United Kingdom

Mikhail I. Rabinovich   BioCircuits Institute, University of California, San Diego, La Jolla, California

Vasily A. Vakorin   The Rotman Research Institute, Baycrest Centre, Toronto, Canada

Bernadette C. M. van Wijk   Faculty of Human Movement Sciences, VU University Amsterdam, Amsterdam, The Netherlands

Pablo Varona   Departamento de Ingeniería Informática, Escuela Politécnica Superior, Universidad Autónoma de Madrid, Madrid, Spain

Marmaduke Woodman   Theoretical Neuroscience Group, Unité Mixte de Recherche 6233, Institut des Sciences du Mouvement, Centre National de la Recherche Scientifique, Marseille, France

Computational Neuroscience

Terence J. Sejnowski and Tomaso A. Poggio, editors

Index

Action-observation, 262–263, 272, 286–288
Active inference, 261–262, 264, 272, 275–276, 280–282, 284–285, 287, 289
Adiabatic elimination, 217, 248
Amari equation, 103, 105–107, 109
Ambiguity aversion, 301
Arnold tongues, 237, 328
Attention, 11, 18, 28–30, 34–43, 86, 142, 177, 262, 286

Background activity, 66, 196
Bayesian brain, 115, 261–262, 267, 269
Bayesian inference, 113, 116–117, 131, 135–136, 261, 269, 272
Bayesian model, 121, 302–303
Biased sampling, 59–60
Bifurcation, 7, 21–22, 78, 84, 114, 162, 219, 237, 240, 241, 248, 251, 316, 320–321
Binding, 209
  dynamics, 153
  heteroclinic, 154, 155, 156
  heteroclinic channel, 156
  information, 141
Brain imaging, 2, 10, 38, 84

Causal analysis, 35–37
Central executive network, 32–38, 41
Cognitive control, 3, 27–28, 33, 38, 40, 43, 146
Cognitive information flow, 142
Complexity, 156, 183–185, 335
  metric, 322–325
  and nonstationarity, 201–202, 206
  semantic, 152
  and spectral power, 197–201
  synaptic, 95
  theory, 2
Computational neurolinguistics, 96
Computing with attractors, 71
Connectivity matrix, 16–17, 19, 80, 82, 118–120, 158, 251
Connectome, 15–16, 66

Context-free grammar (CFG), 93, 97–99, 108
Correlation integral, 187, 190
Cost function, 276–277
Coupling strength, 15, 20, 236, 237, 248–253, 255

Decision making, 11, 32, 40, 84, 87, 141, 156–158, 160, 293, 299, 304, 308–309
Decision theory, 157, 275, 293–299, 301–302, 304–305, 308–309
Default mode
  activation, 176
  network, 32, 34–38, 40, 85–86
Desynchronization, 235, 237–241, 249–255
Dissipative dynamical system, 81, 120, 315, 327
Dissipative saddle, 79, 331
Dynamic cognitive modeling (DCM), 93–94, 96, 109
Dynamic decoding, 143
Dynamic field theory, 101, 103, 106
Dynamical system (DS), 2, 12, 40, 72–73, 79, 81, 88, 93–94, 96, 113–117, 122, 135, 143, 145, 148–150, 153, 192, 211, 214, 217, 222, 235, 261, 313–314, 325, 335

Electroencephalogram (EEG), 10–11, 19, 40, 82, 85–86, 93, 102, 104, 106–109, 113, 165–168, 171–172, 175, 177–178, 183, 186, 193, 195–198, 200–202, 205, 238, 246, 316, 324, 329–330
Ellsberg paradox, 300
Entropy, 20–21, 122, 264, 266, 275
  approximate, 188–190
  conditional, 186
  Kolmogorov, 186–188
  multiscale, 191–201
  Rényi, 185
  sample, 183–184, 188–191, 197–206
  Shannon, 184–186
  topological, 323, 325, 327